Heidi Gier

# *Audiology and Auditory Dysfunction*

**George T. Mencher**
*Dalhousie University*

**Sanford E. Gerber**
*Eastern Washington University*

**Andrew McCombe**
*Frimley Park Hospital*

**Allyn and Bacon**
*Boston • London • Toronto • Sydney • Tokyo • Singapore*

*Executive Editor:* Stephen D. Dragin
*Editorial Assistant:* Christine Svitila
*Editorial-Production Administrator:* Joe Sweeney
*Editorial-Production Service:* Walsh & Associates, Inc.
*Composition Buyer:* Linda Cox
*Manufacturing Buyer:* Suzanne Lareau
*Cover Administrator:* Suzanne Harbison

Copyright © 1997 by Allyn & Bacon
A Viacom Company
160 Gould Street
Needham Heights, MA 02194

Internet: www.abacon.com
America Online: keyword: College Online

***Library of Congress Cataloging-in-Publication Data***

Mencher, George T.
  Audiology and auditory dysfunction / George T. Mencher, Sanford E. Gerber, Andrw McCombe.
    p.    cm.
  Based, in part, on Auditory Dysfunction, published by College-Hill Press in 1980.
  Includes bibliographical references and index.
  ISBN 0-205-16101-4
  1. Audiology.   2. Hearing disorders.   I. Gerber, Sanford E.   II.   McCombe, A.W.
(Andrew Wightman)   III.   Gerber, Sanford E.  Auditory dysfunction.   IV. Title.
  [DNLM:   1.  Hearing Disorders.   WV 270 M536a   1996]
  RF290.M46   1996
  617.8—dc20
  DNLM/DLC
  for Library of Congress                                                      96–26053
                                                                                    CIP

Printed in the United States of America

10   9   8   7   6   5   4   3   2        00   99   98

*Dedicated to*
*Our Children and Grandchildren*
*They, and What We Have Written Here, Are Our Contribution to the Future*

# Contents

# *Preface*

Hearing impairment remains the most common physical disability in North America and, possibly, in the world. It affects more Americans than heart disease, cancer, blindness, tuberculosis, venereal disease, multiple sclerosis, and kidney disease put together. Wilson (1984) observed that on a worldwide basis, hearing impairment of sufficient severity to lead to vocational disability appears four times as often as vocationally disabling visual impairment. It has been reported that 17.4 million persons in the United States are hearing impaired (Wilson, 1985); more than eight million of them have a hearing impairment of sufficient degree to be disabling. Six million of these people have involvement in both ears (DiBartolomeo and Gerber, 1977).

In the United States, and other parts of the world for which we have figures, between 3.5 percent and 5 percent of school-aged children have a hearing impairment. According to the U.S. Public Health Survey (Adams and Benson, 1991), there are approximately 236, deaf individuals in the United States. Among school-aged children, there are approximately 38, in schools for the deaf, and about 100, more requiring intensive special management. Furthermore, there are approximately 250, more who are aurally impaired to an important degree in the regular school environment.

The following definitions, modified from the work of Davis and Sancho (1988), are employed throughout *Audiology and Auditory Dysfunction*. Davis and Sancho based their work on a model of the World Health Organization that they adapted and applied to hearing impairment. We believe the definitions presented here are most important because they provide a point of view of how we think about our patients.

**Pathology:** A disorder of the hearing organ, such as the middle ear, inner ear, hair cell, auditory nerve, auditory cortex, and so forth.

**Impairment:** An abnormal function of the auditory system, such as decreased auditory sensitivity with respect to the population norms.

**Disability:** The reduced abilities of an individual to correctly orient to sounds, to perceive speech in quiet and in noise, and so forth, taking the appropriate developmental norms (age, sex, social class, and culture) into account.

**Handicap:** The adverse effect on a person's life due to the psychosocial and psychological problems associated with auditory impairment and disability and their interaction with nonauditory developmental factors.

The goals of *Audiology and Auditory Dysfunction* are to offer to the beginning student an introduction to hearing disorders and to provide a basic framework from which the more advanced student may proceed. Following three introductory background chapters, the book discusses the auditory system anatomically, progressing from disorders of the sound-conducting mechanism to disorders of the sensory end organ and the neural transduction system. In essence, we progress from the outside in. The final chapter of the text considers assessment of a disability and methods of rehabilitation. The text is designed to be a basic introduction to auditory dysfunction and to provide a ready reference for those future encounters working professionals are bound to have. We hope that someday the reader will say, "Oh yes, I read about that in Mencher, Gerber, and McCombe. Let me look it up there and refresh my memory."

*Audiology and Auditory Dysfunction* has been written with the philosophy that "contemporary otology and audiology are jointly responsible for the diagnosis and management of the ear and auditory system lesions" (Goodhill, 1979). The otologist guides medical management; the audiologist and speech-language pathologist guide communicative resources. Just as the otologist must understand audiological data, procedures, and rehabilitative methods, the audiologist and speech-language pathologist must know and understand the otologist's procedures and methods. Neither is, or needs to be, equipped to practice the other's profession. We are jointly responsible to the patient.

Practicing otologists and audiologists recognize that most hearing-impaired persons cannot expect medical intervention to restore hearing to normal, even when it may alleviate the disease process. Thus, for those patients, the audiologist and/or the speech-language pathologist become the primary source of rehabilitative care. To provide maximum restoration of a patient's ability to communicate acoustically, the clinician must have a comprehensive knowledge of the extent and nature of the impairment and what can be done about it. Fundamental to that knowledge is a general understanding of diseases and disorders of the ear. We need to be able to recognize them, to understand what they are, to know what to expect from medical or surgical intervention, and to know what forms various medical and surgical treatment procedures may take.

The authors hope that physicians and other hearing health care professionals will find this book both interesting and useful. We have adopted the position that the patient is primary, the disorder is secondary. We have endeavored to be explicit about the humanistic concern. We are not dealing with hearing disorders; we are dealing with people who have hearing disorders. We hope that this attitude will be adopted by all our readers. Herein, we stress the ear for those who are interested primarily in hearing (audiologists) and hearing for those who are interested primarily in ears (otologists).

We are, of course, grateful to our wives (Lenore, Sharon, and Tracy) and families for their support, comments, and contributions to the completion of this project. We are grateful to Marilyn Totten for her help in preparation of the text, and to the staff and Board of the Nova Scotia Hearing and Speech Clinic who were so tolerant and understanding during the final preparation of the work. Of course, we are also very grateful to some colleagues for their contributions. We could not have competed Chapter 1 without the assistance of Dr. Tony Jahn. His effort is deservedly recognized as co-author of that chapter. Dr. Dean Garstecki and Dr. Susan Erler contributed Chapter 15. In our opinion it is one of the most outstanding reviews of rehabilitative audiology today. Finally, there is no better photographer of the ear than Dr. Michael Hawke. We are thrilled to have had his assistance. The authors gratefully acknowledge the contribution of Dr. Hawke, Toronto, Ontario, Canada in the preparation of this book. We are honored that he has allowed us to share some of his work within this text. Our deepest appreciation to him, to all our contributors and colleagues, and to those who have granted us permission to include their work within ours.

In 1980, Gerber and Mencher produced a book published by College-Hill Press entitled *Auditory Dysfunction*. This book is based in part upon that original work and could, in some respects, be considered a revision or second edition of that work. However, College-Hill Press and its successors do not exist for us to obtain permission to use our own materials, and this book is certainly not the same as that earlier work. It is significantly enlarged, updated, and modified. We trust that the reader will agree that *Audiology and Auditory Dysfunction* is an exciting new work.

Chapter *1*

# Anatomy and Physiology of the Human Ear[*]

## Introduction

As the organ of hearing and balance, the ear plays a significant role in helping us to orient ourselves. Balance is critical to our movement and our ability to stand upright, and to place ourselves in relation to gravitational forces. Hearing, at the primitive level, is basic to identifying our position relative to other sound-producing structures, including other animals and some objects. At a more advanced level, hearing is the basis for oral and aural communication and higher level language. It also brings us pleasure and pain.

The human ear is a highly specialized paired organ situated on either side of the human head. At its simplest, it is a vibration sensor, but it has developed specific properties that make it most sensitive to airborne vibrations in the frequency range of 250 to 8000 hertz (Hz), that is the perception of sound, and speech in particular. The human ear is traditionally divided into three parts: the outer, middle, and inner ears.

A number of standard anatomical terms must be understood. To do so, the reader must always think of the subject as standing upright and looking straight ahead. The first terms are the following:

Anterior—to the front
Posterior—to the back
Superior—to the top
Inferior—to the bottom
Medial—towards the middle (in this case of the head or ear)
Lateral—towards the outside (of the head or ear).

*Co-Authored by Dr. Anthony Jahn

1

## Outer Ear

The outer ear consists of all the structures lateral to the tympanic membrane. This comprises the pinna and the external auditory meatus (ear canal). The human pinna has a cartilaginous skeleton that provides its convoluted shape, and is covered by normal skin. There is still a number of muscular attachments to the pinna allowing some people to move them, but these are now largely vestigial in function (except for showing off at parties!). The normal pinna protrudes slightly from the head and faces in a slight anterolateral direction. The lower portion of the pinna, primarily fatty tissue and skin, is called the lobule. The pinna also has several curves and ridges that are present in almost all normal ears and that are quite consistent from person to person. These features allow an examiner to note quickly any obvious abnormality of the pinna. The most common landmarks (see Figure 1-1) are called the helix, the inferior and superior crus of the antihelix, the tragus, the antitragus, and the opening to the external auditory meatus (ear canal). This last opening is at the cavum conchae, the deepest part of the pinna.

Because of its shape, the pinna acts as a funnel, gathering sound from the environment and channeling it toward the ear canal. The various channels and hollows formed by the structures of the antihelix, ear canal, and so forth, also act to resonate the higher frequency sounds as they are funneled into the meatus, amplifying those sounds and helping to ensure that they are heard and processed by the inner ear structures.

The pinnae also act to help with directionality. That is, the asymmetric shape of the pinnae and the fact that there are two of them in two different locales sets up the possibility of a difference in the time a sound reaches one ear compared to the time it reaches the other. That time shift allows the listener to directionalize the location of the sound by responding

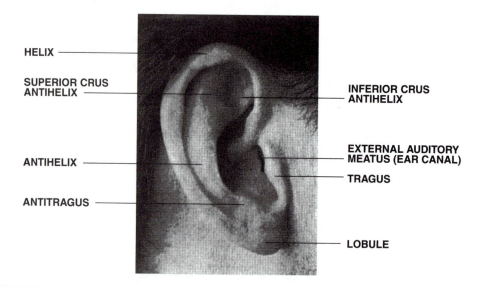

**FIGURE 1-1    A normal pinna with major landmarks indicated. (Sketch of the ear after Starkey, Canada)**

to the closer source of the sound. No matter how minuscule the difference between them, normal ears can perceive that difference, and on both a conscious and unconscious level, the listener learns to use that information for localization.

The normal adult external ear canal is about 2 to 3cm long and oval shaped. The medial two-thirds are surrounded by bone and lined by stratified squamous epithelium. This epithelium has a minimum of glands and no hairs. The lateral one-third is surrounded by cartilage, and the lining squamous epithelium is rich in both hair and glandular (ceruminous—wax producing) elements. The canal passes medially, gently curving in a slightly anteroinferior direction to meet the tympanic membrane obliquely. This means that the anterior wall of the canal is longer and deeper than the posterior wall.

The ear canal displays several properties. The skin lining the external auditory canal is not rubbed off like skin elsewhere in the body and therefore displays the property of migration. Basically the skin of the canal, is like a slow-moving conveyor belt that travels from deep to superficial, carrying with it any overlying debris. At the outer third of the canal, the skin meets the stiff hairs and starts to separate. It then mixes with the secretions of the ceruminous glands to form what we know as wax. The wax and hairs prevent entrance of particulate matter and also combine with the slightly acid conditions that exist on the skin surface throughout the canal to help to kill off microbes and prevent infection.

The outer ear appears to have a functional purpose as well. In addition to being a convenient place for earrings, hanging eyeglasses, and holding on to the ear plugs of personal radios and stereo systems, it begins the process of equalizing the temperature between the outside and the inner auditory mechanisms. The initial cold (or warm) air that reaches the pinna passes through a relatively narrow cavity (the ear canal) where its temperature is moderated, and by the time it reaches the tympanic membrane it approximates normal body temperature. This equalization helps to maximize tympanic membrane function by permitting the structure to be flexible and to respond to sound rather than be affected by temperature. Furthermore, the combined shape of the auricle and canal and the associated cerumen and hair follicles defend the tympanic membrane and the structures beyond from foreign objects that might find their way into the ear.

Finally, as indicated earlier, acoustically the pinna and canal act as a funnel to direct sound onto the tympanic membrane (Ludman, 1988; Pickles, 1988). The outer ear has a natural resonant frequency of about 3000 Hz, and therefore acts to augment or boost sounds around that frequency. Interestingly, that frequency sits nicely in the middle of the speech frequencies (1000–4000 Hz), where the human ear is most sensitive. The convoluted shape of the pinna also leads to resonances of other frequencies. This property is direction-dependent (Fischer and Schafer, 1991; Pickles, 1988), and is important for sound localization. There are, of course, other clues to sound direction, including the time delay between sounds reaching each of the ears.

## Tympanic Membrane

The bridge between the outer and middle ears is the eardrum or tympanic membrane (TM). Technically, a discussion of the TM could be included in a review of either of those structures, but because it is so singularly important a part of the hearing mechanism, a section unto itself seems deserved. A thin, rather taut structure, the TM consists of an outer or lateral surface that is made up of skin, a middle layer of fibrous tissue, and an inner or medial surface of mucous membrane. Generally circular in shape, it sits at a slight angle to the ear canal. It is slightly cone-shaped, similar to a loudspeaker. A portion of the malleus called the handle is attached to the TM. The malleus is one of the three little bones that make up the ossicular chain and are discussed later (see Figure 1-2).

The gross anatomy of the TM is readily visible with an otoscope and should be familiar to the audiologist. The central upper part of the TM is called the *pars flaccida*. The remainder of the structure is called the *pars tensa* and is the active part during sound transmission. The pars flaccida is a shallow triangle, bounded superiorly by the bony rim of the ear canal above and the anterior and posterior malleal folds anteriorly and posteriorly. The malleal folds meet at a knuckle-like bony prominence, the lateral process of the malleus. The main

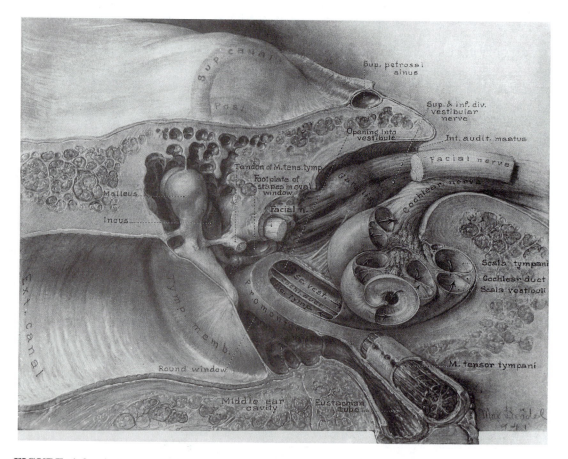

**FIGURE 1-2** **Anatomical illustration of the human ear from the external auditory meatus through the cochlear nerve.**

portion of the membrane is the pars tensa. The handle of the malleus forms a strut that bisects the upper part of the pars tensa, ending just below its center. This point, the *umbo*, represents the deepest part of the loudspeaker cone, and acoustically is the most sensitive part of the membrane. The pars tensa can be subdivided into four quadrants by continuing a line along the handle of the malleus and by then drawing a line at right angles through the umbo. This allows the observer to descriptively locate points of interest as being in the anterosuperior, anteroinferior, posterosuperior, or posteroinferior quadrant.

As already mentioned, the membrane is not at right angles to the axis of the ear canal: It is oblique and curved. Only one segment of the membrane (located in the anteroinferior quadrant) is perpendicular to the ear canal and therefore reflects the light of the otoscope back to the eye of the observer. This phenomenon, known as the light reflex, is often seen and generally suggests that the eardrum is normal (neither retracted nor pushed out). It is not invariably present in normal ears, however, and occasionally may be seen in pathologic cases. The color of the TM varies from patient to patient and depends partly on illumination. It may be pinkish-gray, usually a light shade. Blood vessels are normally present and may be seen coursing down along the handle of the malleus or entering the membrane circumferentially in a radial direction. Examining the membrane at its periphery reveals a whitish thickening of the membrane's substance at its insertion into the bony rim. This condensation of fibrous tissue is the *fibrous annulus*. As already mentioned, the handle of the malleus is clearly visible within the substance of the membrane. If the membrane is particularly translucent, the observer may also see deeper structures, such as parts of the incus and stapes, the other two ossicles of the middle ear. A thin white thread, the chorda tympani nerve, is occasionally detected.

The function of the TM is quite interesting. Because it is sometimes called the eardrum, it is easy for the lay person to think of it in terms of the musical instrument and to have a general understanding of its overall function. However, when TM movement and function are actually compared to those of a snare or kettle drum, it becomes obvious that the analogy is inappropriate. The actual drum is the middle ear, and the membrane is in fact the drumhead. Like a drumhead, the TM vibrates when struck by sound waves. Much of the incident sound energy is dissipated by reflection from the surface, however some of the energy causes a rapid in-and-out vibration of the membrane, This vibration brings the handle of the malleus into motion and converts fluctuations in air pressure into mechanical displacement of the ossicles. Air vibrations of large amplitude impacting on the membrane surface are thus collected over a larger surface and concentrated into small amplitude mechanical vibrations that displace the malleus.

The TM does not vibrate as a unit. It oscillates in segments, and the pattern of vibration depends on the frequency and the intensity of sound. The portions most readily displaced are those least anchored, while segments closer to the annulus and the malleus are stiffer, more resistant to displacement. Low-pitched sounds produce fewer vibrating segments, while higher frequencies result in multiple areas of discrete vibration. Because the TM acts to move the malleus, it seems reasonable that the areas closer to the malleus are more important. As already mentioned, the pars flaccida is not acoustically active, but it is believed that it may act as a counter vent. That is, when the malleus is pushed medially, thus compressing the air in the middle ear, the pars flaccida will move laterally to equalize the pressure.

## Middle Ear

The middle ear is an air-filled space bounded by the TM laterally and the bone surrounding the inner ear as its medial wall. On this bony medial wall can be seen the promontory with the oval window posterosuperiorly and the round window posteroinferiorly (see Figure 1-2). It is important to realize that the middle ear is a cavity within the temporal bone. It is surrounded on all sides by bone, with the exception of the outer (lateral) wall, which is formed in part by the TM. It is the middle ear that forms the drum of which the membrane is the drumhead. In fact, the middle ear is often called the tympanum (drum) or tympanic cavity. Although diagrams often show the middle ear as a box, it is really a slit that continues posteriorly to the honeycombed mastoid. It is wide in its upper and lower parts and narrow in the middle so that in cross section it resembles an hourglass. It contains the three ossicles—malleus, incus, and stapes—and two muscles—stapedius and tensor tympani. The handle of the malleus is fixed in the tympanic membrane and its head connects with the incus in the attic, the space that exists at the top of the middle ear cleft. The long process of the incus passes downward and is connected to the top of the arch of the stapes that sits in the oval window. The middle ear and mastoid air cell system are connected to the pharynx by the Eustachian tube and is filled with air that is replenished several times a minute. The Eustachian tube opens into the middle ear at the hypotympanum, an otherwise empty floor space distinguished by a scalloped, stalagmite-like bony surface. The tensor tympani muscle arises in a tunnel in the Eustachian tube, its tendon winding around the *processus cochleariformis* (a bony hook) to attach to the top of the handle of the malleus. The stapedius muscle arises from the back wall of the middle ear and inserts into the posterior arch of the stapes.

### Ossicular Chain

The ossicular chain is the most important anatomical feature of the middle ear in terms of hearing. This three-bone chain straddles the middle ear, linking the tympanic membrane to the labyrinth. Each of the ossicles resembles the structure after which it is named. The malleus looks more like an Indian war club than a hammer. Its rounded head is separated from its handle by a slender neck. The handle is incorporated into the pars tensa of the tympanic membrane. The head is hidden from otoscopic view, located in the attic of the middle ear. It has a saddle-shaped articulation with the incus. The incus resembles a tiny anvil, or perhaps a molar tooth with two roots. The main portion, or body, articulates with the malleus by a saddle-shaped joint. The peculiarity of this kind of joint is that it allows freedom of movement in two planes (compared to a hinge-type joint, which permits movement in one direction only). The two horns of the anvil are the short and long processes of the incus. The short process, along with the body, rests in the attic, whereas the long process protrudes down into the mesotympanum. It lies medial and parallel to the handle of the malleus and can occasionally be seen when examining a translucent TM with an otoscope. The tip of the long process is flattened into a round disc-like process, which articulates with the head of the stapes. This articulation (the incudostapedial joint) looks like two flat saucers, concave surfaces facing each other. That structure permits a limited amount of movement in every direction. The stapes most resembles its namesake (Figure 1-3). It is the smallest bone in the body, a tiny stirrup as might be seen attached to a cowboy's saddle. It has a head, two limbs (crura), and a footplate. The footplate, a flattened bean-shaped platform, measures only 2 × 3 mm, and sits in the oval window of the labyrinth. Due to the saddle-shaped incudomalleal joint, the incus moves more sideways than in and out. That movement causes the stapes to move, but contrary to expectations, the stapes does not push in and out like a piston, rather, it rocks sideways in the oval window.

To summarize the anatomy, the ossicular chain is made of three tiny rigid bones, connected by two flexible joints (the incudomalleal joint and the incudostapedial joint). The chain is attached to the tympanic membrane (malleus) and the labyrinth (stapes) and is suspended from the walls of the middle ear by folds of mucous membrane. It is further controlled in its movements by two tiny muscles, the tensor tympani and stapedius. The tensor tympani attaches to the neck of the malleus and contracts to pull the malleus medially. It contracts simultaneously with the tensor of the palate, both muscles controlled by the same nerve (trigeminal or fifth cranial nerve). The stapedius muscle attaches to the stapes, and, when contracting, pulls the ossicle posteriorly. It is controlled by the facial (seventh cranial) nerve, and its contraction is triggered by loud sounds. This sound-provoked contraction of the stapedius muscle is called the acoustic (or stapedius) reflex and can be measured by the audiologist using an impedance bridge.

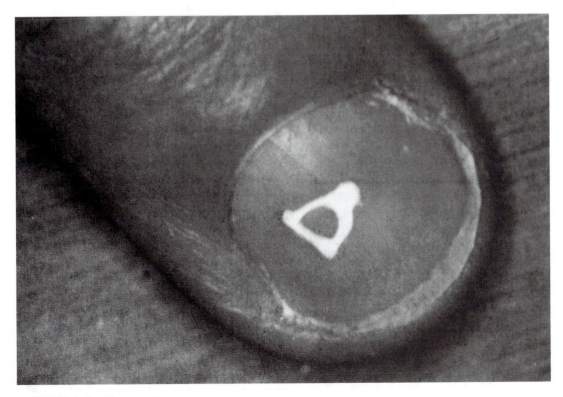

**FIGURE 1-3   Human stapes.**

What is the purpose of the ossicular chain? The middle ear and the ossicular chain help to translate and conserve acoustic air vibrations so that they may effectively stimulate the fluid-filled inner ear. Consider for a moment what would happen if airborne sound waves impacted directly on the fluid of the inner ear. Each medium has a different impedance, a property that resists displacement. If sound waves impacted directly on the surface of the water-like perilymphatic fluid, 99.9 percent of the acoustic energy would bounce off and be lost, due to the great difference in impedance between air and fluid. The ossicular chain acts as a set of step-down gears or an impedance-matching device that converts the wide but gentle oscillations of the air molecules into the narrower but more powerful vibration of the ossicles. The air waves that surround the head and strike the TM are converted by the TM into mechanical vibration that the handle of the malleus collects. The lever action of the malleus and incus further concentrates the force of the vibrations. By the time the vibrations reach the footplate of the stapes, the total effect is such that, per unit area, the force of vibration of the stapes footplate is approximately twenty-two times that of the force of vibration of the TM. That is of sufficient energy to generate fluid waves in the perilymph of the labyrinth.

In addition to transmitting and concentrating sound vibrations, the ossicular chain and middle ear structures protect the inner ear from harmful trauma. Mechanical injury to the eardrum is usually not transmitted directly to the inner ear because the ossicular joints allow a degree of slip, dissipating some of the force of the injury. This protection is relatively unique to higher animals, as in some lower animals the ossicular chain is represented by a single strut called the columella, and consequently, the protective joint mechanisms are not found. Perhaps the most important protective function of the middle ear is in the defense against noise. When high-intensity sound (usually 80–85 dB) is driven through the ear canal and reaches the tympanic membrane, the two middle ear muscles react with protective reflexes. The tensor tympani acts on the malleus handle and affects the tympanic membrane while the stapedius acts directly on the stapes and its movements. The action stiffens the drum and reflects additional sound back down the ear canal, not permitting it to pass through to the inner ear structures. The reflected sound waves may also cancel some energy by creating standing waves. At the same time this occurs in the ear canal, the restriction put on the movement of the footplate of the stapes in the oval window by contraction of the stapedius muscle limits the sound energy entering the cochlea. The action at both ends of the ossicular chain offers some protection to both the middle and inner ears by restricting their ability to respond to high-intensity sound (Henderson, Subramanian, and Boettcher, 1993). The response appears to have a greater attenuating effect on low-frequency sounds (Pickles, 1988). Unfortunately, in today's highly industrialized society, this natural safety mechanism is of only limited value in protecting the ear from noise exposure.

## Mastoid Process

There are one or two other structures to be associated with the middle ear. First, is the facial nerve. This large nerve runs encased through the bony walls of the middle ear and has no importance to hearing, except for its branch to the stapedius muscle. However, as various forms of disease attack the middle ear, the facial nerve may be endangered. The mastoid process, a bony protuberance that can be felt at the side of the head directly behind the ear is another associated structure. If examined in a dry skull, the tip of the outer surface of the mastoid process appears rough. This roughening gives attachment to a large muscle, called the sternocleidomastoid, which rotates the head on the neck. This attachment is probably the main purpose of the mastoid process.

Inside, the mastoid process is excavated to form small air-containing cells. These connect to one another and to the main air cavity of the mastoid, the mastoid antrum. This, in turn, is linked to the attic of the middle ear by a narrow passage, the *aditus ad antrum*. The mastoid air cells and mastoid antrum are lined by a gossamer-thin mucous membrane that is in direct continuity with the mucosa of the middle ear, the Eustachian tube, and eventually the nasopharynx. Interestingly, the air cell system is absent at birth. However, with growth from early childhood, the mastoid portion of the temporal bone grows and becomes pneumatized. The degree of pneumatization depends on the function of the Eustachian tube: a well-functioning Eustachian tube will result in a well-pneumatized mastoid, that is, a large mastoid air cell system. If the function of the Eustachian tube is poor there will be little pneumatization and a sclerotic mastoid will result. The mastoid probably has no role to play in hearing per se, however, it has been suggested that in addition to serving as a muscle attachment on the outside, the air cells act as surge tanks and cushion the air pressure fluctuations that occur with air resorption and intermittent Eustachian tube opening. Of course, the mastoid as a unit serves as a resonator of sound and sound can be transmitted through it by bone conduction.

## *Eustachian Tube*

In the embryo, the middle ear is formed as an outpouching of the pharynx. This outpouching begins as the Eustachian tube and continues as the middle ear and the mastoid process. These structures, while anatomically distinct, are in direct continuity with each other and with the pharynx. They contain air that is frequently replenished from the back of the nose and throat. Indeed, for the middle ear to function properly, it must be filled with air at atmospheric (ambient) pressure. If the air pressure in the middle ear drops (due to poor Eustachian tube function), a hearing loss may develop.

The Eustachian tube is a narrow, obliquely oriented passage that begins in the back of the nose (nasopharynx) and ends in the anterior portion of the middle ear, or inversely, passes in an anteroinferomedial direction from the front of the middle ear space to open in the posterosuperior corner of the nasopharynx (the space at the back of the nose). The tube narrows at its mid-portion to form an isthmus. Even when fully opened, the isthmus of the Eustachian tube is only 2 mm in diameter. The medial two-thirds of the tube (closer to the nasopharynx) is made of cartilage, while the lateral (middle ear) third is bony. The cartilaginous part of the tube forms a narrow slit and is normally closed. It is pulled open by muscles that attach to the cartilage and the soft palate (levator and tensor of the palate). However, when the muscles relax, the cartilage springs shut once more, closing the tube. The cartilage projects slightly into the nasopharynx to form a mound (torus tubarius), which is visible under the mucous membrane. The bony portion is relatively wide and held open by its bony walls. It flares towards the middle ear and narrows toward the cartilaginous tube. The entire structure is lined by mucous membrane, which continues medially as the mucous membrane of the nasopharynx, and laterally as the mucous membrane of the middle ear. The mucous membrane lining the tube itself is thrown up into folds (rugae), further narrowing the passage. One may imagine that any swelling of the mucosal lining might readily lead to obstruction of the passage. The tube is shorter and more horizontal in children and becomes longer and more oblique in adults.

While the tympanic (middle ear) end of the tube opens into an unobstructed area (the protympanum of the middle ear), the nasopharyngeal end is more crowded. Anterior to the torus tubarius is the posterior opening of the nasal passage (choana), with a constant flow of mucus. Medial to the torus are the adenoids, tonsil-like structures which are often prominent and sometimes obstructive in children. The main function of the Eustachian tube is to maintain ambient air pressure in the middle ear. Air trapped within the body tends to become absorbed by surrounding tissues. For that reason, the Eustachian tube opens frequently to replenish the air contained in the middle ear and to equalize pressure between the middle ear and the nasopharynx. The muscles that open the tube simultaneously lift the soft palate. This ingenious mechanism ensures that the tube opens only when the palate is raised, separating the nasopharynx from the back of the mouth (oropharynx). The Eustachian tubes are automatically shielded from food, drink, and saliva in the oropharynx, ensuring that only nasally inhaled air passes through to the middle ear. The Eustachian tubes normally open with swallowing and yawning, several times a minute. They can also be forced open by pinching one's nose and blowing to "pop the ears." This technique, the Valsalva maneuver, is used by divers and pilots to prevent negative middle ear air pressure.

Why did this mechanism for intermittent ventilation develop, and why are the tubes not constantly open? Apart from the dangers of soiling the tubes with food, drink, and mucus, an open tube would also act as a sound conduit, directing the self-generated sounds of talking and breathing up into the middle ear and interfering with the perception of environmental sounds. In the rare instance in which a patient's tubes are constantly open (patulous eustachian tube), patients are aware of these sounds (autophonia) as well as of their tympanic membranes vibrating with inhalation and exhalation. In addition to ventilation, the Eustachian tubes also remove mucus and debris from the middle ears. The mucosal cells have tiny bristles (cilia) that continuously sweep the surface toward the back of the throat, moving mucus, dead cell fragments, and products of any inflammation out of the middle ear into the throat. The mucous membrane also has a protective function preventing throat infections from ascending to the middle ear.

## *Inner Ear*

The bony labyrinth, as the name suggests, is a structure of complex turns, nooks, and crannies. Also called the inner ear, the labyrinth consists of the semicircular canals, which are responsible for the detection of angular acceleration; the utricle and saccule, which are responsible for the detection of linear acceleration; and the cochlea, with which we are particularly concerned, which is responsible for the processing of sound. The entire structure is smaller than the tip of an adult's index finger. The labyrinth is encased in the petrous temporal bone, probably the hardest bone in the body. It is separated into a number of fluid-filled spaces that are created by the presence of a membranous labyrinth within the bony skeleton. It is very important for the reader to understand that these structures, usually shown together as a concrete object in diagrams or classroom models, do not appear in the body as an object that one can remove like a heart or lung. Simply stated, within the mastoid bone there is a series of channels that contain the components of the hearing mechanism. They cannot be removed without destroying them or the skull, nor can they be opened and examined. To drill into the bony structure is to allow the fluids contained therein to leak from the capsule and to destroy the system's integrity.

## Vestibular System

The balance organs of the labyrinth are housed in the vestibule and in the semicircular canals. The vestibule, the central portion of the labyrinth, houses the utricle and the saccule. The balance organs of the utricle and the saccule are the maculae, and these sense linear acceleration and orientation within the field of gravity. In addition, the three semicircular canals arise from the vestibule. They are arranged at right angles to each other, like three sides of a cube, and therefore define the three-dimensional vectors of space (the x, y, and z axes). Each canal has a bulb-like dilatation at one end, which is the ampulla. This contains the ampullary end organs of balance, which monitor acceleration in that particular plane. Among the three canals, any acceleration in any direction (such as head turning) can be analyzed in terms of the three vectors of space. The semicircular canals are the organs of angular acceleration (see Figure 1-4).

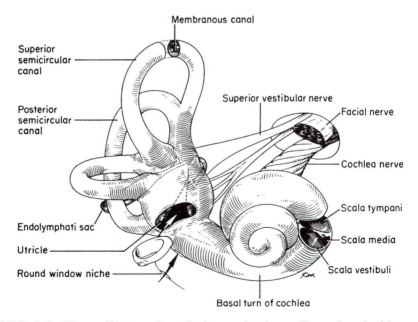

**FIGURE 1-4   The auditory and vestibular mechanisms. (Reproduced with permission of Grune and Stratton, Inc. from Bradford and Hardy, *Hearing and Hearing Impairment*, 1985)**

In the balance portion of the inner ear, there are two kinds of end organs: the otolith organs of the vestibule and the ampullary end organs of the semicircular canals. The utricle and saccule (located in the vestibule) are ovoid and spherical dilatations of the membranous labyrinth. These are seated against the inner wall of the bony labyrinth in appropriately shaped depressions. Each structure contains a densely packed sheet of hair cells. The hair cells project their cilia into a gelatinous sheet, the otolithic membrane. This membrane is studded with tiny multifaceted calcified granules, the otoliths or otoconia. To the naked eye, each otolith organ looks like a white spot, hence its name, macula. The macula of the utricle and the macula of the saccule are grossly similar. Because most of the membranous labyrinth is isodense with water, it therefore has no weight within its fluid bath. The calcium-laden otoconia, however, do have additional mass and will bring weight to bear on the tips of the cilia. Their weight causes the otolithic membrane to shear along the surface of the hair cells, making these hair cells sensitive to the pull of gravity. If the head (i.e., the person) is moving along a straight line, the weight of the otoliths will cause them to lag behind, again displacing the cilia embedded in the otoconial membrane. In this way, the otolithic organs (utricle and saccule) act as sensors of linear acceleration. The sensitivity of the otolith organs is further increased by additional mechanisms that are beyond the scope of our discussion.

The three semicircular canals complete the vestibular labyrinth. They arise from, and recurve into, the utricle. The three ampullary end organs are located at one end of each of the semicircular canals. The dilatation in the endolymph-containing membranous semicircular canal is accommodated by a similar dilatation in the bony canal. A tuft of hair cells sits on the floor of the ampulla on a crest-shaped base (crista ampullaris). The cilia are embedded in a tall gelatinous blob (cupula), and the tip of the cupula touches the ceiling of the ampulla. The entire structure resembles a bar door, free to swing either way, depending on the direction of traffic (flow of endolymph). When the head turns, this acceleration moves the bony and membranous labyrinth promptly. The endolymph, however, lags behind, owing to the inertia of the fluid. The phenomenon is similar to trying to spin a fresh egg. The inertia of the yolk drags on the inside of the shell, and the egg topples over. In the semicircular canal, this drag is represented by the lag of labyrinthine fluid, which causes a relative flow of endolymph past the ampulla in a direction opposite to that of the head motion. This displaces the cupula, deflects the cilia, and triggers an electric signal from the hair cells. Depending on the direction of endolymph flow, the hair cells will depolarize or hyperpolarize. The cupula will remain deflected only while there is a difference in movement between the walls of the labyrinth and the endolymph. Once the endolymph catches up in speed (i.e., the head is moving at constant velocity), the cupula floats back to its neutral mid-position, and the organ stops signaling. Owing to the narrowness of the semicircular canal, each ampullary end organ is highly directional in its response, and is triggered only by head displacement in its own unique direction. On the other hand, any head acceleration, no matter how complex, can be analyzed in terms of the three vectors of space, and this is precisely what the three semicircular canals do. The sensitivity of these canals is further enhanced by input from the other ear and a directional bias that is beyond the scope of this discussion.

The utricle and saccule are both connected to an elongated outpouching of the labyrinth, the endolymphatic duct. This courses posteriorly and ends in the endolymphatic sac. The sac lies inside the head, in the posterior cranial fossa. This ensures that any rapid pressure change inside the head (such as with sneezing or straining) is instantly transmitted to the inner ear, and pressure throughout the system is maintained. This pressure equalization mechanism prevents any damage to the labyrinth due to pressure gradients. Given that this text is predominantly concerned with hearing and its disorders, we now restrict our attention to the part of the bony labyrinth called the cochlea, but the reader is encouraged to further explore the semicircular canals and the vestibular system.

## *Cochlea*

The cochlea is the labyrinthine organ of hearing (Figure 1-5). It arises from the vestibule, where it remains connected to the saccule by a very narrow duct. In the human temporal bone, the semicircular canals lie posteriorly, the utricle and saccule lie in the middle, and the cochlea lies in front. With its 2.5 turns and decreasing width from the base to the apex, the cochlea looks vaguely like a seashell, hence its name. The cochlea is a relatively recent arrival in evolution: fish have no cochleas (they sense motion rather than sound), and even the alligator has no recognizable cochlea rather, it has a simple outpouching at the lower end of its labyrinth, the basal papilla. Neither is the human cochlea the last word in hearing: some rodents' cochleas have more than our 2.5 turns, and others, such as bats, are able to hear well up into the supersonic range.

As already indicated, the cochlea arises as an outpouching from the saccule. It maintains this connection, sharing both the fluids and fluid pressures present throughout the upper (vestibular) portion of the labyrinth. It contains a membranous lining called the membranous labyrinth, which is a delicate fluid-filled sac. The lining floats within the bony casing, the outer surface assuming roughly the same shape as the bony labyrinth. The central or middle room (scala media) of the membranous labyrinth is filled with endolymph, and it floats within the bony labyrinth sandwiched between two other spaces called the scala tympani and scala vestibuli, which are filled with perilymph. The walls of these various rooms are created by their attachments to each other and to the bony labyrinth. Thus, the membranous labyrinth is anchored to the walls of the bony labyrinth, but has a degree of mobility, somewhat like a sea anemone anchored to a reef. Endolymph and

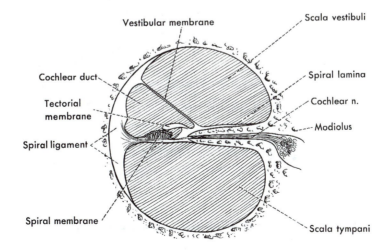

**FIGURE 1-5  Cross section through one turn of the cochlea.**

perilymph are both clear watery fluids that differ from each other only in their concentration of ions. The delicate wall of the membranous labyrinth has the same specific gravity as these fluids, and thus the membranous labyrinth is suspended as if it had no weight.

Thus, internally, the membranous labyrinth is broken up into three spaces as shown in cross section in Figures 1-2 and 1-5. These spaces are the following: the scala vestibuli, which is superior and begins at the oval window; the scala tympani, which is inferior and ends at the round window; and the scala media, which is self-contained in the middle within the cochlea. The scala media contains endolymph. The scala tympani and the scala vestibuli both contain perilymph and are continuous at the distal end of the cochlea, which is called the helicotrema. This means it is possible to trace a course from the base of the cochlea at the entrance to the scala tympani (the oval window), twisting up the 2.5 turns, and when reaching the helicotrema at the apex, passing into the scala vestibuli and traveling back down the 2.5 turns to the basilar end to the round window in a separate channel. The two scalae are connected only at the apical end. The third channel, the scala media, contains endolymph and is separated from the scala vestibuli by the Reissner membrane and from the scala tympani by the basilar membrane. The organ of Corti rests on the basilar membrane in the scala media. Although a coiled structure, the cochlea can be thought of as a U-shaped tube built around a central wall, in this case, the basilar membrane and organ of Corti, with the oval and round windows at each end.

The organ of Corti (see Figure 1-6) is *the* auditory transducer. Its primary function is to convert the mechanical pressure fluctuations of sound, which have passed through the ear

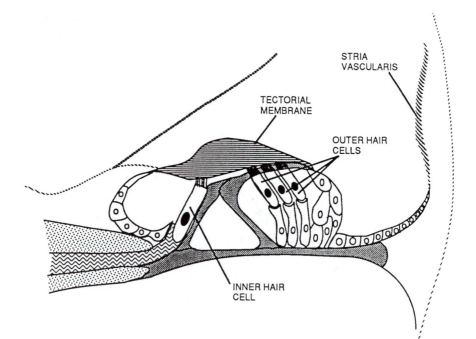

STRIA VASCULARIS

TECTORIAL MEMBRANE

OUTER HAIR CELLS

INNER HAIR CELL

**FIGURE 1-6   Cross section of the organ of Corti. (Reproduced with permission of Dr. Andrew McCombe)**

canal and middle ear to the cochlea, into electro-chemical neural impulses, which in turn will pass up the cochlear portion of the eighth nerve and be processed centrally. Sound waves are transmitted to the cochlear perilymph by vibrations of the stapes, moving with a piston-like action at low frequencies and with a rocking motion at higher frequencies. The basilar membrane varies in width, thickness, and stiffness along its length, being narrower, thicker, and stiffer at the basal end. This physical characteristic gives rise to traveling waves or trains of waves in the perilymph, causing vibration of the basilar membrane. This vibration will reach a maximum amplitude at specific points along the basilar membrane that are frequency-specific and intensity-dependent. Traveling waves caused by high frequencies reach a maximum at the basal end of the cochlea, and those caused by low frequencies reach a maximum at the apical end (von Békèsy, 1960; Pickles, 1988).

To understand how the cochlea processes the traveling waves and converts that mechanical process into electrical energy, it is necessary to understand the anatomy and physiology of the organ of Corti and its surrounding structures. The organ of Corti contains an orderly array of hair cells that wind their way along the scala media, somewhat like the keys of a piano. The array consists of a single row of inner hair cells and three rows of outer hair cells numbered 1 to 3, centrally to peripherally. The cells sit along the basilar membrane and are surrounded and aided by supporting cells (see Figure 1-7). The outer and inner rows of hair cells are separated by the tunnel of Corti, a fluid-filled passage that is triangular in cross sec-

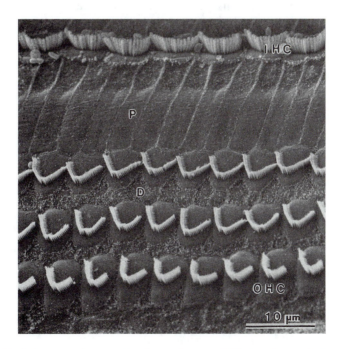

**FIGURE 1-7** **Electron microscopic photo of inner (IHC) and outer hair cells (OHC) of the organ of Corti of a normal cochlea. (Reproduced with permission of Dr. Anthony Jahn)**

tion. The roof of the organ of Corti is the gelatinous tectorial membrane, which forms a canopy over the hair cells, and is tethered both at the modiolus and laterally. The inner hair cells do not make direct contact with the tectorial membrane although the outer hair cells, and particularly those in row 1, are embedded in it (Lim, 1986). Further, the outer hair cells receive efferent innervation via the olivo-cochlear bundle, contain contractile proteins, and exhibit motility, whereas the inner hair cells do not (Figure 1-8). However, the inner hair cells have a richer afferent innervation (Johnstone, Patuzzi, and Yates, 1986; Kemp, 1980; Khanna, 1984; Kim, 1984; Zenner, 1993). Kemp (1980) has reported that the outer hair cells are considered the source of otoacoustic emissions.

### Hair Cell Activity

Although the vestibular end organs and the cochlea differ in many ways, they share the same type of end receptor, the hair cell. It is the hair cell that, when stimulated, converts the mechanical swirling of inner ear fluids into electrical energy, the language of the nervous system and the brain (Figure 1-6). Hair cells, like other cells, are filled with intracellular fluid, which is high in potassium and low in sodium. The hairs, or cilia, protrude from the top (apex) of the cells. The sides and bases of the hair cells are bathed in extracellular fluid, low in potassium and high in sodium. Each of these ions, therefore, has a different concentration on either side of the cell wall membrane. There is, then, an electrical potential difference across the cell membrane, that is actively maintained by tiny ion pumps within the cell membrane. The cilia are sensitive to mechanical movement. They are easily deflected, although the mechanical means of deflection varies depending on which part of the vesti-

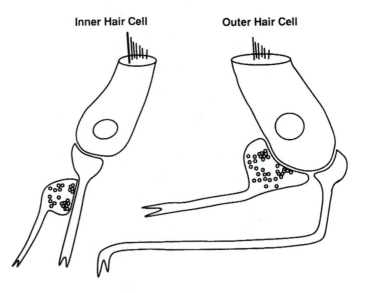

**FIGURE 1-8   Diagrams of hair cells.**

bular or cochlear labyrinth they are found. As the cilia bend, they distort the cell membrane, making it leaky, and allowing for an interchange of ions between the extracellular and the intracellular fluid compartments. This flow of ions depolarizes the cell and generates an electric current. In this way, hair cells act as mechano-electric transducers. Hair cells, however, are even more sophisticated. The row of cilia atop each hair cell are arranged in order of size, starting with the shortest at one end and increasing to the tallest at the other. The tallest cilium, called the kinocilium, has specific properties that are beyond our scope here. It is noteworthy, however, that cilia can be deflected in two directions: toward the kinocilium, and in the opposite direction, away from the kinocilium. Depending on which direction the cilia are bent, the cell will either depolarize (increase the flow of ions across the cell membrane, lower the potential difference), or hyperpolarize (reduce the flow of ions and raise the potential difference). The actual direction varies throughout the labyrinth, but the principle is maintained even in the cochlea, where the hair cells do not possess a kinocilium.

A study of the types and numbers of nerve fibers has revealed a surprising fact: The outer hair cells may not send auditory information to the brain, and it is the inner hair cells that appear to be the actual mechano-electric transducers of sound vibrations. By virtue of their location along the cochlear keyboard (as well as certain intrinsic electrical properties), the inner hair cells are triggered by specific tone frequencies. This tonotopic arrangement of hair cells begins with the highest frequencies at the basal turn, progresses through the mid-frequencies in the middle turn, and ends with the lowest frequencies in the apical turn. At birth, the human cochlea can distinguish a range of frequencies from 20 to 20,000 Hz.

If the inner hair cells are responsible for hearing, what then is the purpose of the triple row of outer hair cells? The outer hair cells of the cochlea have evolved a unique and wonderful adaptation unlike any other hair cells in the labyrinth. These hair cells are capable of movement. They can contract and expand, and they can make their cilia stiffer or more lax. While the inner hair cell cilia do not protrude into the tectorial membrane, but vibrate freely with the currents of endolymph generated by sound pressure, in contrast, the outer hair cell cilia protrude into the gelatinous tectorial membrane and can therefore alter the position and tension of that structure. The mechanism is analogous to tuning a guitar string. By constantly adjusting the tectorial membrane, outer hair cells change the flow of endolymph past the inner hair cell cilia and modulate their sensitivity. Further fine tuning is provided by the outer hair cells acting as the so-called second filter. In essence, as the traveling wave reaches its point of maximum amplitude at some point along the basilar membrane, the action is sensed by the outer hair cells in the region. Active processes and outer hair cell motility then come into play, with the outer hair cells at the region of maximum amplitude acting to increase the vibration up to a hundredfold. As a result, there is a marked increase in the maximum vibration, but it is limited to a very narrow region of the basilar membrane. The inner hair cells at that point may then function in a purely sensory fashion with depolarization leading to stimulation of the cochlear nerve. The overall combined action and results of hair cell movements is relayed to higher centers. The information relayed is how we perceive sound (Johnstone, Patuzzi, and Yates 1986; Khanna, 1984; Kim, 1984; Lim, 1986).

Finally, it is interesting to note that just as the ear canal and middle ear have some built-in protective devices for the hearing mechanism, so too does the cochlea. By their property of motility, the outer hair cells are also thought to offer some protection against noise-induced hearing loss (Henderson, Subramanian, and Boettcher, 1993), possibly by reducing the over-all excursion of the basilar membrane in response to loud sound stimulation (Zenner, 1993).

## *Auditory and Vestibular Nerves and Higher Centers*

The next step in the auditory system is the eighth cranial nerve. Axons from the spiral gan-glion at the base of the organ of Corti join at the modiolus forming what is called the auditory nerve or the auditory branch of the eighth cranial nerve. In addition, the sensory responses of the vestibular system reach the eighth nerve via the vestibular nerve or the vestibular branch. No matter what the terminology, together, the auditory and vestibular nerves form the eighth (vestibulocochlear) cranial nerve. The joining of the two branches has been compared to that of a twisted rope, with fibers from the apical portion of the cochlea forming the core and fibers from the other portions of the cochlea and the vestibular system wrapping around them in a very orderly and systematic fashion (Northern and Downs, 1991). The nerve passes through the internal auditory meatus, an opening in the base of the skull whose sole pur-pose is to allow the auditory nerve to enter the brain stem, and turns into what is called the cerebellar-pontine angle. The eighth nerve shares its passage through the internal auditory meatus with the seventh (facial) nerve. Obviously, this site is one of the most critical for tumors of the eighth cranial nerve and is discussed in greater detail later.

The vestibular branch eventually separates from the auditory nerve and develops its own two branches, which are called the superior and inferior vestibular nerves. They enter the vestibular nuclei of the brain stem. The signal is processed through a series of relays up to the vestibular cortex. Along the way, interconnections occur that tell us to adjust our pos-ture (vestibulospinal tracts), to stabilize ourselves as we move (vestibulocerebellar), and to keep our eye on our environment while turning (vestibulo-ocular pathways). Other connec-tions are responsible for the cold sweat, nausea, and vomiting of motion sickness. The cen-tral vestibular pathways are also paired, and information from the two labyrinths is interchanged and integrated until the vestibular cortex arrives at the realization that the per-son is moving.

There is evidence that the fibers of the eighth auditory nerve are frequency-specific and that their responses can be traced back to individual hair cells within the cochlea (Evans and Wilson, 1977). For the most part, therefore, they carry information from the inner ear to the brain (afferent fibers). Some fibers, however, carry impulses from the brain to the inner ear, instructing it to modify its response to environmental stimuli. Once the auditory fibers leave the eighth nerve and enter the brain stem they become part of a series of relay stations that synaptically send electrical energy up to the auditory processing center in the cortex. The cochlear nerve connects to the cochlear nucleus in the brain stem. Fibers from each of the cochlear nuclei travel upward on the ipsilateral side (the same side), but there is also a num-ber of fibers that decussate (crisscross) to the contralateral (opposite) side (see Figure 1-9).

Leaving the cochlear nucleus, the fibers enter the superior olive, the inferior colliculus, the medial geniculate body and finally, the auditory cortex. At each of these relay points, the electrical signals are processed and the auditory information is passed on. The tonotopic or frequency-specific organization seen in the cochlea continues throughout the central auditory pathways. At each relay station, however, the signal acquires additional degrees of sophistication. For example, the cortex allows the listener to recognize a sound. Specifically, the temporal lobe is identified as the primary area of auditory response in the human brain. Chapter 14 includes a review of the various higher level auditory functions controlled in the midbrain and cortex and focuses on some pathologies seen when those areas cease to behave normally.

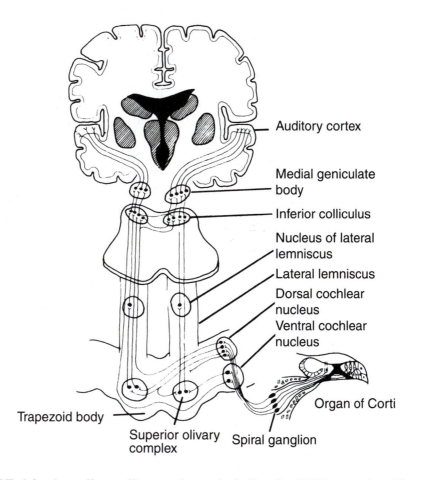

**FIGURE 1-9** **Ascending auditory pathways including the (VCN) ventral cochlear nucleus, (DCN) dorsal cochlear nucleus, (LL) lateral lemniscus, (IC) inferior colliculus, (MGB) medial geniculate body, and the (AC) auditory cortex. (From W. R. Zemlin, *Speech and Hearing Science*, 3rd ed. Englewood Cliffs, NJ: Prentice-Hall, 1988)**

## Comment

In summary, then, sound waves arrive as vibrations at the pinnae. They are filtered, focused, and some are enhanced through resonance. The vibrations continue on their way until they strike the tympanic membrane. Once again, they undergo a modification designed to permit the maximum response from the ear. The vibrations are channeled to the ossicular chain that, through its lever action, serves as an impedance-matching device. When the focused energy moves the stapes footplate in the oval window, it perturbs the perilymph of the vestibule. Because water is incompressible, these perturbations are transmitted throughout the labyrinth and cause a to-and-from movement of the scala media of the cochlea. As the scala media moves up and down, the fluid compartments around the organ of Corti are agitated, displacing the cilia of the inner hair cells. This movement causes a distortion of the cell walls, allowing for a flow of charged ions (sodium and potassium) that generates an electric current. The electric current (cochlear microphonic) generated through numerous cells triggers off a larger discharge (summating potential or action potential). Once an action potential has occurred, it is passed up the eighth cranial nerve to synapse in the cochlear nucleus in the brain stem. This signal then results in further action potentials and the passage of a signal upward through the superior olivary complex, the inferior colliculus, the medial geniculate body, and then onward to the auditory cortex (Pickles, 1988). This discussion of the anatomy and physiology of the ear is only an introduction. We have tried to explain basic structure and function and to impart some of the excitement surrounding this minute but wonderfully sophisticated organ. This brief chapter doesn't even begin to address the sophisticated mechanisms by which the ear achieves temporal, spatial, and frequency discrimination. Indeed, we do not completely understand how this is accomplished, although we do know that there are many discriminatory activities occurring at various levels along the auditory pathway from the auricle all the way to the auditory cortex. By appreciating the complexity of the ear, a clinician gains some appreciation of the limitations inherent in audiological testing. All tests are snapshots in time and can provide only a limited view of this dynamic organ.

# Chapter *2*

## *What We Hear*

It is not possible to discuss hearing loss or impairment without first talking about what it is that we hear. We need to have an understanding of the nature of the signals that stimulate the auditory system, particularly that range of energy we have labeled sound. The study of sound and hearing is shared by the physical science of acoustics and the perceptual science of psychoacoustics. Although we do not need to be a physicist or psychologist to understand the physical and perceptual processes encountered by the human ear, if we are to understand hearing and hearing impairment, we must understand what and how we hear. In essence, to appreciate abnormality we need to have an understanding of the nature of the signals that stimulate the auditory system and how the ear responds normally.

## *Acoustics*

The branch of physics that deals with sound and its properties is called acoustics. Acoustics, in turn, has several branches and sub-branches—such as physiological acoustics, underwater acoustics, industrial acoustics—but we are not concerned with the individual sub-branches here, rather, this discussion is limited to certain physical properties of sound and the units that are used to measure them.

What is sound? Philosophers pose the old question about a tree crashing to the ground in a remote forest where no one was present to hear the tree falling. "Did it make a sound?" they ask. Of course it did. We are talking about sound, not hearing.

Sound is defined quite specifically as (1) a disturbance (2) of the particles of an elastic medium (3) moving forward and backward from their places of rest that (4) radiate outward in all directions from the source. So what does all that mean? It means, first, that there must be a disturbance, an application of some kind of force: for example, the tree hit the ground. Second, the medium through which sound travels must have some elasticity. The obvious example, of course, is air; but sound travels through any elastic medium. It travels through gases other than air; it travels through water; it travels through animal tissue; and so forth. The less elastic the medium—say, concrete or lead—the slower is the speed of sound. Third, because the medium is elastic, the particles can travel only so far from their resting places and then must return. In its travels back and forth, a particle will meet other particles and disturb them away from their resting places, thereby imparting the energy of the initial disturbance to the next particle, and on and on. This oscillation backward and forward will continue both as a function of the amount of elasticity of the medium and of how long the force continues to be applied.

Using a simple analogy, imagine a billiards player rolling one ball into another on the table. The first ball strikes the second and reverses its direction, returning back to the player's hand. If he applies force again (rolls the ball), the journey is repeated again, and again, and again, until the player stops rolling the ball. At the same time, the second ball, which has been struck by the first, is set into motion and moves forward until it strikes another ball. At that point, it reverses its direction and returns to its original location. If the player is still rolling the original ball, the two will meet again, and the entire process will be repeated. If, by chance, the player is still rolling the original ball, but he has moved its location back a few steps, the second ball will continue on its return course, past its point of initial location, and keep moving until it reaches the original ball, strikes it, and then changes direction back past its initial location and forward until it strikes another ball, and then the journey begins again. This will continue on and on until the player stops rolling the original ball.

Of course, what has just been said about how sound travels is true of other forms of radiation as well. For example, we speak of light rays that radiate out from the source. But light travels in straight lines, and so we can't see around corners. The one important difference with sound that differentiates it from any and all other types of energy is that it travels outward in *all* directions. In fact, sound waves travel in a rather spherical path, spreading out as they go. That is one reason why we can hear around corners. To follow along the lines of the earlier analogy, think of the billiards player as the sound source, and his hand throwing balls in 360 different directions all at the same time. Each of those balls strikes another ball, and so on.

There is a number of important parameters that describe the character of a sound wave as it passes a point in space. These parameters are called by common terms that permit professionals such as acousticians, audiologists, and hearing scientists, to communicate easily.

## *Wavelength*

Sound can be represented by a series of compressions and rarefactions in the density of the air that move away from the source of the sound, with no net displacement of the air molecules, that is, areas in which many particles are gathered and striking each other (compression), and areas in which few particles are left because of the movement (rarefaction). If we consider a fixed point in space, the wavelength of a sound will be the distance that the wavefront advances in the time that a solitary particle of the transmitting medium moves from its rest position to that of maximal positive displacement, back past its rest point to its position of maximal negative displacement, and finally back to its resting position (see Figure 2-1). Technically, wavelength is the distance between corresponding points on the waveform.

## Speed of Sound

The velocity of wave propagation (c)—that is, the speed of sound—depends on the density and elasticity of the medium carrying the sound. In air, the velocity is given by the formula: $c = 331 + 0.6t$ where c = the speed of sound in meters per second (m/s), and t = temperature in degrees Celsius. For typical atmospheric conditions, this equates to a speed of approximately 340 m/s or about 1100 feet per second.

## Frequency

Frequency (f) refers to the rate (i.e., the frequency) at which a series of compressions and rarefactions occurs within a period of one second. That is, we can measure the frequency of this action. The word "frequency" is used here in its usual sense: how often did something happen. Each time a complete compression and rarefaction occurs, the movement is called a cycle. Frequency is the number of cycles that occur in one second—the number of cycles per second (cps). A picture of this activity is also seen in Figure 2-1, which illustrates both the wavelength and what is called the sine wave of a single tone. Sine waves, because they are only one frequency, are heard as pure tones. It is important for the reader to understand that the particle is not bouncing up and down as the illustration may lead one to believe. The sine wave is a plot of forward and backward motion which is called sinusoidal motion, and it is measured in Hertz (i.e., cycles per second).

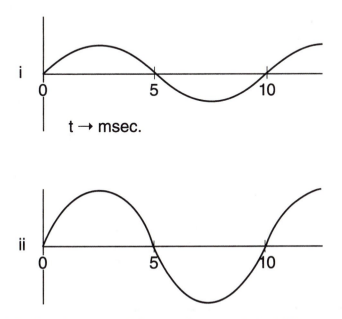

**FIGURE 2-1**    **Two sine waves of the same frequency but of different amplitudes.**

It is equally possible to measure how long it takes for a particle to move away from its place of rest and back again just once. This is the period of the wave. The period T (for time) equals 1/f (for frequency). One may see, then that if f = 1000 Hz, then the period is 1/f = 1/1000 second or one millisecond. If the frequency were, say, 2000 Hz, then the period is 1/2000 or 500 milliseconds. And so on for any value.

As mentioned earlier, frequency is a measure of the number of cycles per second. However, to honor one of the great scientists of the nineteenth century, Heinrich Hertz, the unit of measurement of frequency is called Hertz instead of cycles per second. So, a tone with 1000 compressions and rarefactions in a second produces 1000 cps and, therefore, 1000 Hertz. It is a 1000 Hertz tone, or, if the abbreviation for Hertz is used, it is a 1000 Hz tone. Furthermore, it is important to remember that frequency is a measure of the number of times that particles change direction. This is a physical description of the tone, not a perceptual description. The perceptual subjective correlate of frequency is pitch. The physical property is frequency and can be physically manipulated. How a frequency is heard and interpreted is perceptual, physiologic, and dependent on a listener's ears. That is pitch.

## Amplitude and Intensity

A complete description of a sound requires some indication of its magnitude or *wave amplitude*, something that is subjectively correlated with loudness. Measurement of the amplitude of the displacement of the particles through a transmission medium is difficult; measurement of the average rate of energy flow past a given point in space is much simpler. Consequently, sound intensity and sound pressure level are the measures used.

Sound intensity is defined in terms of the average rate of energy flow per unit area and is measured in Watts per square meter ($W/m^2$), that is, power (in Watts) per unit area (square meters). This measure is based on the principle that sound radiates spherically (outward in all directions) from a point source and will obviously become less intense as it radiates further from the source. This phenomenon obeys the inverse square law: sound intensity is proportional to $1/r^2$ where r = the distance from the sound source in meters. Under typical atmospheric conditions, sound intensity is proportional to the square of sound pressure, which is measured in Newtons per square meter ($N/m^2$) or what are called Pascals (Pa). The ear is a pressure-sensing device, and so it is essential that we understand the concept of pressure (force per unit area) and how it is measured. Note that Newton and Pascal are also names of people.

The range of pressures required for measurement of human hearing is so great that a logarithmic system called the deciBel (dB) scale has been developed to cope. Note again the use of a name. In this case it is Alexander Graham Bell. In the deciBel system, the sound intensity or sound pressure level is expressed as a ratio against a reference value. We are all familiar with reference values. Consider temperature. When it is 0 degrees Celsius, it is cold, but 0 degrees does not mean no heat at all. Zero is a reference. Likewise, the formula Intensity level (dB IL) = $10 \log_{10} I_m / I_{ref}$ (where $I_m$ = the measured intensity and $I_{ref}$ = the reference intensity) really provides a reference for interpreting the amount of acoustic energy used in generating the sound. Hence, the intensity level could be less than zero if the measured intensity were less than the reference or considerably greater if significantly more than the reference. Further, based on the relationship between intensity and pressure, it is also possible to determine: Sound pressure level (dB SPL)= 20 $\log_{10}$ $p_m/p_{ref}$. Note that pressure is denoted by lower case p and power by upper case P. Obviously, these equations are meaningless without their reference values. For sound pressure levels, the reference value is defined as $2 \times 10^{-5}$ Pa and for sound intensity levels it is $10^{-16}$ W/cm$^2$.

Although these measurements will define a pure tone completely, sound as it occurs in the real world is rarely, if ever, a pure tone. Real sounds—such as speech, music, or falling trees—are composed of many frequencies all happening at once. In fact, it is this very mixture that gives various sounds their unique character. The great French mathematician and physicist, Jean Baptiste Joseph Fourier (1768–1830), first described the composition of these complex sounds from multiple simpler sinusoids. Consequently, the breakdown of these complex waveforms into their component pure tones is called a Fourier analysis. Remarkably, this kind of analysis is routinely performed, to some extent, within the human ear in response to virtually every sound in our environment. Fourier observed that complex sounds are composed of a finite set of sinusoids (although sometimes a large set) and that sine waves may be added arithmetically to create a complex wave as illustrated in Figure 2-2.

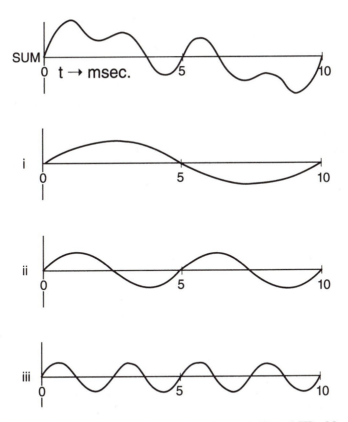

**FIGURE 2-2** **The Fourier transform: Sine waves I, II, and III add to form the complex wave at the top. Similarly, the complex wave at the top may be divided into the three sinusoids.**

## Psychoacoustics

All the preceding is necessary to answer the question raised by the title of this chapter: What do we hear? The term psychoacoustics refers to the human response to acoustic phenomena. We impose our own physiological and psychological rules on the world around us, and it is important to realize that despite the fact that there is relative consistency among humans in response to acoustic phenomena, the rules vary and our response varies from our neighbor.

### Threshold

The concept of threshold is discussed at length in the next chapter. An understanding of threshold allows a basic understanding of many principles involved in psychoacoustic tests. The hearing threshold of any individual is not at a fixed point but exists more as a narrow range (Moore, 1989). Threshold estimation involves presentation of an appropriate acoustic signal and asking a listener to respond when the signal is heard. The threshold is taken as that level at which the subject responds correctly to 50 percent of the test presentations. For any listener, then, there will be a level at which the test signal will never be heard and, at a slightly louder level, at which the signal will always be heard. The true hearing threshold lies somewhere in this range, and the actual point at which the subject responds will therefore depend on many factors. These include the degree of motivation and arousal of the subject, his or her personality, the instructions given by the tester, the attitude and encouragement (or lack of it) by the tester, and the technique used. The recorded threshold will also be influenced by the presence of background or environmental noise during the testing and by any calibration errors of the machinery used. On this basis, threshold measurement would appear to be a fairly crude tool with a standard error of the order of 3 to 5 dB (Burns, 1973). Given the inherent variability of any biologic system, this is probably the best that can be achieved. It is also important to note that threshold defined in this way refers to the value of the stimulus at which a listener responds half the time. It is sometimes said to represent a stimulus bias rather than a response bias.

### Pitch

Pitch is said to be the perceptual correlate of frequency, and it very nearly is. Human sensitivity to tones of various frequencies is not uniform. The structure of the cochlea does not allow a one-to-one match with frequency. Figure 2-3 illustrates the relationship between pitch and frequency for a normal human ear. Note that the unit of frequency is the Hertz and the unit of pitch is the mel.

There are two ways to construct such a scale and fortunately they tend to render pretty much the same curve. These are called the method of fractionation and the method of bisection. In the method of fractionation, a listener is presented with a tone of a given frequency (usually 1000 Hz) and then asked to adjust a second tone so that it is half or double the pitch of the reference tone. Once that has been done, the new tone is halved or doubled, and so on. Interestingly, if a subject is asked to halve the pitch of a tone and then double it, it rarely gets

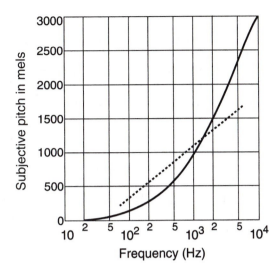

**FIGURE 2-3** **A pitch function showing how pitch (in mels) varies with frequency (in Hz).**

back to the original tone. In the method of bisection, a listener is presented with two tones of different frequencies and asked to adjust a third tone so that it falls between the two original tones. In both methods, the mel scale closely corresponds to the frequency scale, but not perfectly with either. Most importantly, note that the scale of pitch is not linear with the scale of frequency. Our ability to make pitch discriminations is not as finely tuned at extreme frequencies, so the close relationship between the physical presentation of the sound and the psychological interpretation of that sound is less predictable and reliable at the extreme ends of the frequency spectrum.

The ear has a functional frequency range of roughly 20 to 20,000 Hz, but is not equally sensitive to sounds in this range. It exhibits maximal sensitivity to sounds in the speech frequencies, that is, between about 500 Hz and about 4000 Hz, and progressively less sensitivity at increasingly high and low frequencies. This is also demonstrated in Figure 2-3 by the bends at the ends of the curves.

Experiments to measure these phenomena are usually done at a sound pressure level of 40 dB. It might be easier to suppose that if the sounds were made louder, a listener would be able to overcome any insensitivities. Unfortunately, that is not true. In fact, the further we get from 40 dB, the more the pitch scale diverges. In other words, there is also an effect of sound pressure on the perception of pitch.

## Loudness

Just as pitch is almost a correlate of frequency, so loudness is almost a correlate of sound pressure level. The unit of measurement of loudness is the sone, and it can be measured in the same way as pitch, by either fractionation or bisection. Loudness measurements must be made one frequency at a time. Examination of Figure 2-4 shows that, in the middle frequency range, frequency has relatively little effect on loudness. That is not the case at the extremes. In other words, just as with pitch, our ability to make loudness discriminations is not as finely tuned at extreme frequencies, so the close relationship between the physical presentation of the sound and the psychological interpretation of that sound is less linear, less predictable, and more unreliable at the extreme ends of the spectrum. Notice also in Figure 2-4 how rapidly loudness grows with sound pressure. At low pressures, it takes a rather small pressure change to produce a large change in loudness perception. At high pressures, the ear becomes incapable of perceiving further pressure increases, probably because we are approaching or have arrived at the threshold of pain.

It is noteworthy that the human ear seems to respond to both frequency and intensity in a geometric rather than arithmetic fashion. Indeed, a doubling of the presented frequency is perceived as an octave and a 10 dB increase is usually perceived as a doubling of sound intensity (Moore, 1989).

## Loudness Level

In the discussions of pitch and loudness, there was frequent reference to the effect of loudness on pitch perception. The generalization is that neither is uniform in relation to the other. To illustrate this point, it is necessary to construct a scale of loudness levels. The

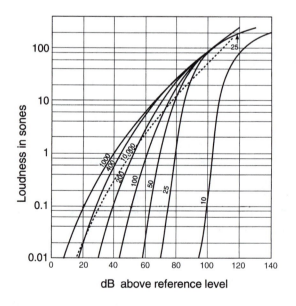

**FIGURE 2-4    A loudness function showing how loudness (in sones) varies with sound pressure level (in dB).**

unit of measurement on that scale is called the phon. Figure 2-5 illustrates a family of loudness levels or equal loudness contours. Phon curves are considered very reproducible and reliable across time and populations (Churcher and King, 1937; Fletcher and Munson, 1933).

Phon curves are constructed by presenting a tone of 1000 Hz at 40 sones. Then a tone of another frequency is presented, and the listener is asked to adjust it to be as loud as (equally loud to) the 1000 Hz tone. When that is completed, another tone of a different frequency is presented, and again the listener is asked to adjust it to be as loud as the 1000 Hz tone. This is continued over a wide range of tones (i.e., sinusoids) until the customary frequencies have been covered. Then, when the points for each frequency passing through 40 sones at 1000 Hz are connected, the result is a 40-phon contour. It is not flat, once again illustrating that our sensitivity, and even our relative discrimination ability, is not perfect.

If the procedure is repeated at 30 sones and at 50 sones, and so on, the result is a family of curves called "equal loudness contours." The contours are not parallel. They are quite bowl-shaped at low loudness levels and rather flat at high loudness levels. The bowl shape illustrates our inability to hear very low sound pressures, while the flat shape reflects our inability to discriminate at high pressure levels. The bottom of the set of equal loudness contours is sometimes called the "curve of zero loudness."

To find a curve of zero loudness, one can also do an experiment to determine the lowest level of loudness sensitivity or the minimum audible pressure (MAP). In such an experiment, a listener is placed in an anechoic chamber, a room with no sound wave reflections

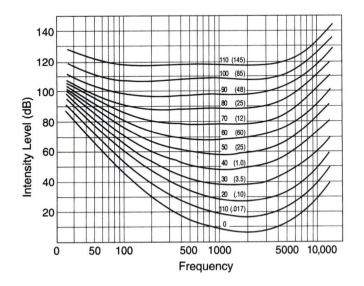

**FIGURE 2-5** **Loudness level (or equal loudness) contours. Any point on one curve is as loud as any other point on the same curve. Loudness level is measured in units called** *phons.* **Zero phons represents a curve of the minimum audible pressure.**

and no sound admitted from outside. An earphone is placed over one ear and a microphone is placed between the earphone and the opening to the ear canal. The sound pressure level (at a given frequency) is adjusted so that the listener reports an ability to hear on only half the presentations (Remember the term *threshold*?). The microphone is then used to measure the sound pressure at the threshold. The process is repeated for several different frequencies, and in this way the MAP is defined for that individual (Figure 2-6). Notice that the curve of minimum audible pressure corresponds very well with the curve of zero loudness.

Figure 2-6 also illustrates a curve called the minimum audible field (MAF). Humans do not go through life wearing earphones. The head is virtually always in an acoustic field. Therefore, it is appropriate to repeat the MAP experiment without headphones, with the listener's head in an acoustic field. However, the head itself reflects and diffracts sound. Simply stated, it gets in the way. To do this experiment properly then, it is necessary to find the minimum pressure at which the subject responds in the field, remove the subject from the field, and put a microphone where the listener's head had been. An azimuth of 0 degrees means that the loudspeaker was pointed at the listener's nose; random azimuth means that it was pointed somewhere else. Examination of Figure 2-6 reveals that the MAF is lower than the MAP. This is primarily due to the fact that two ears (binaural) were used. The difference between curves 2 and 3 suggests the way in which a listener's head gets in the way. This is called a head shadow, just as your head would cast a shadow when a light was pointed at it from some angle and the shadow would change as the angle (the azimuth) would change.

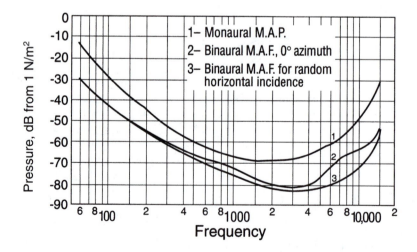

**FIGURE 2-6    The minimum audible pressure (MAP) and the minimum audible field (MAF).**

## *The Acoustics of Speech*

Obviously, speech is an acoustic signal. Consequently, all the things said above about sound apply equally to speech. Speech, though, is not just another acoustic signal. It is, unquestionably, the single most important acoustic signal for the human to hear. For that reason it is important to understand the acoustics of speech. Moreover, in audiometry (Chapter 3), one of the most important measures is how well a listener understands speech. It is important to know and understand, then, how the acoustics of speech relate to a listener's ability or inability to comprehend it. How is a listener's understanding of speech affected by a hearing loss?

A spectrum is the frequency and amplitude content of a signal. If a sound contains all possible frequencies at the same amplitude, then the signal is called white noise (analogous to white light). Most acoustic events, including speech, contain only some frequencies and those at different amplitudes. A line spectrum indicates what they are. Figure 2-7 is a line spectrum of speech. Observe that the lines are of various heights and that some in particular stand out. It is these peaks in the spectrum of speech that make it intelligible. They are called formants. How can we tell if someone said "beet" or "boot"?—because the formant structure of /i/ (as in beet) differs from the formant structure of /u/ (as in boot).

Figure 2-8 shows the formant structure of three syllables, /da/, /di/, and /du/. In this picture, the formants are shown as a function of frequency and time, and only the first two formants are shown. In reality, there can be as many as ten formants associated with any speech sound. However, usually it is only the first two or three that carry the information the listener requires to discriminate between speech signals (words or sounds). Normally, it is the frequency of the second formant that permits the discrimination of vowels. The

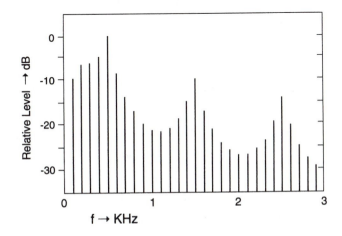

**FIGURE 2-7    A line spectrum of speech. The peaks are the formants.**

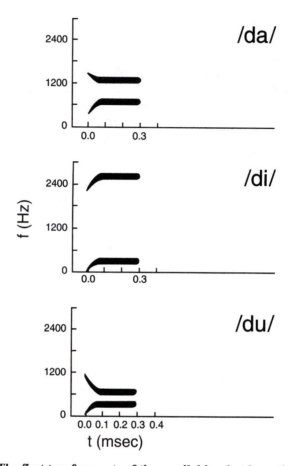

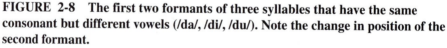

**FIGURE 2-8    The first two formants of three syllables that have the same
consonant but different vowels (/da/, /di/, /du/). Note the change in position of the
second formant.**

first formants do not change appreciably. Notice that the frequency of the second formant
of the /a/ in /da/ is at a considerably lower frequency than the second formant of the /i/ in
/di/. It is this difference that permits us to know what was said. Similarly, the second formant frequency of the /u/ in /du/ is still lower than the /i/. It is the exact same thing, the
frequency of the second formant, which allows us to tell the difference between "beet"
and "boot".

The same thing applies to consonants as to vowels. How can we tell if someone said
"dot" or "got"? The formant transition from the consonant /d/ into the vowel /a/ differs from
that of the consonant /g/ into the vowel /a/. Figure 2-9 shows that the vowel formants didn't
change; the sounds all use the same vowel, /a/. What changed was the bend of the second
formant into the vowel and that is a function of the consonant. One discriminates /ga/ from

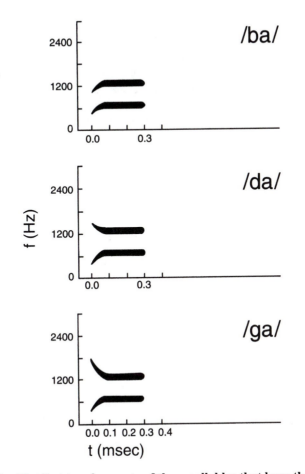

**FIGURE 2-9** **The first two formants of three syllables that have the same vowel but different consonants (/ba/, /da/, /ga/). Note the change in the shape of the second formant.**

/ba/, for example, because the second formant transition of /ga/ falls to the vowel formant whereas the second formant of /ba/ rises to it.

These acoustic phenomena, formants and transitions, characterize speech as different from other acoustic phenomena. Formants appear only with voiced sounds, that is, those in which the vocal folds are vibrating—vowels and voiced consonants. There are no formants in voiceless sounds, such as /s/ or /t/, and their spectra are aperiodic or noise-like. Furthermore, the brain is peculiarly sensitive, by a process of pattern recognition, to the various regularly recurring features of speech. We see, again, that speech is not just another acoustic occurrence, but in fact the auditory phenomenon to which the human ear and brain seem most acutely tuned. As clinicians, we need to be alert to differences that may appear between patients' abilities to hear tones and their abilities to hear speech.

## *Comment*

Given this cursory introduction to acoustics and psychoacoustics, the reader is now ready to embark on the study of audiometry: the measurement of hearing for clinical purposes. Undoubtedly, it may be difficult to understand how all this relates to hearing loss. A listener with a high frequency hearing loss may not be able to discriminate /di/ from either /da/ or /du/ or /i/ from /u/. A listener with a middle ear pathology will respond differently from one with cochlear pathology. The fundamentals discussed provide a foundation for understanding what is normal. It is important to understand normal before trying to understand abnormal. The next chapter calls upon the ideas introduced up to this point and moves to a study of auditory dysfunction.

# Chapter 3

# *Basic Audiometric Testing*

Thus far the emphasis has been on the physical attributes of hearing: anatomy and physiology, acoustics and psychoacoustics; and, of course, theories of audition and perception. In this chapter we expand into a new dimension, adding the mechanical processes to measure hearing and the psychological factors affecting those measures.

## *The Audiometer*

To measure hearing, we need instruments that reliably and efficiently produce and reproduce the same sounds every time. Not only must each instrument itself be reliable, but for testing to be comparable among sites, common standards in terms of both frequency and intensity are necessary for the sounds these instruments produce. Electronic devices called audiometers fulfill this role. To ensure that audiometers meet common standards, they are calibrated to protocols established by the International Standards Organization (ISO) or by the American National Standards Institute (ANSI) (1969). The difference between the standards of these two bodies is of a very small magnitude, and consequently, either is acceptable with some countries adhering to one and others using the other.

An audiometer consists of certain basic components, no matter which company produces it and how plain or fancy it appears on the outside. These parts include a source for generating the sound, an amplifier to increase the energy (intensity) of the signal, a potentiometer or "volume control" to allow this energy to be increased or decreased at will, and some sort of speaker unit in the form of earphones or loudspeakers. Figure 3-1 illustrates the typical component structure of an audiometer.

### *Frequency Characteristics*

Remember that the human ear is sensitive to the range of frequencies from 20 to 20,000 Hz. However, the most critical frequencies for speech are located between 125 Hz (the average lowest fundamental of the human voice) and 8000 Hz (the point at which the impact of hearing loss upon the understanding of everyday speech diminishes significantly). That is why audiometers are designed to produce pure tones at discrete frequencies within

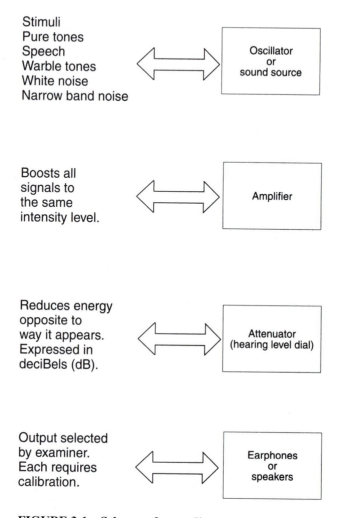

Stimuli
Pure tones
Speech
Warble tones
White noise
Narrow band noise

Oscillator
or
sound source

Boosts all
signals to
the same
intensity level.

Amplifier

Reduces energy
opposite to
way it appears.
Expressed in
deciBels (dB).

Attenuator
(hearing level dial)

Output selected
by examiner.
Each requires
calibration.

Earphones
or
speakers

**FIGURE 3-1    Schema of an audiometer.**

that frequency range, specifically at those points that permit examination of hearing along the lines of harmonic structure. Most audiometers generate signals at 125, 250, 500, 1000, 2000, 4000, and 8000 Hz. Some also include 1500, 3000, 6000, and 10,000 Hz, while others do not include 125 or 250 Hz. These differences are related more to the setting in which the equipment will be used than to any philosophy. For example, measures of extremely low or very high frequency may be required more often in a medical setting, while general measures of the mid-frequency range may be sufficient during educational hearing screening in the schools. These subtle differences are discussed in more detail throughout the text.

## *Intensity Characteristics*

Once the sound is generated and amplified to a level equal to the maximum output of the audiometer system, the potentiometer attenuates or reduces the sound energy being passed to the earphones or loudspeaker. What this means is that each time the output level of the audiometer is lowered, the examiner is preventing a greater amount of energy from the amplifier reaching the earphones and not really reducing the actual energy level produced by the sound generator as it may appear from the manipulation of the controls. Conversely, when the sound level is increased, the examiner is in fact taking less sound away from the amplifier and allowing a greater amount of energy to reach the earphones. This means that what is happening inside the audiometer is the opposite of what the examiner sees on the control panel. To reduce sound levels, greater energy decrement is required and to increase sound levels, less energy decrement is required. This is one of the reasons why the "volume control" on the audiometer is called the attenuator—it attenuates the signal from the sound generator to the output transducer.

The audiometer is designed to allow attenuation at each of the tones included on the frequency selector dial. There is a catch however. A "0" (zero) on the attenuator dial does not mean that no energy is being passed to the transducer. In fact, this is a reference zero and represents the amount of sound energy that can just be heard (i.e., threshold) by the average, healthy ear of an average eighteen-year-old. The level is strictly specified in a number of international standards. What this also means is that persons with better than average hearing may be able to respond at levels below zero on the audiometer. Those with particularly sensitive ears may respond at –10 dB or even lower. Again, just for review, audiometric zero at a given frequency is the least audible level of sound pressure required for normal ears to respond to that frequency. The sound pressure level required for each frequency has been determined by research and is an integral part of the ANSI and ISO standards to which audiometers are calibrated. Because the human ear is more sensitive in the mid-frequencies (1000–4000 Hz), relatively greater energy is required for zero at the higher and lower frequencies than in the mid-range. Once the reference zero is set for each frequency, the additional amount of energy required to increase by 5, 25, or even 100 dB is the same for all frequencies. A 5-dB difference at one frequency is the same as a 5-dB difference at another.

## *General Audiometer Controls*

Besides the two main controls for frequency and intensity, all audiometers have an on–off switch, an interrupter switch, and some mechanism for determining where the output is channelled (Figure 3-2). Audiometers today are transistorized and usually do not require long warm-up periods before usage. However, once the unit has been plugged in and turned on, it is a good idea to wait a few minutes and to let the unit stabilize. Furthermore, those who use portable audiometers and move them frequently from car to office will find it beneficial to allow the audiometer to warm (or cool) to room temperature before turning on the power. This will prolong the life of the equipment. The interrupter switch allows the examiner to choose between two signal presentation modes. Either the sound can be off until the

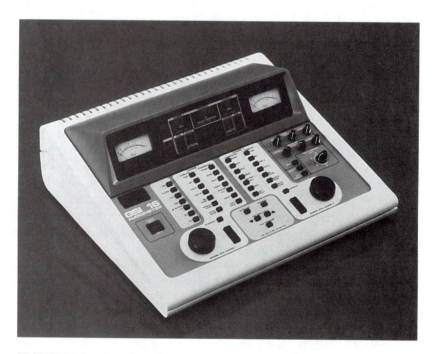

**FIGURE 3-2    A typical two-channel audiometer. Note the various stimulus options, the output selector, and the intensity selector (attenuator). (Photograph courtesy of Grason-Stadler, Inc.)**

interrupter switch is activated or it can be on until the switch interrupts it. It is standard convention that sound is kept off until the examiner uses the interrupter switch to initiate the signal.

Even the simplest audiometer has a selector switch to direct the signal to the right or the left earphone. The more complex the equipment, the more options available on the output selector switch. A full two-channel clinical diagnostic audiometer will include options for left or right ears for air conducted stimuli, bone conduction presentations, and sound field options for left or right speakers. Sometimes, one stimulus may go to one ear while another goes to the opposite.

### Alternative Stimuli

Previously we discussed the various frequencies used as stimuli in pure tone audiometry. There are many other stimuli used for hearing testing. In fact, any sound can be presented through an audiometer. However, such things as music and the sounds of noisemakers and animals are generally used in more elaborate clinical settings and calibrated specifically for their test environment. Our discussion here is limited to those sounds likely to be encountered and employed in basic audiometric settings. Among the alternative stimuli available on audiometers are various types of narrow bands of noise, warbled tones, white noise, sawtooth noise, and speech. The ability to use each of these stimuli may be built into an audiometer or played via audiotape or compact disk through the audiometer at calibrated levels, depending on the model selected. Although some of the stimuli may appear redundant in their usage, each has a separate function and offers an additional tool in differential diagnosis and hearing measurement.

### Narrow Band Noise

One commonly utilized non-pure tone stimulus is narrow band noise (NBN). These are bands centered around the same frequencies as the pure tones. For example, a 1000-Hz pure tone and a 1000-Hz NBN have their peak energy at the same frequency. However, the pure tone is limited to that frequency while the NBN contains energy from frequencies surrounding 1000 Hz (e.g., 999, 998, 1001, 1002, etc.). The range of frequencies involved with each narrow band varies according to ANSI standards and is generally around 5 percent of the peak frequency. Narrow bands of noise are most frequently used as stimuli with specific types of patients, notably children, adults with tinnitus (a ringing or buzzing in the ears), and those unable to respond to something as abstract as a pure tone. They are also used as a masking noise when testing a specific frequency in the other ear.

### Warble Tones

Warble tones are another variation on the pure tone. Instead of using a specific tone (e.g., 1000 Hz), a signal of that frequency is varied continuously (i.e., frequency modulated) over some range, for example, 5 percent. If, for example, there was a 5 percent modulation of a 1000-Hz tone, it would vary continuously from 950 Hz to 1050 Hz at a rate usually around 40 Hertz; that is, forty times each second, the tone would "warble" or sweep from 950 to 1050 Hz. Audiometers are usually built to present warble tones at each frequency calibrated to specific ANSI or ISO standards. Just as narrow band noise is useful with specific test populations, warble tones serve a similar purpose and provide excellent alternative signals. For example, because of their distinctive auditory characteristics, which usually focus a listener's attention, warble tones are frequently used as emergency or warning sounds. While in the hearing clinic, they are often particularly useful with children who report that the warbling tone resembles a bird's song, and find it far less frightening than bands of noise. Warble tones are also especially useful when a patient has tinnitus because they permit the patient to distinguish between the frequency of the tinnitus and the test frequency.

### White Noise

White noise contains all the frequencies perceived by the human ear at exactly the same intensity. Physicists define white noise as all frequencies at equal energy. Thus, a white noise signal of 80 dB SPL contains 125 Hz, 126 Hz, 127 Hz, and so on through 1000 Hz, 1001 Hz, and so on through 7866 Hz, 7867 Hz, and so on, to approximately 8000 Hz, at 80 dB SPL. This makes it the signal most likely to be heard by everyone, including the most severely hearing impaired. Unfortunately, because it is so easily heard, white noise is one of the least effective test stimuli. It is used in some hearing screening procedures based on observation of a startle reflex in response to sound. However, its primary use is as a masking sound during some clinical tests; that is, to mask or hide sound reaching the non-test ear so that it does not interfere with measures in the ear under examination. White noise may be the only masking signal available when the audiometer is not equipped to produce narrow bands of noise. Of course, narrow bands are superior for masking, being less overwhelming for the listener and just as effective. Nevertheless, white noise is a very effective masker and may be employed with excellent success.

### Sawtooth Noise

Some audiometers use a variation of noise called sawtooth noise for a masking stimulus. This is a noise consisting of a fundamental frequency and then all its harmonics, usually up to approximately 10,000 Hz. Thus, a typical sawtooth noise might begin with a fundamental frequency of 125 Hz and then include 250, 375, 500, 625, 750, 1000 and so on, up to 10,000. Sawtooth noise is not as effective a masker as narrow bands of noise. It may also be used as a broad frequency stimulus when testing special populations.

## Speech Stimuli

Speech is one of the most important stimuli for the evaluation of human hearing. Not only do speech test results provide important clinical diagnostic information, but in the end, the final question is always, "How well does the patient communicate?" Speech testing goes a long way toward answering that question. No matter what the pure tone results say, a patient's responses to speech are what actually reflect how well that person functions in the real world. Whisper tests can be considered a very basic form of speech audiometry. However, in general, speech audiometry implies the formal qualitative assessment of a subject's perception of speech. These measures are useful in a variety of contexts including assessment and diagnosis of peripheral and central hearing disorders, rehabilitation of hearing aid users, and medicolegal assessment.

The presentation of speech stimuli requires a microphone circuit for live voice or some system for including speech signals previously recorded on CD or audiotape. Therefore, the input selector of most clinical audiometers includes both microphone and prerecorded audio options. In general, testing is performed in a soundproof room using a cassette player or microphone for live voice tests with the signal intensity controlled through the audiometer to present speech material to the subject via loudspeakers or headphones. The specific speech signals and the methods used to present them depend upon the test administered. Basic to all speech testing are two procedures called the speech reception threshold and speech discrimination test. These are discussed below.

## Calibration

Finally, and before beginning a detailed discussion of audiometric test procedures, it is important to recognize that all of these test procedures are performed with electronic equipment. Considering the state of the art of today's circuitry, it is reasonable to expect that the equipment will remain in good working order for quite some time. Similarly, the old adage, "If something can go wrong, it will go wrong" is not just a joke. Sudden surges of electricity, changes in temperature and humidity, jostling of equipment, dust, and so on, all take their toll. Every piece of electronic equipment should be examined every time it is used. Such an evaluation is called calibration. Sometimes calibration involves very sophisticated electronic analysis of the frequency and intensity systems, the stimulus generators, and so on. At other times, it is merely a quick personal evaluation by the user, a biological calibration, to ensure that all is well and the system is functioning properly. This former check is akin to listening to the car when starting it in the morning to ensure it is not making unusual sounds. One listens to the sound of the engine, pumps the brakes, turns the wheel, and so forth. With an audiometer, the procedure is not so different. You listen to the frequency changes, check out the interrupter switch, and sweep up and down with the attenuator controls to monitor changes. Every audiometer should have a daily biological check. A simple recipe for this type of calibration follows:

1. Plug in and turn on the audiometer.
2. Do a self-threshold for pure tones at 500, 1000, 2000, 4000, and 8000 Hz in both ears the first time the equipment is started on any given day. Results should be compared to previous threshold results obtained from the same examiner. Failure to obtain comparable results demands a formal calibration check before any clinical testing.
3. A final biological check is to listen to and memorize the sound of a 1000-Hz pure tone at 40 dB. Every time the audiometer is turned on, the examiner should listen to a 1000-Hz, 40-dB tone and compare it to the memorized signal. Any variance should result in a formal calibration check of the equipment.
4. Clinical testing should not be done until formal calibration is completed with satisfactory results if any of the biological checks are failed. Remember, testing in the face of known equipment error renders test results invalid. This puts the client at risk for misdiagnosis and you, the examiner, at risk for malpractice.

## Test Procedures

Up to this point we have considered the physical characteristics of the machine (the audiometer) and the materials (tones, speech, noise, etc.) used to test hearing. These can and should be rigidly controlled and monitored. There are clear and definitive standards to be followed that make such a requirement reasonable and possible. Now, however, the discussion shifts to something that is also well-structured but is subject to greater variation and less control. Test procedures are only as good as the clinician who uses them. All the equipment standards in the world fail if the examiner ignores test protocols and procedures. For that reason, there are specific methods of testing pure tone thresholds taught all over the world. Theoretically, a threshold examination in Oshkosh will follow the same technique as an examination in Inuktituk or in Irkutsk.

The most common method used to establish auditory thresholds is called the method of limits. The most common clinical process used within that psychophysical measurement paradigm is called the "The Ascending-Descending Technique." The idea is quite simple and is based on a bracketing technique. When a subject responds to a sound, the examiner will decrease its intensity until the sound is no longer heard and the client fails to respond. Next, the examiner increases the sound until there is a response. This up and down (bracketing) procedure is repeated until a reasonably reliable figure for threshold is established. The technique can be applied to all threshold measures including pure tones, bands of noise, and speech (Carhart and Jerger, 1959).

## The Ascending-Descending Technique

The following detailed approach to obtaining a pure tone threshold from a cooperative adult patient is an easily followed protocol and should yield consistent and appropriate results. For the purposes of the illustration, it is assumed that a full physical examination of the ear has been performed and that there is no obstruction preventing an accurate test. It is also assumed that the test environment is a quiet room or sound chamber specifically designed for hearing testing.

### Step 1: The Instructions
The patient must be given instructions that are clear, brief, and easy to follow. For example: "I am going to put these (earphones) on your head. Next, I will present a sound to your right (left) ear. It will not be difficult to hear. When you hear it, raise your right (left) hand. I will then turn the sound off. When you no longer hear the sound, put your hand down. We will repeat this two or three times until you are comfortable with the process. I will gradually make the sound softer. No matter how loud or soft the sound is, whenever you hear it, raise your hand, and when the sound goes away, put your hand down. Do you understand?

### Step 2: The Earphones
Place the earphones on the patient's head, ensuring they are not pressing on the tragus and causing a collapsed ear canal. Be sure earrings, headbands, and the like, are not displacing the phones or blocking the ear canal. One common error made by beginners and one that even occasionally happens to experienced clinicians, is placing the earphone on the wrong ear. Manufacturers produce earphones with color-coded bands. The "red" goes on the "right" and test results from that ear are marked on the audiogram with a "round" circle. The left ear is identified by a blue band and results are marked with an X on the audiogram. If the examiner recalls: Red = Round = Right, the left is automatically identified as the alternative. Problems occur when the examiner sees the red phone in his or her own right hand and places the phones on the patient's head. You see, if the examiner is standing in front of the patient (face to face), the examiner's right hand is on the patient's left ear. It is vital the examiner ensure that the Right–Red combination refers to the patient's ears and not his or her own side.

### Step 3: A Word of Caution

When the client is instructed and the earphones properly placed, the examiner is then ready to begin the actual test procedure. Before discussing the step by step process, a few cautionary words are in order. Hearing-impaired persons are very sensitive to visual clues in the environment. This is a learned behavior that helps to compensate for their auditory deficits. Consequently, a hearing-impaired person may be able to "read" the examiner and thus invalidate the test results. For example, if the examiner pauses and looks at the audiometer after every frequency or intensity change or just before presenting a test stimulus, the subject soon learns to wait for that telltale movement, wait a few seconds, and respond. Similarly, if the patient perceives the tone presentations are regular, say about every five seconds, the patient may soon start raising a hand automatically every five seconds. If the examiner is not careful, the patient's responses will be accepted at face value and his or her hearing will appear much better than it really is. Thus, be sure not to invalidate the test procedure by accidentally presenting behavioral or visual clues.

### Step 4: The Test Process

The first few sounds are presented at an intensity high enough to ensure that the client understands the instructions and to verify appropriate response behavior. The clinician selects the intensity level of the initial tones on the basis of several factors. Generally, normal conversation is thought to be at about 60 dB. Therefore, for a normal (or near normal) ear, a 60-dB initial presentation is quite comfortable and appropriate. The greater the loss, the greater the intensity of the initial signal. Another word of caution here. If the patient has reported a sensitivity to loud sounds (a phenomenon called recruitment), it is advisable to be caring and cautious when increasing the intensity level of sounds.

For purposes of this discussion we will assume the patient has near normal hearing. Thus, the initial tone would be presented at about 60 dB (near the intensity level of normal conversation). We usually start testing with examination of the better ear, if it is known. That information should be available from the case history, interview, or medical or other test records. If the better ear is unknown, then the choice is arbitrary. The better ear is selected because it is easier to examine and helps in verifying the validity of the test process. Each tone is usually presented for about one to two seconds. This is sufficient time to allow the subject to hear and respond, although older and very young folks may need longer. Bear in mind that the longer the tone is on, the greater the opportunity for error because the patient may respond by chance. Usually, the patient's hand will be raised or in motion before the two seconds of tonal presentation are completed. If not, the examiner should be very cautious in interpreting results and suspect a false positive response. Verify the result by repeating the process. Once the examiner is comfortable that the patient has heard the initial tone and responded properly, the intensity of the reference tone should be reduced (ideally by 20 dB) and another, less intense reference tone presented. Let us assume our client responded to the initial tone at 60 dB. Our next presentation would be at 40 dB. If a proper response is noted to 40 dB, a third tone would be presented at 20 dB. This 20-dB descent in intensity would continue until the patient fails to respond. Let us say our patient did not respond at 20 dB. We have responses at 60 and 40 dB, but not at 20 dB.

### Step 5: Exploring Threshold

The ascending-descending technique follows the simple rule of down by 10 and up by 5. In other words, once the initial reference tones have ensured that the test procedure is satisfactory and have located the approximate point of the patient's hearing threshold, the actual threshold level is determined using smaller decibel variations. In our example, we have determined that our patient does not respond at 20 dB. So, following the test rules, we would present the next tone at 20 dB + 5 dB or 25 dB. Our patient responds. Following test procedures, the next tone should be presented at 25 dB – 10 dB or 15 dB. Our patient fails to respond to 15 dB. The next tone is presented at 15 dB + 5 dB or 20 dB. Our patient didn't respond to 20 dB the first time it was presented, but responds this time. Why? Please recall that threshold is that point at which a tone is heard 50 percent of the time and not heard 50 percent of the time. Furthermore, keep in mind that the first time a 20-dB tone was presented we had decreased the signal from 40 dB to 20 dB. Sometimes that large a decrease is so great that the patient may not be listening carefully for a very soft tone at or near threshold and may miss its presentation. This was illustrated in our example.

Thus, our patient did not respond the first time the tone was presented, but did the next. Because our patient has now responded at 20 dB (as we ascended in 5-dB steps), the next presentation should be at 20 dB – 10 dB, or at 10 dB. There is no response. We increase the tone by 5 dB to 15 dB. There is no response. We increase the tone by 5 dB to 20 dB. This time there is a response. We now know our patient never responds to 15 dB, always responds at 25 dB, and sometimes responds (and sometimes does not respond) at 20 dB. What is the threshold level?

The answer is presented in Table 3-1, which illustrates the procedures outlined above and includes an extra ascending-descending sequence to verify that threshold has been obtained.

**TABLE 3-1    Exploring threshold using the ascending-descending technique.**

| | | | *Down by 10 and Up by 5* | | | |
|---|---|---|---|---|---|---|
| Intensity | Descend | Ascend | Descend | Ascend | Descend | Ascend |
| 60 dB | ⇓R | | | | | |
| 55 | | | | | | |
| 50 | | | | | | |
| 45 | | | | | | |
| 40 | ⇓R | | | | | |
| 35 | | | | | | |
| 30 | | | | | | |
| 25 | | ⇑R »»» | | | | |
| 20 | ⇓NR »»» ↗ | | ↘ | ⇑R »»» | | ⇑R - Threshold |
| 15 | | | ⇓NR »»» ↗ | | ↘ | ⇑NR »»» |
| 10 | | | | | ⇓NR »»» ↗ | |

One final note in passing is that there are other ways of performing this measure. The intensity steps may be smaller or larger and/or one can approach threshold from the bottom up as well as the top down. However, the method outlined here is the one in most common usage and seems to afford the most control over the testing process. In essence, we believe it is the best method, but it is certainly not the only one.

## Masking

When the difference between the hearing of the patient's ears is 40 dB or more, there is a very good chance that when a sound is presented to the poorer ear, the better ear may be able to hear it. Sometimes this is because the sound leaks out from the earphones and is intense (or loud) enough to be heard by the other ear. Sometimes this is true because the difference is so great that the sound can actually travel through the head and stimulate the cochlea on the opposite side. When testing via bone conducted stimuli this problem is even greater. Remember that the principle of bone conduction is that the bones of the skull will be set into vibration and directly stimulate the fluid in the cochlea. Clearly, both cochleas will be stimulated by a vibrating skull. The only way to know which ear is responding is to mask out the sound in the non-test ear. Masking is the phenomenon by which one sound impairs the perception of another. In the context of pure tone audiometry, masking is used to raise the threshold in the contralateral (non-test) ear using air conducted sound. This overcomes any cross hearing and allows an accurate assessment of the true threshold of the test ear for either air or bone conduction. Because masking is most effective when the frequency of the masking noise overlaps the test tone, narrow band noise with a center frequency identical to the test tone is most often used.

## Frequency Choice

Our discussion thus far has focused on the intensity of the signal. The next question to be asked is which frequencies should be tested and in what order? Unfortunately, this choice is much less clearly defined. In part that lack of clarity is due to the wide variety of auditory pathologies discussed throughout this text. In an ideal world, the examiner would face a mature, cooperative, willing and eager patient. In the real world, there are many different patients—a child, a malingerer, a terminally ill patient, a voluntary test required for entry to a desirable program, and a school screening test—which makes the audiologist's work interesting. Some of those differences require a variation in test procedure. For example, when testing a very ill patient undergoing chemotherapy and trying to determine if the patient's medication is affecting hearing, the test might begin with 1000 Hz to determine the response to the important frequencies for speech and to establish a baseline level of hearing. The next frequency might be 8000 or 12,000 Hz, frequencies most likely to be affected first by chemotherapy. The patient may not be physically able to tolerate much more testing than that. On the other hand, when seeing another adult for a routine reassessment, the protocol might call for the examiner to begin with 1000 Hz and then move to 500

Hz, 2000 Hz, 4000 Hz, and 8000 Hz in that order. There is no right or wrong in these choices. They are just choices based on the minimal information required and what is most important. When pure tone testing is complete, all frequencies will have been tested using the ascending-descending technique. The audiogram will have been properly marked with Os for the right ear (round = red = right) and the responses of the left ear will have been illustrated in blue with Xs.

## Tests of Middle Ear Function

The reader will recall that the ear is divided into the outer ear (pinna to the tympanic membrane), the middle ear (the tympanic membrane through to the footplate of the stapes), and the inner ear (the cochlea and vestibular structures). Hearing tests done via earphones depend upon the transmission of the sound energy through the tympanic membrane and middle ear to the cochlea via a medium directly dependent upon or affected by air. Thus, that approach is called air conduction testing. When the ear is normal, the response to air conduction testing will reflect hearing levels between 0 and 10 dB at all test frequencies (see Figure 3-3, left ear). When either the outer or middle ears (or both) are functionally abnormal, whether because of disease, fluid, abnormality, blockage, or tympanic membrane dysfunction, the patient may suffer an interruption in the conduction of sound via the air medium. A hearing loss caused by that type of disruption is called a conductive hearing loss. The initial audiogram will show responses outside of normal limits (see Figure 3-3, right ear). Unfortunately, the examiner cannot tell from the initial audiogram if the problem is in the conductive mechanism or if it is beyond and in the cochlea or auditory nerve. A deficit in those structures is called a sensorineural hearing loss. Thus, an important aspect of hearing testing is determining the location of the problem or the site of lesion, be it conductive or sensorineural .

To test for the presence of a conductive hearing loss, two techniques can be used. One is an indirect measure of middle ear function called bone conduction, while the second is a more direct measure variously termed tympanometry, impedance, or immittance testing.

### Bone Conduction

In addition to standard air conduction procedures, tones may be presented by a device placed over the mastoid process that produces vibration of the bone overlying the cochlea. These vibrations are conducted through the bone directly to the cochlea. This is termed bone conduction and although not an exact measure of cochlear function, it provides a reasonably good approximation. The difference between the results obtained by air and bone conduction is called the air-bone gap. The gap reflects the efficiency (or inefficiency) of the auditory mechanism from the opening of the external auditory meatus on the outer aspect of the ear through to the footplate of the stapes at the vestibule. In the normal ear there is no air-bone gap. In the ear with significant middle ear pathology, the air-bone gap may be as high as 60 dB. That is, responses to sound presented by air conduction may be as much as 60 dB

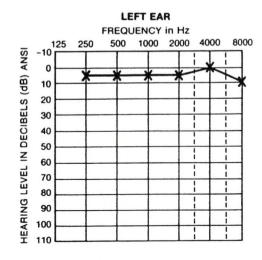

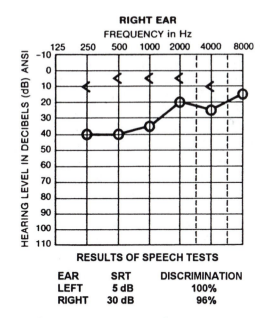

RESULTS OF SPEECH TESTS

| EAR | SRT | DISCRIMINATION |
|---|---|---|
| LEFT | 5 dB | 100% |
| RIGHT | 30 dB | 96% |

**Figure 3-3   A typical audiogram format. Note that the frequency and intensity levels are marked on the graph. The left ear is within normal limits. The right ear has a mild conductive hearing loss with an air-bone gap. All speech test results are in agreement with what would be expected from this audiogram.**

poorer than those presented via the vibrating oscillator placed on the mastoid bone. In most cases the difference is not that great, but it can be so.

An audiogram obtained by bone conduction follows the same procedures and protocols as air conduction testing, except that instead of stimulus presentation via earphones, the patient is fitted with a bone conduction oscillator and the sound energy transmitted via that medium. The ascending-descending test protocol is virtually the same. Masking is essential when testing by bone conduction. Finally, it should be noted that not all audiometers are designed to permit this test procedure.

## *Immittance Testing and Tympanometric Screening*

The middle ear and mastoid system exists as an air-filled system that communicates with the nasopharynx via the Eustachian tube. As a closed system, air is being continually absorbed by the lining mucosa but is periodically replaced when the Eustachian tube opens during the act of swallowing. Sound transmission from the external to the inner ear is optimal when the compliance of the middle ear system is maximal. This normally occurs when the pressure in the middle ear is equal to the pressure in the external auditory meatus. Compliance is a measure of the system's ability to allow the passage of sound energy through it and is inversely related to impedance, which is a measure of the system's resistance to the passage of sound energy. In order to evaluate the impedance-compliance paradigm in all its aspects, an electroacoustic impedance instrument is used for impedance audiometry or immitance testing, terms that are used interchangeably. This device, sometimes called an "Acoustic Bridge," may be used to examine middle ear pressure, tympanic membrane mobility, Eustachian tube function, the presence or absence of acoustic reflexes and their level of activation, and the integrity of the middle ear ossicular structure. The test instrument, which for the sake of brevity we will call a tympanometer, consists of an oscillator, an air pump, an electrically controlled balance meter, and a probe tip with three channels in it. The exact function of each of the components is not important here, and the reader is referred to Katz (1993), Jerger and Northern (1980), and Northern (1988) for a more detailed explanation.

We are concerned here, however, with some general test procedures and with the specifics of tympanometric screening. No matter which test or screening process is being performed, the process begins when a three-channel probe is placed at the opening of the external auditory meatus. The probe has a rubber tip so when it is properly seated, there is an airtight seal in the external auditory meatus. The three channels are used as a sound producer, a sound receiver, and a device for altering the air pressure within the meatus. The sound producer does not actually produce the sound, but rather, it is connected to the oscillator and is used to channel the signal it generates into the ear channel. The sound receiver is really an opening to a microphone that records sound coming back toward the probe tip, and the third channel is connected to the air pump and permits the examiner to alter the air pressure in the ear canal by increasing or decreasing pressure. Such a change in pressure will normally impact on the tympanic membrane allowing inward (proximal) or outward (distal) movement.

A test tone of 220 Hz at 65 dB is projected into the EAM via the sound-producing channel. Some of that signal will be absorbed (admitted) by the middle ear system (drum and ossicles) and some will be reflected. The reflected sound energy is measured by the probe microphone located in the sound receiver channel. The examiner can alter the relationship of the structures within the conduction system by changing the pressure in the EAM. At that point another signal can be sent from the sound producer. Changes in the structural relationship prior to the second tone presentation will alter the compliance of the system and, in turn, the amount of reflected sound energy. The difference is measured by the immitance instrument and interpreted as the amount of change in reflected sound energy. The pattern of change yields significant diagnostic information.

In the specific case of tympanometric screening, the process is typically initiated by pumping air into the ear canal at a pressure level equal to approximately +200 mm of water. This places the tympanic membrane at a point of poor mobility, normally pressing it slightly inwardly (proximally). The compliance of the tympanic membrane is measured. When the air pressure in the canal is reduced slightly the structural relationships are altered and the mobility of the membrane is improved. Once again, the compliance is measured. This process is repeated until the air pressure in the canal allows maximum mobility of the membrane, and then it is continued to gradually create a negative pressure situation in the ear canal. Once again, this unbalances the equalized air pressure on both sides of the tympanic membrane and adversely affects eardrum compliance. The measures taken all along the continuum are plotted as a graph called a *tympanogram* and can be interpreted by the clinician. Jerger (1970) developed a classification system that forms the basis for the interpretation of typical tympanometric patterns (Figure 3-4). It is important to point out that screening tympanometry sounds far more complicated than it is in actual application. Most testing is done with a screening tympanometer that is equipped with an automatic testing device. The clinician ensures that a tight seal is present at the opening of the ear canal by checking that a green light or similar device is lit on the probe. Once the seal is obtained, the machine automatically pumps in the air and records compliance. When the entire process is completed, usually in a matter of seconds, the screening tympanometer prints out a tympanogram. It is up to the examiner to interpret the results.

The Type A curve is found in ears with normal middle ear function. Note that the peak response or compliance occurs when the pressure level in the ear canal is normal or the same as it is in the test room. Compliance is reduced as pressure is increased and decreased relative to normal. In other words, the pressure on both sides of the tympanic membrane is normal at room pressure, and the conductive system is not being impeded or restricted by any stiffness, mass, or weight in the middle ear.

The Type $A_S$ curve is found in ears with normal middle ear pressure, but with limited compliance. How could that happen? If the pressure on both sides of the tympanic membrane is equal, the mobility of the drum reflects that state. However, if there is something causing a stiffness to that movement, say a thickened or scarred eardrum, it would be less compliant even though it was fully pressurized and mobile. That reduction in compliance would be reflected in a lowered compliance reading on the tympanometric form. The curve is an A but *s*hallow ($A_S$) compared to a normal ear.

The Type $A_D$ curve is found in ears in which only the slightest air pressure change results in a major change in compliance. This can occur when there is no resistance against the tympanic membrane, as would be the case in a disruption in the ossicular chain. It might also occur if the response was being obtained from something other than the eardrum itself.

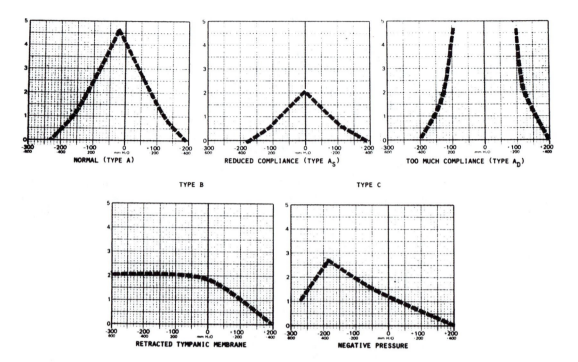

**FIGURE 3-4** **The classification system for tympanograms as proposed by Jerger (1970) and in common clinical use.**

For example, some persons develop an extra membrane (called a monomeric membrane) that sits directly in front of the eardrum in the ear canal. On quick visualization the clinician may believe it is the tympanic membrane, but it is not. Because it has no weight, mass, or stiffness associated with it, because there are no structures attached to it, it is extremely compliant and will yield a Type $A_D$ tympanogram. In any case, whether it is due to a disarticulated ossicular chain or a monomeric membrane, the response indicates a flaccidity in the presence of equal air pressure. Thus, the curve is an A but *d*eeper (Type $A_D$) or more compliant when compared to the normal ear.

The Type B curve is found in ears in which there is essentially no change in compliance as the pressure in the ear canal is altered. This can occur when the tympanic membrane cannot move because it is restricted by a massive fluid buildup in the middle ear (otitis media) or by a malformation or even when the membrane itself is affected by cerumen or a foreign object, for example. Generally, Type B tympanograms are associated with a conductive hearing loss. Simply stated, no matter how much pressure is put into the ear canal or taken from it in an effort to equalize pressure between the canal and the middle ear space, the response will be noncompliance.

The Type C curve appears when compliance is near normal, but there is significant negative pressure in the middle ear. There is some controversy about when this occurs, although there is strong evidence that when it appears there is a three times greater chance of the presence of middle ear fluid. In any case, Type C curves are often the result of poor Eustachian tube function that does not allow the air pressure in the middle ear to equalize to that of the pressure on the ear canal side of the tympanic membrane. The normal ear may experience a similar phenomenon when descending in an aircraft. The pressure on the tympanic membrane is increasing as the plane descends, eventually reaching a maximum at ground level. If the Eustachian tube is blocked or is temporarily dysfunctional, the pressure inside the middle ear is less than the increasing pressure in the canal. The result is often pain or discomfort and a temporary mild hearing loss. The difficulty with interpreting a Type C tympanogram is that it usually must be taken in the context of ongoing treatment and disease. If the ear is in the process of filling with fluid the curve will probably move from a C to a B. On the other hand, if treatment has been instituted, or if the ear is spontaneously resolving back to normal, the curve may go from a C to an A. Furthermore, a Type C may be representative of only a temporary state such as described earlier in an aircraft. The Type C requires *C*aution when interpreting it!

## *Speech Audiometry*

The two procedures basic to speech audiometry are the speech reception threshold (SRT) test and the speech discrimination test (SDT). The SRT is the sound intensity at which the subject scores 50 percent correct responses. Thus the procedure starts at a comfortable loudness level, and then the signal is gradually decreased in intensity until the patient's threshold for speech is reached. On the other hand, the SDT is a measure of the subject's optimal responses to speech stimuli if the sound is loud enough all the time. In essence, it measures the clarity of the person's hearing ability. Responses will be 100 percent when hearing is normal. Both of these procedures are based on presenting word lists to the patient and scoring by correctly identified phonemes, words, or sentences. The SRT is scored as a deciBel level of hearing while the SDT score is a percentage of words understood and interpreted with reference to the sound level used during the testing. Speech stimuli can be presented live voice by the tester using a microphone, although this method is prone to variation in both intensity and accent. Standardized, prepared speech material presented by audiotape or compact disc and controlled by the audiometer is preferable. The speech can be presented in the sound field by way of loudspeakers or headphones. Use of headphones allows each ear to be tested individually and, if required, to provide masking to the non-test ear. Masking sounds in speech audiometry are chosen to recreate an appropriate noise background such as speech, cocktail party, and babble noise. Pink noise (equal energy for each octave over the hearing range) is often used when these are unavailable.

## *Speech Reception Threshold*

The purpose of the SRT test is to determine a hearing threshold level for speech in deciBels and to relate that level to the same response from normal ears and to the listener's own response to other auditory stimuli. For example, generally speaking, the SRT for each ear correlates very highly with the pure tone average in deciBels for that ear at 500, 1000, and 2000 Hz.

The administration of the SRT test may appear deceptively simple. However, like all audiometric procedures, success is based on a variety of factors beyond the obvious. Variables such as patient cooperation and motivation, perception of instructions, linguistic integrity, earphone placement, calibration, and examiner bias may influence the results to a greater degree than the patient's actual hearing loss. For these reasons, it is necessary to take a rather cook-book approach to testing procedures and protocols and to follow that recipe precisely every time the test is administered. Once the procedure for speech reception testing is well understood and accurately practiced, not only is it quite easy to generalize to other audiometric test processes, but all persons and institutions involved can be assured of a uniform calibrated test process that eliminates many of the variables associated with human behavior and the errors leading to misdiagnosis and litigation.

The primary stimulus for testing the SRT are words called spondees. These are words of two syllables with equal accent on both syllables (e.g., baseball, airplane, toothbrush). The spondee words are always preceded by a carrier phrase such as: "Say the word." Instructions to the patient might begin with: "I am going to say some words to you. Please repeat the words you hear. The words will become softer, but you must still repeat the words you hear." The examiner would then begin with the carrier phrase and a spondee word (e.g., Say the word "baseball.") presented at a very comfortable loudness level, usually at 40 dB above the pure tone average of 500, 1000 and 2000 Hz. When the patient responds correctly, the next word would be presented in the same fashion. Once the examiner is sure the client understands the process and is responding appropriately, the intensity level of the words of subsequent presentations will be decreased in 10-dB steps. Once again, the ascending-descending (bracketing) approach to obtaining a threshold should be used to obtain the SRT. Even though the stimulus is different from testing with tones, this time including a carrier phrase and changing spondee words, the test technique is really identical. This ensures control over as many variables as possible and helps the patient to feel comfortable with the process. In the end, just as a pure tone *threshold* is obtained, so is a speech reception *threshold*. As indicated, generally speaking, the SRT for each ear correlates very highly with the pure tone average in deciBels for that ear at 500, 1000, and 2000 Hz. If, when the final SRT is obtained, there is a significant variation (greater than 5–10 dB, depending on the configuration of the audiogram) between it and the pure tone average, the test procedures and the test results should be carefully rechecked.

## *Speech Discrimination Test*

Speech discrimination really means speech understanding. The speech discrimination test is designed to answer one simple question: If the speech is loud enough for the person to hear it, how much will be understood? Perhaps the simplest analogy is that of a motion picture that is out of focus. The picture may be bright enough to be seen, but the lack of focus makes it impossible for the viewer to visualize it accurately and to interpret the image. In the case of hearing, poor speech discrimination means that the person hears the sound loudly enough, but simply cannot make sense of it. This is not a problem within the brain, but rather, it is a function of the inability of the ear and its associated auditory tracts to accurately process energy received at the hair cells or to transmit it without error to the auditory cortex. The results of speech discrimination testing are interpreted in terms of a percentage score, with 100 percent being perfect.

Speech discrimination material is chosen to provide a representative balance of all the sounds (phonemes) in a language. These are the building blocks of speech and represent the smallest unit of recognizable speech sound (e.g., ay, aw, ah, etc.). Test materials are usually presented as lists of real or synthetic words. A number of lists have been developed in a variety of the world's languages ranging from French to Spanish to Hebrew to Arabic to Chinese and Japanese. There are forty-nine phonemes in the English language, and in Canada and the United States the Central Institute for the Deaf (CID) and the Northwestern University NU-CHIPS word lists are well accepted, while in the United Kingdom the Medical Research Council and the Boothroyd and Manchester Junior word lists are well used. The CID lists are typical examples of these types of materials. Originally developed at Harvard University and adapted by the Central Institute for the Deaf, each of the fifty-word lists is designed to include all the sounds of the English language in the initial and final positions. Each is an independent list and can be spoken either live or presented as prerecorded materials.

The procedure for determining a speech discrimination score is quite different from that used for the various threshold measures considered earlier. For one thing, the materials in each list are presented at the same intensity level and that is usually 25 to 30 dB above the SRT or pure tone average. The patient would be instructed in a manner quite similar to previous tests. That is: "You are going to hear some words and I want you to repeat those words back to me. Once again, you will hear the phrase 'Say the word . . .' before each word you are to repeat." The examiner may also wish to reassure the patient by indicating that the words will not decrease in intensity. The examiner then sets the attenuator on the audiometer to a level approximately 25 to 30 dB greater than the client's SRT and presents the first word. While listening to the response, the examiner marks a correct or incorrect next to each word on the list.

While the SRT is measured in terms of a deciBel level, speech discrimination results are expressed in terms of a percentage of words understood. If the patient understands and repeats all the words correctly, the score is 100 percent. Because there are fifty words on each list, a patient who responds correctly to forty-five words has a (45 × 2) 90 percent score. A patient with thirty correct has a (30 × 2) 60 percent score, and so on. The examiner should also note the pattern of any errors. That is, are they all high frequency sounds? Low frequency sounds? In the final position? The pattern of errors is sometimes more informative than the number of errors.

A number of specialized audiological procedures utilize speech discrimination testing as their basis, and it may be necessary to retest with subsequent intensity presentations at +10, +20, –10 or –20 dB from the basic test level. Results will be scored by percentage for each test, the percentage scores plotted on a graphical display, and an articulation curve drawn. However, that is beyond the scope of this introductory text. Our purpose here is to introduce you to the basic concepts and to let you know that this is only the beginning.

## *Comment*

The combination of pure tone thresholds, bone conduction, tympanometry, speech reception threshold, and speech discrimination score is called the "Basic Battery." This battery of tests forms the baseline for all further audiometric tests. The ability to understand these procedures and their interpretation is essential to the understanding of all hearing disorders.

*C h a p t e r* **4**

# *Acquired Disorders of the External Ear*

Speech–language pathologists, public health nurses, industrial hearing technicians, hearing aid dispensers, and others, should be especially alert to alterations in the appearance of the external ear because they may be the first persons to observe them. External ear problems are usually disorders or skin diseases caused by irritative reaction, fungus, or the presence of a foreign body. The prefixes "ot," "oti," and "oto" refer to the ear; while the suffix "itis" refers to inflammation or infection, as in tonsillitis or appendicitis. Hence, otitis refers to any infection of the ear, while otitis externa is limited to an infection of the external ear. Problems that arise from pathology limited to the external ear usually have greater significance otologically than audiologically. That is, the extent (in frequency) and degree (in deciBels) of a hearing loss that results from an external ear problem are usually limited. However, these conditions require medical treatment and, if left untreated, can result in far more serious complications than the initial difficulty. For example, some forms of otitis externa have the potential to lead to an otitis media (infection of the middle ear) or to spread by themselves and damage the tympanic membrane and other structures.

## *Infective and Inflammatory Disorders of the Pinna*

The pinnae are often the site of irritating or traumatic disorders. Generally, they are not well protected from cold, trauma, or disease, and they are often used for functional purposes (earrings, eyeglasses, etc) that may trigger a variety of disorders. Among the frequent pathologies seen around the pinnae are irritative reactions caused by constant rubbing, insect bites, contact with chemical substances, or the introduction of foreign objects (keys, beans, cigarette filters, cotton swabs, etc.). Irritation may also be caused by improperly fit ear defenders or ear molds. If the skin is broken, the risk of infection is markedly increased. Generally, the problem is rapidly relieved by treatment with a topical application of appropriate medication. Hearing loss does not usually accompany any of these problems; however, marked swelling can result and can occlude the canal and cause a minimal temporary loss.

## *Trauma*

Occasionally, a clinician will encounter a case of direct trauma to the external ear. This might be a serious gash or cut, a hematoma or blood bruise caused by a blow to the auricle, or even a human bite. Usually the surgeon's skill can restore a respectably normal appearance, and there should be no permanent effect on hearing. If, however, the trauma is associated with underlying trauma to the side of the head, cosmetic surgery will not repair damage to the middle and inner ear structures within the temporal bone, and hearing loss may very well be present. For a further discussion of this important point, refer to Chapter 9. On occasion, even a simple trauma to the auricle can result in a significant swelling of the tissues around the injured region. The resulting edema can project into the external auditory meatus and cause an interruption in sound transmission. The most obvious example of that type of repeated trauma is the cauliflower ear of the boxer that is the result of blood collecting next to the cartilage skeleton of the ear (Figure 4-1). The hearing loss in such a case is conductive and usually quite mild.

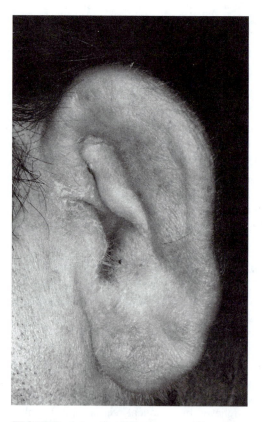

**FIGURE 4-1   Cauliflower ear. (Courtesy of Dr. Michael Hawke)**

Trauma to the ear canal or the tympanic membrane can be a much more serious matter. Usually the result of introducing an object into the canal, the most common sign is a hematoma. Because the skin of the canal is relatively thin and vascular, scratches and bleeding tears are also frequently seen. Sometimes, when the object is pushed to the extreme, the trauma extends to the tympanic membrane causing extreme pain, an occasional puncture, a substantial hematoma, and a hearing loss. Some patients have even suffered from vertigo as a result of that type of trauma. Obviously, the extent of the trauma will determine both the short- and long-term effects. A simple tear along the floor of the canal can heal. If it does not heal easily, however, the canal area is subject to bacterial infection and all that that entails. If the tympanic membrane itself is traumatized, a hematoma may cause a mild low-frequency hearing loss that, as the wound heals, will disappear of its own accord. A seriously damaged drum may result in long-term effects, such as a persistent perforation that can lead to recurrent middle ear cavity infection and a more substantial hearing loss. Surgical repair is then frequently required.

## *Seasonal Temperature Variations*

Temperature variation can also cause significant irritation and discomfort. In the winter, frostbite is a thermal injury to the pinna occurring after prolonged exposure to temperatures below freezing (Figure 4-2). It is usually characterized by four degrees of injury. The first degree consists of numbness and swelling of the pinna, while the fourth entails a loss of the auricle due to necrosis. In the early stages of frostbite, a gradual warming and the use of antibiotics to prevent infection usually succeeds in relieving the condition. In the later stages, the physician applies medical and surgical techniques appropriate to the damage and the effects of the cold. Any hearing loss associated with frostbite will be in direct proportion to the degree of damage sustained due to exposure. First stage trauma may not affect hearing, while loss of the entire pinna as the result of a stage four exposure may cause serious scarring, ear canal trauma, tympanic membrane damage, and significant conductive hearing impairment.

In the spring, children who have been kept indoors all winter may be exposed to too much sun rather suddenly. The result can be a rash called a juvenile spring eruption, which occurs behind the pinna and on other parts of the head and neck. The rash itches and usually results in scratching and associated infections. Keeping the skin dry and proper medical treatment will alleviate the difficulty, but the potential for complication is great if the child is not monitored and prevented from irritating the situation. The infamous baby rash seen behind the ears of many tiny tots in summer can be a similar source of itching, pain, and infection; if untreated, serious complications can result.

In the fall, exposure to cold air may cause some people to develop a disorder commonly called chilblains. The auricle swells, vasoconstriction occurs, and small blood vessels near the surface of the ear are deprived of their normal oxygen flow. This is quite similar to patterns seen in the early stage of frostbite. If this continues over many years, the result is that the normal resiliency of the pinna is affected, and it seems to harden or become calcified. Eventually, skin sensitivity, appearance, and color are all affected. When exposed to the cold, use of ordinary ear protection can help to prevent this disorder that is common in persons who work outdoors in cooler climates. Those who work in the fishing, lumber, and con-

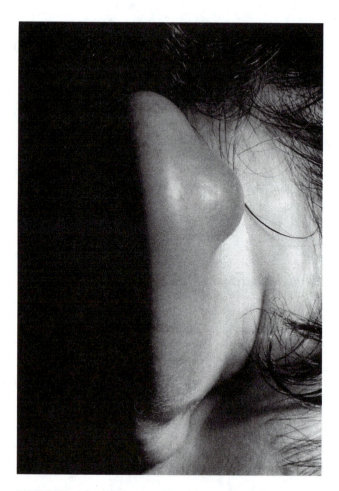

**FIGURE 4-2    Mid-stage frostbite on the left pinna.
Note the swelling and discoloration associated with the
disorder. (Courtesy of Dr. Michael Hawke)**

struction industries most often appear in our clinics with symptoms of this problem.
Because the pain is not felt, the danger is in not realizing how cold the ear is. The pinna may
sometimes show cracks or tears in the skin surface, but there is no pain associated with it.
Hearing loss is usually not present in chilblains. However, the nature of these employment
settings certainly puts those who work in them at risk for noise-induced hearing loss (see
Chapter 11) and further investigation is certainly warranted. Another possible long-term
complication of this disorder relates to the loss of flexibility of the pinna with aging. For
those with a history of chilblains, the "cardboard" appearance of the pinna becomes problematic with aging and it appears to elongate and enlarge. Furthermore, should such persons

require use of amplification—which is not out of the question because of noise exposure—the shape, sensitivity, and resiliency of the pinna can become a significant issue in hearing aid choice and user satisfaction.

## Otitis Externa

Otitis externa is far and away the most common single condition to affect the external auditory canal. It is an inflammatory condition of the skin lining the external canal and has many causes. It may be acute or chronic and also diffuse or localized.

### Acute Diffuse Otitis Externa

Acute diffuse otitis externa is an infective condition in which the external auditory canal becomes invaded by some microorganism, usually bacterial and commonly *Pseudomonas auriginosa*, although many other species may be responsible. Although this condition may occur spontaneously, it is more common to find the presence of some predisposing factor such as local trauma, frequent swimming, or previous chronic otitis externa. This condition causes acute swelling of the canal, which may be severe enough to close the external meatus, watery secretion from the canal, and hyperkeratosis (excess skin production). The patient will typically complain of pain, which is often severe, decreased hearing, and a whitish, watery discharge. The mainstay of treatment is aural toilet to remove all the infected debris. This procedure should be performed by an otologist. Analgesics and topical antibiotic–steroid combination drops also are helpful.

### Acute Localized Otitis Externa

Acute localized otitis externa, another of the otitis externa group, exists in two main forms. The first, called *furuncle*, is seen as a spot in the external canal and is invariably the result of infection of a hair follicle by *Staphylococcus aureus*. Although exquisitely tender, it will usually resolve, even if untreated, in a few days. Analgesics may be required to ease pain and discomfort. The second form of acute localized otitis externa is called *bullous myringitis*. It is a localized viral infection of the tympanic membrane and deep auditory canal that results in blood blisters of variable number and size. It is also very painful, but again, is self-resolving in a few days. Symptomatic treatment is all that is necessary. If the deep canal is filled with debris, local cleansing by an otolaryngologist may be required.

### Chronic Otitis Externa

Chronic otitis externa is the final example of generalized otitis externa. The condition is fairly common and is usually diffuse in nature. It is in essence a chronic eczematous-like dermatitis of the skin of the external auditory meatus (Figure 4-3). Pain is less of a feature and itching is much more frequent. The lining skin usually appears red and scaly, and wax is rarely seen. In the hypertrophic variant of this condition, the skin may thicken until there is almost complete occlusion of the meatus. A watery discharge and acute exacerbations are common. Treatment of this condition involves regular aural toilet and topical steroids and

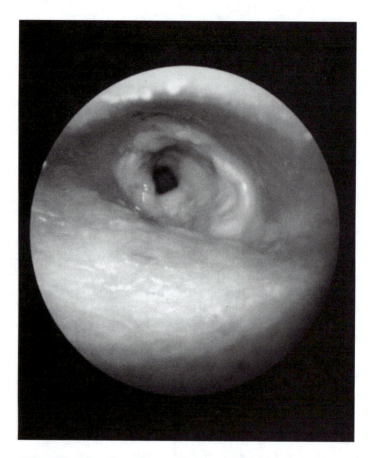

**FIGURE 4-3   Chronic suppurative otitis externa. Note the gradual closing of the ear canal. (Courtesy of Dr. Michael Hawke)**

usually demands the skills of an otolaryngologist. Complications of this condition include stenosis (a closing) of the canal or the development of a false fundus or monomeric membrane. A false fundus is a membrane that forms across the canal and obscures the drum and significantly impairs sound conduction. This causes a marked conductive hearing loss.

Figure 4-4 is another good example of otitis externa. In this case, however, it has resulted from lupus vulgaris, a variant of tuberculosis. If undetected, this disease can progress to complete destruction of the pinna. However, in today's medical environment the disease is rare on the American continent, and when it appears, it can be treated with antibiotics.

### Malignant Otitis Externa

This uncommon condition is most frequently seen in elderly diabetics. It is classified as a form of otitis externa, but more specifically it is an osteitis of the temporal bone. Left

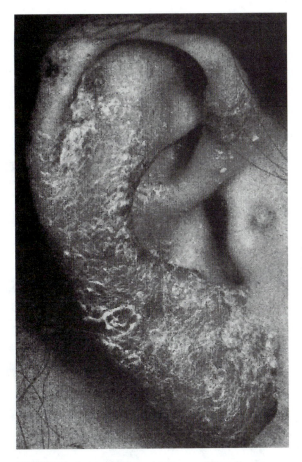

**FIGURE 4-4**    **Otitis externa resulting from lupus vulgaris. (With permission from Edward Arnold, Ltd.)**

untreated there is a high mortality because it leads to palsies of the last four cranial nerves, which can then lead to difficulties with swallowing, aspiration pneumonia, and ultimately death in an already compromised group of individuals. Treatment requires hospitalization, intravenous antibiotics, and occasionally surgical debridement of the necrotic portions of the temporal bone.

## *Fungal Infections (Otomycosis)*

Given the compromise of the canal's normal defense mechanisms and the frequent use of topical antibiotic preparations when a chronic otitis externa is present, superadded fungal infections of the canal are a common complication. This is frequently termed otomycosis

(Figure 4-5): in its literal meaning "oto"—ear, "myco"—fungus, "osis" —state or condition of. In other words, otomycosis means the condition of having a fungus in the ear. Although many varieties of fungi may appear, the three most common are *Aspergillus fumigatus*, *Aspergillus niger*, and *Candida albicans*. They may be very colorful, ranging from blue-black to green and yellow to white. These fungal infections produce a great deal of debris within the ear canal. Patients often complain of some hearing loss and a wet feeling inside the ear as well as discomfort and frequent itching. Fungal infections also may arise de novo. Ironically, fungal infections may be the result of a medical treatment. Overzealous use of an antibiotic can eliminate most of the body's natural bacterial defenses and destroy the delicate balance between bacteria and fungi that exists in all of us. That is one reason why physicians are careful about dosage and administrative patterns of antibiotics and are distressed when patients ignore instructions.

The danger of a fungal infection is its ability to gradually eat its way through the walls of the auditory canal. Much the same as a fungus eats through a tree trunk in the forest, a

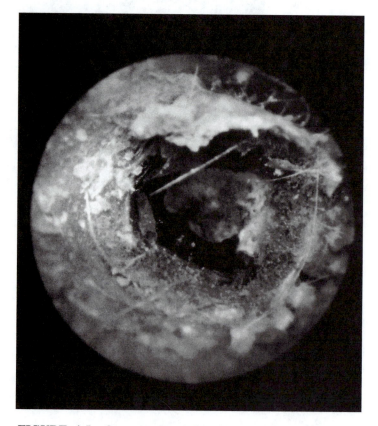

**FIGURE 4-5   Otomycosis—A fungal growth in the ear canal. (Courtesy of Dr. Michael Hawke)**

fungus eventually can destroy the ear canal sections of the mastoid bone. If continued unchecked, it can form the basis for even more serious complications such as meningitis and even death. This takes time and is a long-term negative result, but the point is, the presence of fungus in the ear canal should be taken seriously. This is clearly a medical problem and treatment is difficult and involves regular aural toilet and antifungal agents.

## Herpes Infection

The herpes family of viruses include those causing chicken pox and shingles (*Varicella zoster*) as well as simple cold sores (herpes simplex). Herpes infection of the ear usually begins with a burning pain in the affected ear and no visible pathology. The infection declares itself with the development of vesicle formation. This infection usually involves the facial nerve on the affected side and will often lead to a facial palsy, the Ramsay Hunt syndrome. In severe cases, the labyrinth and eighth cranial nerve may be involved leading to temporary dizziness and a permanent and often profound sensorineural hearing loss (Nahmias and Norrild, 1979). Treatment demands on early recognition and the use of antiherpetic medications, often by the intravenous route initially, as well as supportive treatment for the labyrinthitis. There is a much more detailed discussion of these viruses, which may affect the cochlea and central auditory pathways as well as the external ear, in Chapter 8.

# Obstructions

## Collapsed Ear Canals

Because of unique differences in the structure of the ear, there are patients with enlarged tragi that are easily flattened when pressed. In the normal situation, the ear canal is opened and the tragus projects out, away from the opening of the ear canal. When a finger is pressed against the tragus, or more importantly, an earphone presses against the ear, the tragus is flattened across the opening of the ear canal. The result is an occluded ear canal and an associated hearing loss, sometimes as much as 50 dB. A collapsed ear canal may occur from evacuation of air from the ear, which occurs when placing the earphones on a patient (especially a very young or very old person) who has an extremely narrow isthmus or highly compliant canal walls. A collapse will often account for significant differences between results obtained during testing in the sound field and those obtained via earphones. Sometimes a child with a suspected hearing loss will be referred from a school screening to an audiology center. This suspicion of hearing loss may be due to a flattened tragus or a collapsed ear canal. The audiologist should always be alert to that possibility.

If the patient has tragus or collapsed ear canal problems, the difficulty will usually be relieved by gently pulling upward and backward on the pinna as the earphone is placed over the ear. If that does not work, it may be necessary to hold the earphone against the head and not to fix it in place with the headband. Ingenuity and caution are appropriate.

## *Wax Impaction*

The external auditory canal is lined by squamous epithelium (i.e., normal skin), which exhibits the unusual property of migration. On all other parts of the body, the dead superficial layers of skin are usually shed as a result of local friction with items such as clothes and brushes. This is not possible in the external ear canal. In this site, the skin slowly moves laterally, like a conveyor belt, from the tympanic membrane to the outer part of the external canal where it starts to separate (desquamate) and mix with the secretions from the ceruminous glands. Ear wax, or cerumen, is a mixture of secretions from pilosebaceous and ceruminous glands, desquamated skin, dust, and other foreign materials. The wax and contained skin are carried out of the external auditory meatus by the process of migration.

The ceruminous glands are found in the skin of the outer two-thirds of the external acoustic meatus and secrete a liquid material. After secretion, evaporation occurs to leave a sticky, waxy substance that is able to trap dirt, squama, and microbes with relative ease. Wax can be secreted in one of two forms. Wet wax is produced by most blacks and whites and is familiar as being moist, sticky, and honey-colored. The dry type is more common in Oriental races and tends to be grayer in color, less sticky, granular, and brittle. The gene for wet wax is dominant. Regardless of type, ear wax tends to become drier with age as a result of reduced glandular numbers and activity. Wax production is sensitive to the presence of other local skin conditions and tends to be reduced in the presence of local inflammatory pathology. There is also great individual variation in the amount of ear wax produced. Wax secretion and the relatively acidic conditions on the superficial skin cells provide an effective protection against infection in this site.

The natural process of wax secretion and export can be upset by a number of factors and can cause wax impaction (Figure 4-6). Impaction is commoner in males due to the presence of thicker and coarser hairs in the lateral part of the EAM. Narrow canals, zealous use of cotton buds, and even a hearing aid mold can impede the normal flow of wax to the periphery. In some people, no obvious cause is found to account for their impaction and it has been suggested that desquamation of the superficial layer of the meatal epidermis is impaired.

Impaction of wax can cause a sensation of obstruction, mild conductive hearing loss, otalgia, vertigo, and coughing (via auricular branch of the vagus), although wax impaction is a relatively rare cause of hearing loss. Most of these symptoms are improved by removing the wax, which usually can be accomplished easily by syringing. On occasion it will be expedient to soften the wax beforehand with a ceruminolytic. Olive oil is a useful agent because it is relatively effective, cheap, readily available in most households, and does not run the risk of causing otitis externa from local irritation, unlike some other proprietary ceruminolytics. In general though, water-based solvents, such as sodium bicarbonate, are more effective on wax than are oil-based solvents.

Today, many audiologists practice cerumen management as part of their practice. In addition, of course, general physicians and specialists in otology and nurses and hearing aid dispensers include that procedure in their practice. There are commercial products available that are used and sold by those individuals or that are available through the local pharmacy. Before anyone puts anything in an ear, even for so noble a purpose as cleansing

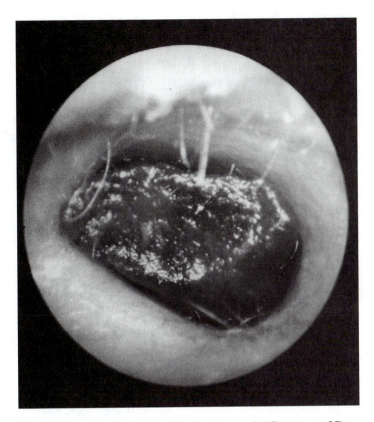

**FIGURE 4-6** **Cerumen plug in ear canal. (Courtesy of Dr. Michael Hawke)**

it to improve hearing, a proper otoscopic examination is mandatory. If the tympanic membrane is ruptured or inflamed, or if there is a disease process or foreign object in the canal, when a strong chemical is applied, the results can be disastrous. Caution should precede cleansing. Look in the ear before you put anything into it! Children seem to enjoy putting foreign objects in their ears, and even adults sometimes find the strangest objects lurking in that dark, warm, moist, environment (Figure 4-7*A*, Figure 4-7*B*). Syringing involves directing a jet of warm (body temperature) water along the roof or posterior canal wall so that it passes behind the wax and forces it outward. Although relatively safe, complications may occur and include coughing, pain, local trauma, otitis externa, and rarely tympanic membrane perforation and otitis media. Contraindications to syringing include frequent previous episodes of otitis externa, a known or suspected perforation and, a "difficult" ear, which is often due to a narrow and/or tortuous external meatus. In these cases, removal under direct vision with an operating microscope using microsuction or wax-hooks is a

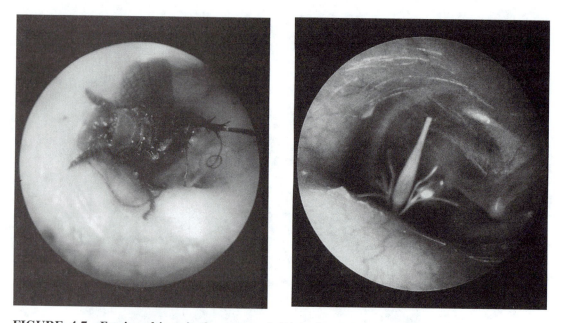

**FIGURE 4-7** **Foreign objects in the ear canal. (*A*) An insect has found refuge. (*B*) Seeds and plants take root. Look before testing, before syringing. Look before beginning any procedures. (Courtesy of Dr. Michael Hawke)**

more appropriate and safer alternative. Overzealous use of a jet stream or the wrong water temperature can induce nausea and vomiting resulting in a less than happy patient and an embarrassed clinician.

## Neoplasms

Neoplasms, or literally "new tissue," are seen in two basic forms, benign and malignant. Among the most common are exostoses, osteomas, and granulomas. Occasionally hemangiomas (blood-filled tumors) or hygromas (water-filled tumors) are also found (Figure 4-8). The danger to the auditory system lies in the disturbance of the normal location of the facial and auditory structures. Furthermore, rupture of the structure carries risk of infection and serious complications.

### Exostoses

Exostoses are bony growths and the commonest benign tumors of the external ear. They are in fact localized hyperplasias, usually due to irritation of the overlying periosteum or to some idiopathic cause. These may take the form of a single growth or multiple bony masses

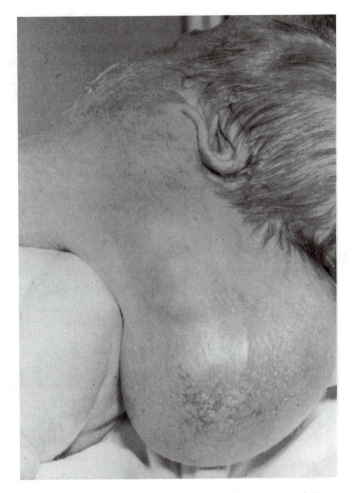

**FIGURE 4-8** **A hygroma or water-filled tumor of the neck that has displaced the auditory peripheral organs.**

(Figure 4-9). One thing that seems to lead to, or at least to aggravate the growth of, an exostosis is what has been called swimmer's ear. Persons who swim regularly in cold salt water repeatedly present an irritant to the lining of the ear canal that may develop into an exostosis, but when these become large, they may interfere with the normal process of migration and lead to a variety of symptoms. Thus the patient may not initially report pain or discomfort, but a conductive hearing loss may be present in 40 percent of the cases. Eventually, the symptoms may include tinnitus and associated infections such as acute otitis externa and pain. Exostoses are frequently bilateral, although DiBartolomeo (1979) reported that 80 percent of his cases started with unilateral symptoms. Treatment is medical and surgical,

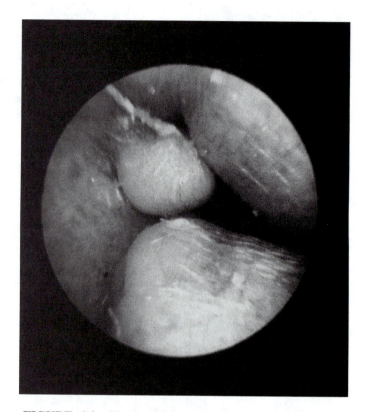

**FIGURE 4-9    Exostosis of the external auditory meatus. Note how the bony growth is gradually filling in the ear canal, eventually occluding it completely. (Courtesy of Dr. Michael Hawke)**

depending on the extent of the growth and the associated complications, including antibiotic therapy for ear canal infections. Surgery generally involves cutting or grinding away the bony growth to provide a patent ear canal. This is one of those pathologies that might be initially detected during the first hearing screening because of a mild complaint of hearing loss. The good clinician looks in the ear and knows what to see and what not to see . . . and when to refer.

### Osteomas

Osteomas vary significantly from exostoses. They are, literally, a tumor composed of bone. Exostoses tend to be irregular and often appear as multiple masses, and osteomas are smooth, firm masses that usually appear singly and represent a true benign bone tumor of the external canal. Where exostoses may be initially treated medically, an osteoma is more likely to require surgical treatment and will far more frequently cause symptoms, although the symptoms may be identical to those of the exostoses. If either mass enlarges sufficiently enough to hinder the normal migration of cerumen or to block the canal directly, hearing loss may occur. Both exostoses and osteomas are more frequent in adolescents than children and both may be associated with congenital disorders or a family history of a similar problem. Obviously, the audiologist must be alert to recognize an abnormality of the external ear canal when viewing the ear before audiometry.

## Granulomas

Granulomas are small rounded benign tumors made of granulation tissue. Think of a granule of sand and extend that thought to imagine small tissue masses forming at the healing edge of a wound. They can interfere with the healing process by blocking the blood supply to the leading edge, or they can form an uneven and rough surface at a point that has already healed. Granulomas may develop in the canal following injury or trauma. These are harmless, unless of course, they grow to unusual size or are, themselves, damaged or traumatized by introduction of foreign objects. Sometimes they develop their own layer of skin and become papillomas. If they arise from a mucous lining of the ear or any part of the body, they are called polyps. If they are cyst-like or develop around a central core, such as infected hair follicles, they may be more susceptible to infection and may also indicate a more serious underlying pathology. In any case, they are a medical problem with hearing loss almost never present.

## Malignant Tumors

According to DiBartolomeo, Papparella, and Meyerhoff (1991), some 90 percent of skin cancers appear in the head and neck region, and 6 percent of all skin cancers occur on the ear (Figure 4-10, Figure 4-11). Basal cell carcinomas and squamous cell carcinomas are the two commonest tumors to affect this region and most commonly follow prolonged sun exposure. Both may present as either a raised scaly lesion or a slowly growing ulcer. Treatment may be by either radiotherapy or excision surgery. Other tumors affecting this area include malignant melanoma and with the advent of AIDS, there have been a number of cases of Kaposi sarcoma of the external auditory meatus (Flower and Sooy, 1987). These kinds of problems are not primarily auditory nor are they exclusively otologic. They often require the services of an oncologist (a physician who specializes in tumors) and a facial plastic surgeon. Many forms of tumor may arise or invade the ear canal, although this is extremely uncommon, and may present with a hearing loss. The audiologist should be alert to this possibility and, if so, should immediately refer the patient for treatment.

## Comment

The clinicians' responsibility (be they a speech pathologist, a nurse, hearing aid dispenser, or industrial hearing screening technician, etc.) is to look at the outer ear and in the ear canal to do two basic things. First, a visual inspection and an otoscopic view are necessary to ensure

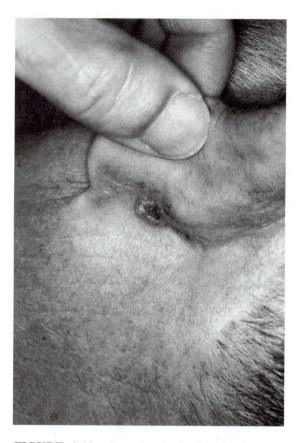

**FIGURE 4-10    A postauricular basal cell carcinoma. (Courtesy of Dr. Michael Hawke).**

that there is no obvious condition or disease requiring medical evaluation and treatment. Clearly, appropriate and prompt referral is an integral part of that responsibility. Second, the clinician must ensure that nothing in the ear or on the ear will interfere with audiometric testing or compromise the health of the patient or the standards of the test facility.

A physician or an audiologist examines an ear with an otoscope to look at the shape and health of the external auditory meatus and the color and mobility of the tympanic membrane. Once it has been established that the canal is clean, dry, and healthy, the focus shifts to the tympanic membrane. The drum is normally gray in color. If there is disease, especially in the middle ear, the membrane will mirror that in an alteration of its basic color or in its ability to reflect light. For example, the membrane may be pinkish or red from severe irritation. It may be purple or black from an old scar that has necrotized. In a rare situation, it may even appear to have white plaques due to tuberculosis, a disease that can occur in any part of the body except the teeth and nails. In short, the color of the tympanic membrane is an important clue in the diagnosis. And, if not visible at all, it may be obscured by cerumen or a neoplasm.

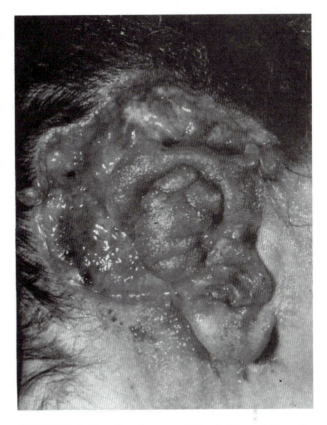

**FIGURE 4-11** **Carcinoma of the right auricle and extension into adjacent soft tissue. (With permission of Dr. R.C. Bryarly)**

In one otology clinic, the physician peered through the otoscope and discovered the tympanic membrane to be a beautiful shade of royal blue. An audiologist colleague concurred that was indeed the color. Gray is normal; pink, red, yellow, and black all occur under various pathologic conditions. Royal blue does not appear, even in the ears at Buckingham Palace! The otologist asked the patient's mother if the family had been painting the house. An affirmative reply indicated that the garage was being painted blue.

The clinician must also ensure the cleanliness of the audiometric equipment and the safety of the patient. Many of the diseases discussed to this point, and to be discussed later, are highly infectious. It is essential therefore, that the earphone cushions, the ear inserts and impedance tips, and the specula used with the otoscope are sterilized to obviate contagion to other patients. In fact, many audiology clinics wisely disinfect equipment and instruments after every patient. This may be done by ultraviolet radiation or by chemical sprays. The cushions need to be removed from the earphones if they are to be sprayed so that the spray does not contact the earphone diaphragm.

Finally, one does not expect to see a significant hearing loss or threshold shift with disorders of the external ear, although exceptions in which the canal is actually occluded have been noted. The audiometric contour will usually approximate normal, or if a loss is present the contour will typically be flat or slightly rising (better) in the high frequencies. Speech discrimination should be normal. Given that an aural inspection has revealed the presence of pathology before testing was initiated, it is likely that the clinician would not have attempted tympanometry.

Chapter *5*

# Anomalies of the External Ear

## Embryology

A great principle of embryology is that ontogeny recapitulates phylogeny: Embryologic development follows the same course as evolutionary development. An individual animal, in its prenatal life, repeats the development of the species. The phylogenetic scale begins with single-celled creatures, then two-celled creatures, four, eight, and so on. We start out looking very much like those two- or four- or eight-celled animals. Based on gross anatomy, one could not distinguish a human embryo of a few hours gestation from the embryo of any other animal. Even after a few days—and, sometimes, weeks—we look very much like our brothers and sisters in the animal kingdom. Ontogeny, the development of the individual, really does repeat the development of the species homo sapiens from the one-celled animals through the invertebrates and the rest of the vertebrates and eventually mammals.

The second great principle of development is that ontogeny proceeds in two directions, cephalocaudal (from head to tail) and proximodistal (from near to far). Observe very young infants. Cephalocaudal development is evident from the fact that the head appears to be quite large with respect to body length; this is because, in fetal and early postnatal life, growth has proceeded from top down, from head to tail. In a human adult, the head accounts for perhaps one sixth of total body length; in an infant, it is substantially more than that (Figure 5-1). This is important for the present purpose because of its implication for the development of aural anatomy. Proximodistal development is literally from near (proximal) to far (distal).

### Ontogenic Development

Ontogenic development starts at the time a one-celled structure (an ovum) is fertilized by another (a sperm) and promptly results in a two-celled creature. It is literally a matter of minutes in which that two-celled creature becomes a four-celled animal, and so on by a process of cell division and multiplication. The process of human prenatal development

73

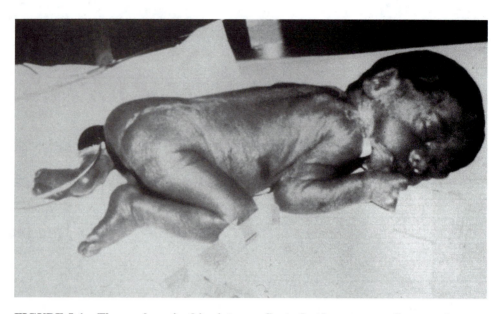

**FIGURE 5-1**   **The newborn in this picture reflects that human growth proceeds cephalocaudally (from head to tail). Note the size of the head in proportion to the rest of the body. Compare that to older children and adults. Growth of the embryo begins primarily with the head and proceeds distally.**

takes a rather short period, normally 38 to 40 weeks. Hence, it is essential that some developments occur simultaneously. The sequence and timing of antenatal developments may be important for later diagnosis. A skilled clinician brings a knowledge of embryology to bear on diagnosis in the sense of "if this, then that." If there is some interruption in prenatal development that results in an observable defect or alteration in a given structure, then one may assume that another structure could also be affected because of the time or place of interruption.

Certain structures develop from the same *anlage*, that is, the same primordial tissue. This fact has consequences for the clinician as a diagnostician. For example, a persistent dry cough is a symptom that sometimes accompanies otitis externa. Why? The ear canal, the auricle, the mandible, and the hyoid bone all develop from the same anlage. Think of it as the same as the concept of referred pain. The pain or the cough occur at a place seemingly remote from the site of the difficulty, but not really so, since developmentally the two locales are closely associated. Hence, two things are important in pathology and therefore in diagnosis. One is time. If something disrupts or interrupts development at a particular time, then it can disrupt everything else developing at the same time. Second, if there is disruption in a given place, one should look for a disruption in another place on the body arising from the same anlage. This is especially obvious for those hearing impairments occurring with craniofacial anomalies. If there is disruption of a certain structure at a certain time, the result could very well be alteration of other structures of the middle ear, the external ear, and the mandible. For example, later on there is a discussion of *mandibulofacial dysostosis*, known as Treacher Collins syndrome. These patients have conductive hearing impairments with microtia, atresia, and alterations of the ossicles plus anomalies of the eyelids and the mandible, all structures of an associated anlage. It is said that if you see a child with an unusual facial appearance because of the associated anlage, assume the child is hearing impaired until it can be demonstrated otherwise (Stool and Houlihan, 1977).

## *Auditory System Development*

One of the best ways to determine the gestational age of a normally developing fetus is to equate postconceptional age with crown–rump length. Table 5-1 details the expected growth patterns for a normal fetus. However, it is not only the length of the fetus that is critical. Other growth aspects are simultaneously underway. By three weeks of development, an embryologist can identify an otic anlage that, early on, develops into an otic placode. The placode will slowly invaginate and become an auditory pit. At that point, it is possible to see the first development of an auditory ganglion, as yet still disconnected from the auditory pit. It will eventually connect the cochlea with the auditory nerve. The auditory pit approaches the ganglion as it changes into an auditory vesicle at about the third week of the prenatal period.

Early in the fourth week, one can identify a tubotympanic recess, arising between the first and second branchial arches, that will eventually connect the cavity of the middle ear with the nasopharynx via the Eustachian tube. At the same time, six small cartilaginous hillocks can be seen forming in the region of the future pinna. These will go on to form the various convolutions of the adult pinna. At eight weeks, the vestibular system starts to appear including the semicircular canals, saccule, and spiral ganglion. In addition, the start of a cochlear nerve as well as a vestibular ganglion may be found. In a nine-week fetus, the stria

**TABLE 5-1   Crown-rump length and gestational age.**

| Length (in mm) | Age |
|---|---|
| 9.0 | 33 days |
| 9.8 | 35 days |
| 18.7 | 37 days |
| 21.2 | 41 days |
| 22.0 | 43 days |
| 26.0 | 45 days |
| 29.0 | 47 days |
| 32.5 | 8 weeks |
| 42.0 | 9 weeks |
| 54.7 | 10 weeks |
| 82.7 | 12 weeks |
| 107.3 | 13–15 weeks |
| 138.8 | 16–18 weeks |
| 184.5 | 19–21 weeks |
| 368.5 | Newborn |

vascularis may be seen along with the beginnings of the cochlear structure with inner and outer ridges that become hair cells, a primitive tectorial membrane, and other related structures. By ten weeks, one can recognize a middle ear cavity, a cochlear duct, a stapes, and a relatively large vestibular system. Also by ten weeks the developing cochlea has succeeded in achieving its expected 2.5 turns. By twelve to fourteen weeks it will separate into the scala vestibuli and scala tympani. At sixteen weeks the two scalae are separated by a primitive basilar membrane. In addition, the ossicles may be seen, having developed from the mesenchyme of the first and second branchial arches.

Auditory anatomy develops quickly after that. In the final trimester, the external auditory meatus, middle ear, and Eustachian tube recanalize, having been occluded with mesenchymal material prior to this point. By forty weeks—that is, full term—the inner ear structures are nearly adult size (Fritsch and Sommer, 1991) and the rest of the auditory system is about 75 percent of its eventual size. Shape and position change in postnatal life as a function of head growth. Figure 5-2 illustrates how the adult face develops from the embryonic face, demonstrating the anlage concept and the importance of understanding developmental sequencing and processes.

Figure 5-3 shows a comparison of the newborn's ear with the adult's ear over time. Note that the neonate's ear canal is almost horizontal and has virtually no isthmus. With head growth, the meatus bends in anterior and inferior directions and the isthmus narrows, and with age, a crease develops in the lobule and the entire structure enlongates.

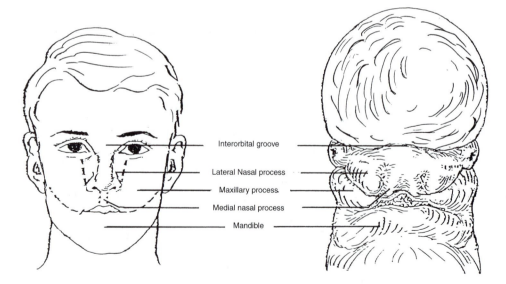

Interorbital groove

Lateral Nasal process

Maxillary process.

Medial nasal process

Mandible

**FIGURE 5-2    Comparison of the embryonic face and the young adult.**

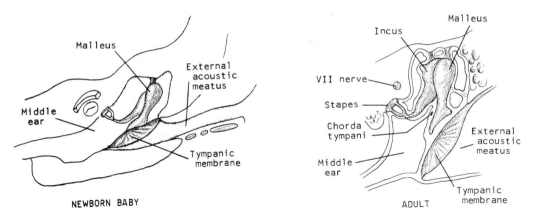

**FIGURE 5-3    Comparison of the angle of the external auditory meatus in a newborn with that of an adult.**

## *Irregularities of the External Ear*

Anomalies of the external ear may be classified under the general heading of aural agenesis or dysgenesis—a total or partial failure to develop. If it is the pinna that has failed to develop, the condition is described as microtia if partial, or anotia if completely absent. If it is the external auditory meatus that has failed to develop, the appropriate term is atresia, which indicates absence of an opening. When atresia occurs in the external auditory meatus, it is called aural atresia (Figure 5-4). If an opening is present but abnormally narrow, it is called a stenosis.

## *Microtia and Atresia*

Given what is known about embryology, it is reasonable to expect that microtia and atresia will occur together, and they usually do, but not always. The prevalence is about 10,000 to 20,000 persons in the United States (Bordley, Brookhouser, and Tucker, 1986). Atresia occurs with severe microtia, but may also occur with a normal pinna (Mattox, Nager, and Levin, 1991). Microtia may be due to interruption of development at a vulnerable period in utero or it may be an inherited trait. There are some rather interesting and peculiar things about microtia that are not easily explained. Microtia and atresia are usually unilateral by a ratio of four to one, occurring more often on the right side of the face than on the left. Further, the problem occurs more frequently in males than in females (Bordley, Brookhouser, and Tucker, 1986).

A university clinic reported one family in which the mother and all three of her sons had congenital aural atresia without microtia. The members of that family all had moderate conductive hearing impairments due to the atresia; yet they had no immediately obvious signs (because there was no microtia) of external ear anomaly. Clearly, the problem was a genetic disorder—one that also occurred in the mother's sister. However, the malformation did not appear in the grandparents, nor did it appear in the sister's children. One should assume, therefore, that the problem in that family is due to either a recessive mode of inheritance or to a dominant inheritance with variable expression.

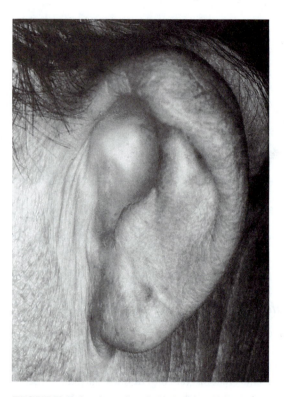

**FIGURE 5-4    Atresia of the left auditory meatus. (Courtesy of Dr. Michael Hawke)**

Another recent case involved K.M., a two-year-old exhibiting Goldenhar syndrome (hemifacial microsomia). She had an initial evaluation in a doctor's office and was referred for further evaluation. Results indicated she could localize to speech in the sound field at 55 dB with the signal on her right and at 50 dB with it on her left. A startle to speech was elicited at 70 dB. When a bone conduction vibrator was held to her left mastoid and a signal of only 20 dB HTL was presented, she stopped sucking on her bottle and lateralized appropriately. These data corroborated the conductive nature of her hearing impairment. A hearing aid with a bone conduction vibrator was prescribed and a program of auditory habilitation begun. She will be assessed for a possible middle ear construction or bone conduction hearing aid implant within a year.

## Facial Anomalies

It is quite surprising that disorders of embryological development are not seen more frequently. Congenital anomalies present a broad spectrum of severity from simple skin tags, preauricular pits and fistulae, to the extremes of complete anotia (absence) and severe microtia (Figure 5-5A–F).

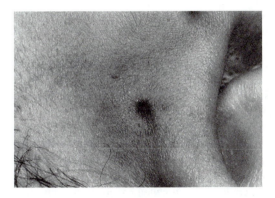

**FIGURE 5-5***A*    **Preauricular sinus. (Courtesy of Dr. Michael Hawke)**

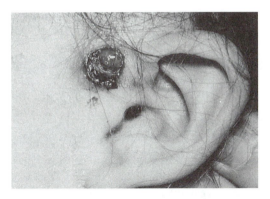

**FIGURE 5-5***B*    **Preauricular sinus with fistula.**

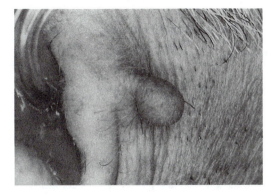

**FIGURE 5-5***C*    **Preauricular skin tag. (Courtesy of Dr. Michael Hawke)**

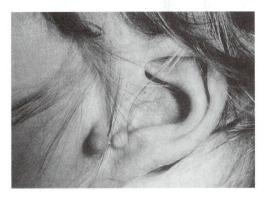

**FIGURE 5-5***D*    **Preauricular skin tag.**

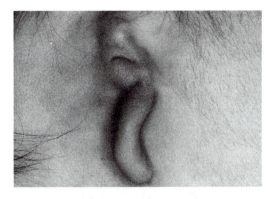

**FIGURE 5-5***E*    **Microtia. (Courtesy of Dr. Michael Hawke).**

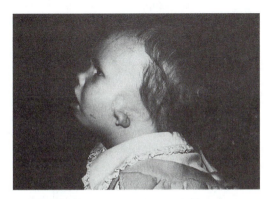

**FIGURE 5-5***F*    **Microtia.**

The importance of recognizing minor anomalies is their frequent association with other potentially more serious anomalies. For example, one clinic reported the case of a preauricular pit on a grown woman who had always thought it was a type of dimple. The woman complained of a sudden hearing problem that had been related to her middle ear. Otologic examinations revealed that this pit was a $1\frac{1}{2}$–inch canal that was migrating into the middle ear. She was actually having severe middle ear problems because the unrecognized canal had become infected and was allowing contaminants to reach the middle ear. Surgical correction was required.

Just as the pinnae may be too small or even missing, they can also be too large (macrotia); low set; or even placed at unusual angles (lop ear) on the head. Probably the most common congenital anomaly of the external ear is the failure of the normal antihelical fold to develop normally with a resulting protuberant appearance, so-called bat ears. The important point to remember here is not the specific placement of the pinnae but the concept of anlage and to recognize that this unusual placement can mean an associated malformation in the ear canal or middle ear and thus the patient should be evaluated carefully for hearing impairment.

### *Additional Terminology*

Before proceeding further it is important to review a few common epidemiological terms likely to be encountered in the reading. Understanding their meaning helps to clarify the relationships among the various pathologies discussed and also provides some basic clues to their etiology. For example, thus far the terms *malformation* and *deformation* have been used. What is the difference? A malformation is, literally, the poor or inappropriate formation of a structure. It is "any morphologic defect caused by an error in the developmental process beginning at its most elementary level" (Siegel-Sadewitz and Shprintzen, 1982; Gerber, 1990). It could be genetic or due to administration of a toxic substance. For example, if a woman takes a pharmaceutical product during pregnancy and that product has negative effects on the development of the fetus, the results are considered a malformation due to mechanical interruption at a particular time during the pregnancy. A deformation, on the other hand, is caused by a mechanical interference with development, such as an unusual fetal position or small uterine space.

Another set of terms that often causes difficulty is endemic and epidemic. When a disease or disorder is *endemic* to a population it is something that is present in that community at a higher level than normal and for a long period of time. For example, in many small communities in rural locales there is a strong tendency toward marrying within a family. While consanguinity, the marriage of first cousins or closer, is outlawed in many areas of the world, that practice still does exist. If the family happens to have strong genetic traits for a particular disorder, the prevalence of that disorder will be higher than in the general public at most times, and it can be said that the disorder is endemic to that population. That is, the problem will not simply cease in a few weeks and the population will always show a higher number of cases. In contrast, an *epidemic* is something that attacks many people in a community, but is not continually present. For example, if the flu visits a city we can say there is a flu epidemic. But that problem will cease in a few weeks and things will return to normal.

Three very frequently used terms are syndrome, sequence, and association. Since all these terms describe a group of anomalies or symptoms, on the surface, they may appear to be the same. But they are not. A *syndrome* is a collection of anomalies or symptoms resulting from a single pathogenic process or cause. In other words, all the problems are related to the same exact causative factor. The term *anlage* should come to mind. A *sequence* is a series of multiple anomalies resulting from a single defect or mechanical event, but each is a consequence of another. For example, something mechanical (e.g., body position) is forcing the fetus to form with only a very small mandibular space, which, in turn, might force the tongue away from its normal position on the floor of the mouth and up into the palatal space. The result could be a palatal cleft or other oral deformation. Each event has triggered another and the final event is the cleft. That would be called a sequence. Finally, an *association* is a collection of disorders or anomalies that consistently occur together, but that are not caused by the same pathogenic process nor has one triggered the other in a sequence. The concept of anlage is inappropriate when considering an association because no common cause is apparent for the associated characteristics.

## Complex Craniofacial Anomalies

Especially important anomalies of the external ear are those that are among the several stigmata of certain craniofacial anomalies. An encyclopedic discussion of the hundreds of complex craniofacial anomalies falling into the category is found in Konigsmark and Gorlin (1976). The reader is also referred to Gerber (1990), Gorlin, Cohen, and Levin (1990), and Jaffe (1978) for additional information. Presented here are two of the more common and apparent forms of these disorders (Treacher Collins syndrome and Crouzon syndrome).

### Treacher Collins Syndrome (Mandibulofacial Dysotosis)

Treacher Collins syndrome is properly called mandibulofacial dysostosis, which means a failure of bony development of the mandible and the face. It occurs in about 1.5 percent of congenital hearing losses. It results from a dominant mode of inheritance, which means that it may be passed along to half the offspring (see Chapter 8). It is characterized by (1) microtia (85 percent) and atresia (30–40 percent) with accompanying conductive hearing impairment (although a sensory hearing loss has been noted in some patients); (2) a notch of the lower eye lid called a coloboma; (3) a characteristic facial appearance caused by maldevelopment of the bones of the face, especially those associated with the temporomandibular joint; and (4) occurrence more often in males than females (see Figure 5-6).

According to Konigsmark and Gorlin (1976), radiographic and surgical investigations of Treacher Collins patients have shown sclerosis of the middle and (rarely) inner ear, with poor delineation of all structures. There may be fixation, fusion, malformation, or absence of any one or all of the ossicles or the oval window. Furthermore, abnormalities of the labyrinth have been found in 25 percent of the patients. In short, conductive or sensory hearing loss, and a host of other sequelae, may be present. Of course, these all accompany an unusual facial structure.

### Crouzon Syndrome

Crouzon syndrome is another relatively common example of a complex craniofacial disorder. It is a member of a group called cranial dysostoses. Patients with Crouzon syndrome, unlike those with Treacher Collins syndrome, usually do not have microtia, but are likely to have bony anomalies of the middle ear. A striking feature of Crouzon syndrome is an anom-

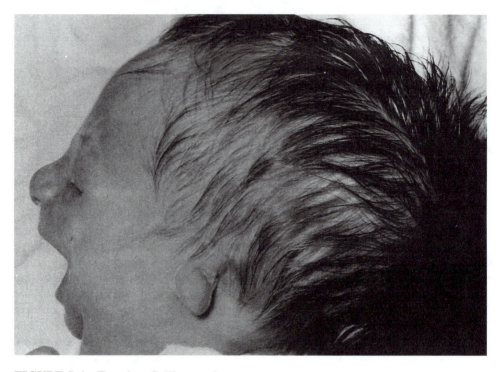

**FIGURE 5-6    Treacher Collins syndrome.**

aly of the orbit that produces a characteristic bulging of the eyes called exophthalmos (Figure 5-7). This is accompanied by other ocular deformities such as hypertelorism (increased distance between the eyes) and strabismus (cross-eye). There are also anomalies of the nose and maxilla that contribute further to a characteristic appearance. Such patients are likely to have normal intelligence and normal emotions, unless the cranial dysostosis has inhibited brain growth, and must be treated accordingly. When the stigmata of Crouzon syndrome are accompanied by anomalies of the hands or feet (the so called lobster claw anomaly), it is known as Apert syndrome.

Most notable among the defects associated with Crouzon syndrome that affect hearing are an infrequent deformity of the acoustic meatus, ossicular ankylosis (fixation) or anomaly, and (rarely) atresia of the ear canal. Occasionally, the atresia is bilateral. Patients have been reported to have an absence of a tympanic membrane and middle ear structures. The most prevalent finding is fixation of the stapes to the promontory (Konigsmark and Gorlin, 1976). Fraser (1976) reported a case in which Crouzon syndrome was mistaken for otosclerosis. Hearing impairment is present in approximately one third of the cases (Boedts, 1967). In the majority of cases, the impairment is conductive. However, because microtia or other similar anomalies of the pinna rarely present in this syndrome, although the patient may exhibit no overt or outward signs of ear anomaly, a bilateral malformation of the ear canal or middle ear structures and an associated hearing impairment still may be present.

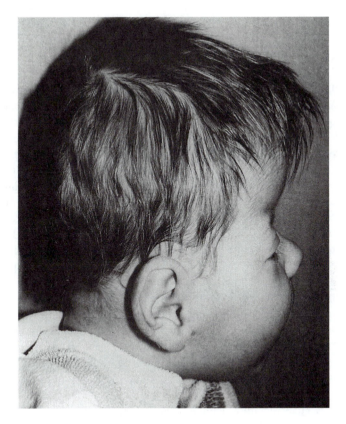

**FIGURE 5-7    Crouzon syndrome.**

### *Other Complex Craniofacial Disorders*
Other complex craniofacial disorders number in the hundreds (Konigsmark and Gorlin, 1976). Most incorporate conductive hearing loss, but a few are characterized by sensorineural pathology (Gorlin, Cohen, and Levin, 1990). The examples cited here are quite typical and provide some insight into the problem. However, they only touch the surface. Consider the Otofacialcervical syndrome, which consists of facial anomalies including ear malformations, cervical fistulas or nodules, and a hearing loss. Consider a syndrome with lop ears, imperforate anus, triphalangeal thumbs, and hearing loss. It would be impossible to list and discuss all the various complex craniofacial disorders known. What is important is to know that they exist, that any syndrome can include a hearing problem, and how to recognize one. The clinician should always keep in mind that as the fetus develops, it develops as an entire structure. Anything that interferes with that development, no matter what the cause or what the obvious site along the body structure, can also interfere with other structures that are developing at the same time in other sites along the same body structure. Thus, a syndrome that includes deficits in hearing and abnormal digits, or one that includes a hearing loss and an imperforate anus, is quite reasonable, plausible, and not all that unusual.

## *Treatment for Complex Craniofacial Disorders*

### *Surgical Approaches*

What is to be done? This question has to be answered on an individual case basis. The majority of anomalies are minor (e.g., skin tags, low set ears, preauricular pits, etc.) and consequently, rarely require any treatment beyond reassurance. For many of the other anomalies, the problem is primarily cosmetic and will usually be treated by plastic surgery to provide a more normal looking pinna. Fortunately, many of the more severe cases of microtia or anotia are unilateral and accompanied by a normal ear on the contralateral side. This means the individual will usually have at least one normal hearing ear and so the problem becomes essentially cosmetic. Unfortunately the reconstructive surgery for these types of deformity is complex, difficult, demanding, and not always successful, particularly when a new external meatus is created. Before creating a new meatus, the surgeon must know the extent of cochlear function, and what structures will be found within the middle ear cavity at the end of the new canal. For this, simple skull x-rays are inadequate. What is required is a procedure called high-resolution computerized tomography (CT scan), a process that uses very thin (1-mm) slices to construct an image of the temporal bone anatomy. The actual surgery involves drilling a hole where there is the best pathway. Ironically, it is a situation of going against nature to cure a problem that is unnatural, by creating a natural structure, unnaturally. If an arm or a leg, or any other bone in the body, is broken, it heals. The same may be true for temporal bone tissue that has been drilled out to create an ear canal. Thus, a newly formed ear canal has been known to fill in. The failure rate of this surgery had actually been very high because of this natural regenerative process. For example, the family referred to earlier, in which four members had atresia, underwent a series of individual operations to cure the problem. Four ears underwent operation, one on each head. Three of the four failed simply because it was so difficult to keep the ear canals open. Modern surgical techniques are certainly improving the success rate of these types of procedures. In fact, there have been some reports of a failure rate as low as 1.5 percent.

Another new surgical advance is the substitution of a prothesis for an abnormal pinna, one that either has developed that way or been damaged in an accident. An interesting and very useful development was the technique of bone anchoring. In simple terms this technique uses special platinum screws onto which bone can adhere, resulting in a very rigid fixation. The screws are used to anchor a bone conduction hearing aid, a prosthesis or both. This technique is very useful for dealing with a severe deformity in which the individual also has a significant conductive (or mixed) hearing loss. The quality of bone-conducted sound using the technique is excellent. Figure 5-8 illustrates how a prosthesis is attached with bone implanted clips.

Figure 5-9 illustrates several prosthetic pinnae in place, illustrating that this technique has a wide range of applications. In fact, these surgical reconstructions are remarkable in their ability to recreate a normal looking appearance to the ear. In the past the only choice was long hair, although age, sex, and current fashions certainly influenced that choice. There is no question that, in the case of craniofacial anomaly, cosmetic surgery may be more important than anything else.

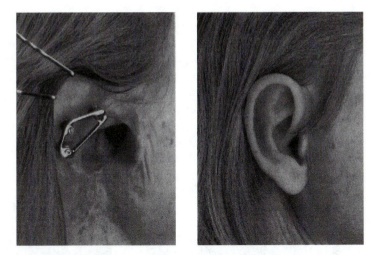

**FIGURE 5-8   Surgical procedure to attach a prosthetic pinna. (Courtesy of Nobelpharma, Canada—manufacturer of the prosthetic devices)**

Of course, reconstructive surgery is not limited to the pinna. It is used in a variety of situations involving complex craniofacial disorders, many of which count hearing loss among their sequelae. When the procedure succeeds, it succeeds strikingly. For example, Figure 5-10*A* and *B* illustrates the pre- and postsurgical appearance of a patient with extreme Apert syndrome. There would undoubtedly be significant agreement that the surgery greatly improved this young man.

## *Audiological Approaches*

When dealing with a patient who has a microtia or an atresia, several things must be considered. The significance of the patient's disability is determined not only by the degree of any hearing loss, but also to what extent the anomaly is part of a more complex disorder. If the patient lacks an ear canal or conductive mechanism on one side, then that ear has the maximum amount of hearing loss possible (55-60 dB HL) due to the failure of the sound conducting mechanism. However, while it is true that some patients who have unilateral hearing losses may have trouble hearing in a theater or church or lecture, for most adults, there is no significant auditory handicap if only one side is affected and the problem is almost entirely cosmetic. For children, on the other hand, there can be educational consequences. Bess and his colleagues (1984) have shown that children with unilateral hearing impairments often display educational difficulties that could not have had other causes. It becomes important, therefore, to ensure that proper amplification is provided (when indicated) and that teachers are made aware of how to ensure maximum communication with such a child. On occasion, children have been held back in school because of failure that could have been avoided by

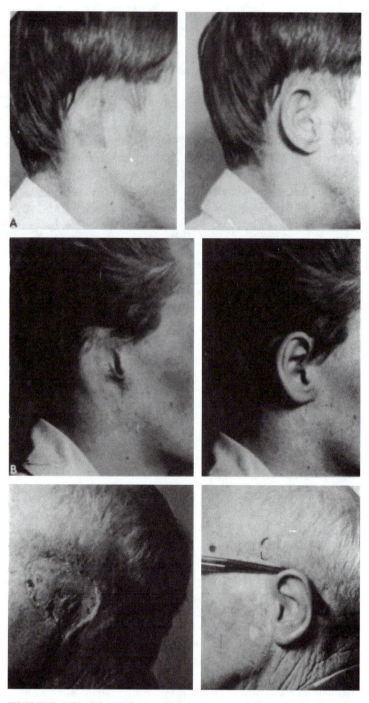

**FIGURE 5-9    Multiple prosthetic pinnae. (with permission of W.B. Saunders Co.)**

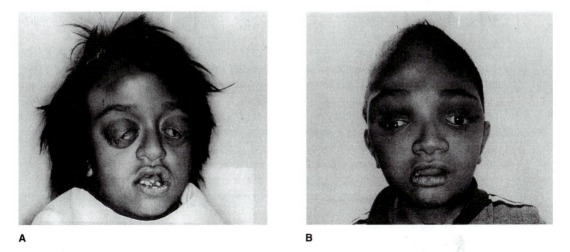

**A**                                                                      **B**

**FIGURE 5-10(*A*, *B*)     Pre- and postsurgical appearance of a patient with Apert syndrome.**

better attention to a unilateral impairment. If the atresia is bilateral, the patient will have a hearing impairment that could be truly disabling. Because these disorders are congenital, a child born with bilateral atresia of the external auditory meatus may have difficulty learning spoken language. In such cases, the audiometric configuration is usually flat, with equal impairment across most frequencies. Some patients may have slightly better hearing in the higher frequencies (2000 Hz and above) than in the lower frequencies.

Speech reception thresholds are usually at 45 to 55 dB. Speech discrimination scores should be very high, often nearly 100 percent if the stimulus is intense (loud) enough, because the problem is one of conduction and not one of sensory function. An audiologist may recommend a bone-conduction hearing aid for patients with bilateral conductive hearing impairments because such aids provide signals that bypass the middle ear and stimulate the cochlea directly. As previously discussed, a bone-anchored hearing aid (plus or minus a prosthesis) is particularly useful in these situations.

## *Comment*

Something else needs to be introduced here. It is all too easy to see a child with Treacher Collins syndrome or some other craniofacial anomaly and come to incorrect and dangerous conclusions. The harmful, old term "a funny-looking kid" is a classic example. First, no one wants to be considered funny looking. Second, the fact that people may have a peculiar appearance should elicit great sympathy and not embarrassment in those of us who observe them. Third, and most importantly, the vast majority of patients with craniofacial anomalies have normal intelligence and normal emotions. It is wrong to deal with such patients as though they suffer from profound mental retardation or severe emotional disturbance. They do not. They know how they look, and they know how others look at them. It is essential to recognize that these patients are normal human beings who happen to have anomalies of the face, and they can and will be improved over time by some rather marvelous surgical procedures. These folks do have hearing impairments, however, and audiologists must assume full rehabilitative responsibility. Sometimes that means the clinician must be able to go beyond the hearing impairment and, if necessary, be a counselor for a person with an anomalous face. If an audiologist is not able to be that counselor—perhaps because of a lack of sufficient training—the patient must be referred to a psychologist or other appropriate therapist as required. Further, these patients often require supportive services from speech–language pathology as well. Poor use of muscle structure, abnormal dentition, poor vision and hearing, and a host of other factors often result in speech and language delays and serious articulatory disorders that require treatment. In short, modern medicine, surgery, and rehabilitative procedures have improved the lives of patients with craniofacial anomalies. Cosmetic surgery, hearing aids, and speech therapy may allow such persons to take their proper places in the community.

*C h a p t e r* **6**

# *Otitis Media*

Otitis—meaning an infection or inflammation of the ear—is qualified in this case by the additional word "media," referring to the middle ear. Any inflammatory condition of the cavity of the middle ear, basically disease of the mucous membrane, is properly described as otitis media. It occurs far more frequently in children than in adults with its incidence decreasing with increasing age (Shambaugh and Girgis, 1991). It is second only to the common cold as childhood's most prevalent disease (Diefendorf, Leverett, and Miller, 1994). Shambaugh (1967) claimed an 80 percent incidence in children under three years of age. The severity of this disease's sequelae have finally been fully appreciated in that the potentially negative implications for speech and language development in children have been recognized.

The orientation of this chapter encompasses two themes. First, we adopt the otological perspective of Goodhill (1979b) that we are considering a continuum of disease processes, all of which may be subsumed under the title "*otomastoiditis.*" Second, we view diseases of the middle ear from the audiologist's perspective as changes in the stiffness or the mass of the middle ear contents.

## *The Middle Ear Transformer and Conductive Hearing Impairment*

The primary purpose of the middle ear system in the human animal is to affect an impedance match between a gas medium (air) and a fluid medium (the cochlear fluids). A sound wave traveling through air and striking a liquid surface would be almost totally reflected. The middle ear mechanism affects an air–fluid interface by providing a mechanical amplifier that transduces the airborne sound to the cochlea for fluid-borne transmission. Hence, the middle ear system "facilitates the transfer of sound in our environment to the cochlea" (Feldman and Wilber, 1976) and is, therefore, an impedance matching transformer. When a sound wave travels the length of the ear canal and strikes the tympanic membrane, some of its energy will be transmitted to the ossicular chain and some will be reflected. This depends in part upon the frequency of the tone, but depends primarily upon the stiffness encountered at the drum membrane. Obviously, the stiffer the membrane, the greater the amount of the reflection, and the poorer will be the hearing for that ear. Hence, any pathologic condition of the middle ear that increases the stiffness of the ossicular chain will be reflected by increased resistance of the drum membrane to a sound wave striking it. The terminology in current use would describe such an ear as having a high impedance (i.e., the energy transfer is impeded) or a low admittance (i.e., little energy is admitted into the middle ear system). The opposite can occur also. If, for example, the incus were to become disarticulated from its connection to the stapes, the stiffness of the system would decrease markedly; this is a condition of low impedance or high admittance. Normally, the system's impedance lies between such extremes.

Stiffness is the principal component of the middle ear impedance. However, changes of the mass of the contents of the middle ear also will be reflected in changes of impedance. Clearly, the main source of the mass component is the ossicles themselves, and changes of their mass caused by disease or injury also will change the stiffness of the system. In general, changes of the mass will not be reflected as changes of impedance except for frequencies lower than 600 Hz (Simons, 1979).

## Pathology and Etiology

Goodhill (1979b) views otomastoiditis as a continuum of tubotympanitis–otitis–mastoiditis. All steps in this continuum do not necessarily occur, but the sequence is necessary. That is, not everyone with tubotympanitis gets otitis media, and certainly not everyone with otitis gets mastoiditis, nor do they necessarily occur in rapid order; however, otitis follows tubotympanitis, and mastoiditis follows otitis. One conceptualization (Table 6-1), adapted from Goodhill (1979b), exhibits the sequence and provides a comprehensive outline for the condition.

For more information about these various disorders, the reader is also referred to Hawke's *Clinical Pocket Guide To Ear Disease* (1987) and Hawke and McCombe (1995) for full color illustrations of all the outer and middle ear pathologies considered in this text.

Another far more simple model than that presented in Table 6-1 is found in Figure 6-1. As can be seen from that figure, the continuum ranges from acute to chronic otitis media with each of those major categories having subpatterns. Note that acute otitis media progresses from suppurative to serous, while chronic progresses in what appears to be the opposite sequence. This pattern reflects treatment intercession whereby a suppurative process may be interrupted by an antibiotic, but not completely abated. The end result is a return to a serous state that becomes a chronic condition with continued exposure to ongoing bacterial infection and disease.

The key to the function of the middle ear and consequently its diseases is the Eustachian tube. The middle ear–mastoid system is an air-filled cavity. As with all enclosed body cavities, air is continuously absorbed by the mucosal blood supply. Because optimal middle ear function requires the pressure on both sides of the tympanic membrane to be equal, some mechanism must exist to allow the middle ear cavity to be regularly re-aerated. The Eustachian tube is opened by the levator palatini muscle during the act of swallowing and allows direct communication between the nasopharynx and the middle ear. This provides aeration of the middle ear, equalization of pressures, and optimal function of the middle ear mechanism. Impaired function of the Eustachian tube inevitably leads to problems in this

**TABLE 6-1    Sequential patterns of the tubotympanitis–otomastoiditis continuum.**

1. Acute and subacute patterns
   a. Transitory tubotympanitis (mild mucositis, negative pressure, no middle ear fluid)
   b. Acute tubotympanitis (mucositis, negative pressure, serosanguineous middle ear fluid or clear serous fluid)
   c. Acute purulent otitis media (tubotympanic mucositis, negative pressure, seropus)
   d. Subacute or chronic secretory otitis media (tubotympanic mucositis, tubal blockade, sustained otitis media, negative pressure, seromucoid fluid [glue ear]
   e. Acute otomastoiditis (tympanomastoid mucositis plus osteitis, mucopurulent middle ear and mastoid exudate)
   f. Acute otomastoiditis with complications (labyrinthitis, lateral sinus, meningitis, thrombophlebitis, etc.)
2. Chronic: Type A
   a. Chronic otomastoiditis with tympanic fibrosis (healed osteitis, no middle ear fluid, middle ear and mastoid fibrosis, tympanic membrane perforations)
   b. Chronic purulent otomastoiditis (mucosal polyposis, granulomatosis, osteitis, ossicular necrosis, purulent exudate, tympanic membrane perforation)
3. Chronic: Type B
   a. Chronic purulent otomastoiditis with tympanosclerosis (otomastoiditis, osteitis, mucositis, tympanosclerosis, ossicular necrosis, and/or fixation, mucopurulent middle ear exudate, tympanic membrane perforation)
   b. Chronic purulent otomastoiditis with cholesteatoma (keratoma), (otomastoiditis, osteitis, granulomatosis, polyposis, ossicular necrosis, cholesteatoma, and tympanic membrane perforation)
   c. Chronic purulent otomastoiditis with tympanosclerosis and cholesteatoma (keratoma)
   d. Chronic purulent otomastoiditis with cholesteatoma (keratoma), and/or tympanosclerosis, and complications (cranial nerve involvement, meningitis, sigmoid sinus thrombophlebitis, brain abscess)

Adapted from Goodhill, 1979b, p. 295 ff, with permission of the author and Harper & Row.

system. For a variety of reasons, Eustachian tube function is poorest during childhood. Important influences include the childhood anatomy: the tube is shorter and more horizontal than in the adult, adenoidal hypertrophy, the occurrence of frequent *upper respiratory tract infections* (URTIs), and poorer muscle function than adults. Cleft palate is an important cause of Eustachian tube dysfunction and is due to failure of function of the levator palatini. It is also temporarily impaired in adults during an URTI (as we can all testify!) and some individuals are unfortunate enough to have no obvious cause for their impaired Eustachian tube function—so-called idiopathic dysfunction. If the Eustachian tube does not function properly, there is reduced pressure in the middle ear cleft that results in an inflammatory response. What happens next will depend on a number of factors that are best considered in terms of each of the otitis categories.

## *Acute Suppurative Otitis Media*

Almost exclusively a disease of children, acute suppurative otitis media starts with an URTI that leads to impaired Eustachian tube function as described earlier. The impaired Eustachian tube function triggers a natural response in which the membranous lining of the

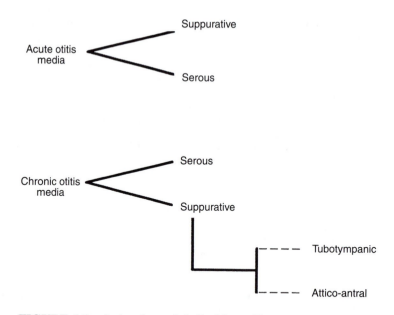

**FIGURE 6-1    A simple model of otitis media.**

middle ear secretes a clear fluid in an effort to cleanse the cavity and force open the tube. If the blockage and associated URTI continue, and the initial natural response of the body is unsuccessful in restoring normal function, what follows is the formation of an inflammatory exudate in the middle ear and mastoid cleft. The exudate is a thick fluid rich in proteins and cellular material. If the disease process continues, the fluid eventually becomes secondarily infected by the bacteria present. This acute infection then leads to the formation of pus in the middle ear and a series of fairly classic symptoms. The infection itself and the fluid buildup in the middle ear and its pressure against the tympanic membrane lead to pain, which is usually the main feature. The child is always systemically unwell with loss of appetite, malaise, and fever. The fluid in the middle ear often results in a conductive hearing loss that is rarely noticed amidst the other features. Otoscopic examination reveals a red and bulging eardrum. If antibiotics are given in the early stages, the infection may well resolve. Often however, the eardrum will burst and the pus will discharge through the perforation and out of the external auditory meatus. This type of perforation usually heals spontaneously but occasionally it may persist as a chronic perforation, leading to another type of chronic suppurative otitis media. Fortunately, other complications of this condition are relatively rare, the most common is an acute mastoiditis occurring when the infection in the mastoid air cells starts to come through the temporal bone and form a subperiosteal abscess over the mastoid process. Other complications include spread of the disease superiorly, leading to meningitis or even brain abscess. Fortunately such complications are uncommon.

   Given that this condition is the consequence of an infective process, antibiotics are the mainstay of treatment, along with appropriate analgesia to relieve pain and fever. This treatment normally leads to a rapid resolution, but if it does not, the physician may opt to perform a myringotomy. According to Shambaugh (1967), a myringotomy should be done if the drum membrane is thickened and bulging. The prefix *myringo-* refers to the tympanic membrane. The suffix *-otomy* refers to the "cutting of." A myringotomy is a relatively minor surgical procedure in which a very tiny incision (2 or 3 mm) is made in the tympanic membrane and the fluid in the middle ear is withdrawn by vacuum. In acute suppurative otitis media, this is done primarily for the relief of the pain produced by the rather considerable intratympanic pressure associated with the disease process and its resultant fluid-based distention of the tympanic membrane. If there are complications, either acute and intracranial, or chronic such as a residual perforation, specialist medical care will be required.

## Acute Serous Otitis Media

This is most commonly seen in adults as barotrauma. The typical story is of an individual flying or diving either during or shortly after an URTI. When the rapid pressure changes associated with these activities occur, the reduced function of the Eustachian tube does not permit those changes to be transmitted to the middle ear. The problem is a reduction in middle ear pressure relative to the outside world, and Eustachian tube "locking" may occur. Should this happen, a rapid pressure differential is created across the tympanic membrane that leads to an acute inflammatory response with the production of a serous transudate, often with associated hemorrhage, into the middle ear cleft. The affected individual typically describes a pressure change followed by severe otalgia and then deafness. The hearing loss is obviously conductive and due to middle ear fluid interfering with sound conduction. Although any pain may settle quickly, often within a few hours, the serous fluid, and consequently the hearing loss, may persist for days or even weeks

Treatment for this condition is largely the use of an expectorant to promote secretion from the mucous membrane and to facilitate its expulsion, allowing the body's natural defenses to gain control. In other words, with the passage of time, the condition usually resolves spontaneously. Unfortunately, this time period is variable and unpredictable. Measures to hasten resolution include the use of topical or systemic decongestants or, if the illness or consequent hearing loss is particularly protracted, a myringotomy and aspiration of fluid can be performed. If the condition continues to recur and is interfering with the patient's lifestyle (e.g., flight attendant, frequent flyer businessperson), it may be wise to place a ventilation tube (grommet) in the tympanic membrane. While the tube is in place and patent, it effectively prevents recurrence of the condition.

## Chronic Serous Otitis Media

Sometimes called otitis media with effusion, OME, chronic mucinous otitis media, or glue ear, this is also primarily a disease of children. If Eustachian tube dysfunction should persist chronically, but without acute superadded (bacterial) infection, then a chronic low grade middle ear inflammatory response will result. This chronic inflammation results in the middle ear cleft filling with a thick, gelatinous inflammatory exudate, comprised of inflammatory proteins, glycoproteins and cellular debris: the "glue" of glue ear. The exact character of the exudate varies among individuals. However, its occurrence is remarkably common, especially in younger children, with figures for prevalence of 40 percent at age 2 and only 1 percent at age 11. Prevalence also varies with the efficiency of Eustachian tube function and thus tends to be much less in the summer months. Generally, the condition tends to be more common in boys, in patients who have cleft palates, and in children with Down syndrome. It is a capricious condition with intermittent resolution and reinfection. In the longer term, however, spontaneous resolution is usually the ultimate outcome (>90 percent). The presence of fluid in the middle ear cleft leads to a conductive hearing loss of variable severity and is responsible for most of the clinical features. Hearing impairment, whether persistent or intermittent, noticed by parents, relatives, teachers, or identified at routine screening, is the presenting symptom in over 80 percent of cases. Learning difficulties and speech delay account for the bulk of the remainder. In an unfortunate minority of these children, the chronic negative middle ear pressure leads to retraction of the tympanic membrane and ultimately the formation of retraction pockets and the development of bone erosion. That process will ultimately lead to chronic suppurative otitis media.

Diagnosis should be based upon pneumatic otoscopy, tympanometry, and audiometry. Further, if a sustained or recurrent problem is diagnosed, in addition to medical and/or surgical treatment, educational intervention should be applied in the form of language stimulation programs or low level amplification.

What constitutes a sustained or recurrent problem? When should the primary health care provider refer the patient with ear disease to an otologist? The answer to this question varies with the condition. The primary medical consideration is eradication of the disease; the secondary goal is restoration of hearing. Clearly, eradication of a disease process that threatens audition is itself a means to restore hearing. Participants at an International Conference on Early Diagnosis of Hearing Loss (Gerber and Mencher, 1978) and the U.S. Joint Committee On Infant Hearing (1994) have both suggested that because middle ear effusion may persist chronically for months or years, resulting in a mild bilateral hearing loss with associated speech, language, educational, and behavioral problems, particular attention should be paid to those children likely to have sustained middle ear effusion. The effusion should be considered a problem and referral to a specialist should follow if it is sustained (more than three months) or is recurrent (over 50 percent of the time for six months).

Management of the problem should be appropriate to the severity of the condition and should always bear in mind the natural history and its tendency towards spontaneous resolution. For many patients, explanation and reassurance are all that is required. In more severe cases, and for those whose hearing is in doubt, a review visit after three months is useful to establish the persistent nature of the patient's condition. Medical treatment has little role to play in this condition although some physicians have used long-term low-dose antibiotics.

Autoinflation of the Eustachian tube using the Otovent device (essentially a balloon on a nasal speculum) has been shown to give useful results (Figure 6-2). Previously this technique was known as Politzerization. It is a simple technique by which air is forced up the Eustachian tube by insufflation through the nose. The purpose of such a procedure is to ventilate the middle ear. In more severe cases, ventilation tubes (grommets) are inserted in the opening created by a myringotomy (a procedure called myringotomy and tubes) and improves hearing and shortens the overall duration of the pathologic condition. The tubes work on the principle that they provide ventilation and pressure normalization in the middle

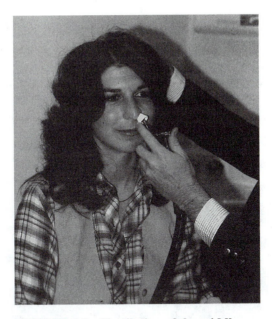

**FIGURE 6-2    Ventilation of the middle ear using politzerization.**

ear (Figure 6-3). This effectively abolishes the inflammatory stimulus and allows resorption of the "glue." Once the middle ear is re-aerated, function and hearing usually return to normal. Unfortunately, grommets remain in situ for an average of nine months, with a typical range of three months to two years (Figure 6-4). Once they extrude (fall out) there is a risk the otitis condition will recur. A sizable proportion of affected children (25 percent) will require subsequent tube insertion. The benefits of ventilation tubes may be augmented by combination with adenoidectomy. The benefits of adenoidectomy are greatest between the ages of four and eight years. Tonsillectomy does not seem to influence the condition.

Grommets require little aftercare. There is no good evidence that swimming with unoccluded ears increases the risk of infection although some form of earplug should be worn when shampooing. The main complications of grommets are infections, granulated tissue forming on the surface of the tympanic membrane, and the development of tympanosclerosis. Infections are treated by aural toilet and antibiotic–steroid eardrops in the first instance, but grommet removal may be required if the infection fails to settle. There is little that can be done to prevent the occurrence of granulomatous tissue or tympanosclerosis, found in 30 to 40 percent of children one year after grommet insertion. It has been noted that the use of minigrommets seems to improve the situation and produces fewer of these complications. Fortunately, apart from its dramatic appearance, tympanosclerosis seems to have little adverse effect on hearing except in rare cases in which there is involvement of the middle ear and ossicles leading to a significant conductive hearing loss.

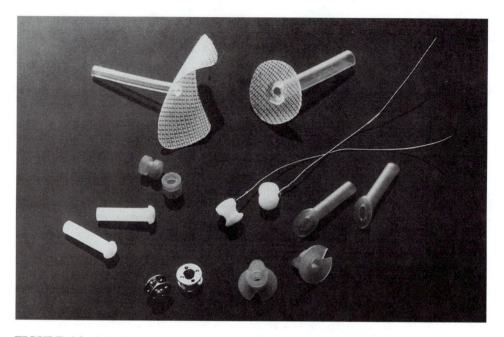

**FIGURE 6-3    Myringotomy grommets. (Courtesy of McGhan Medical Corp.)**

M.P. is a typical school-aged child with this disorder. She was referred for a complete audiological evaluation when she did not respond within normal limits to an audiometric screening at school. She had a history of bilateral otomastoiditis and five months previous an otologist had placed polyethylene tubes in both tympanic membranes. The tubes were still in place, although it could not be confirmed that they were open and patent. M.P.'s father observed that she listened to the television at quite high levels and that she did not seem to hear quiet conversation. Pure tone air and masked bone conduction thresholds revealed a mild, bilateral conductive loss, slightly worse in the right ear at low frequencies. Speech reception thresholds (27 dB on the right and 25 dB on the left) were consistent with the pure tone average, and word discrimination scores were normal bilaterally. Tympanometry was not attempted at the initial visit due to the presence of the tubes. The child was referred back to the otologist for further medical treatment. At the time of the medical visit, tympanometry was employed and the tubes were found to be blocked. The blockage had resulted in continued middle ear complications. New tubes were inserted and the child improved rapidly.

## *Chronic Suppurative Otitis Media*

This condition is almost invariably the legacy of childhood ear disease. It exists in two broad forms, so-called tubotympanic and atticoantral (cholesteatoma) disease. Tubotympanic disease describes a perforation of the tympanic membrane, most commonly toward the inferior part of the eardrum. It is often the residue of previous episodes of acute otitis media in which a perfo-

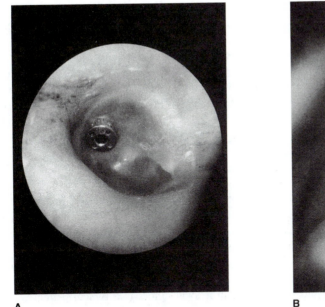
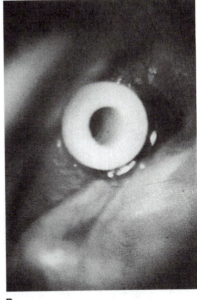

**A**  **B**

**Figure 6-4(*A*, *B*)  View of grommets (commonly called "tubes") in place in a tympanic membrane. (Figure 6-4A courtesy of Dr. Michael Hawke)**

ration fails to heal. Although in many cases the presence of a perforated eardrum may be completely asymptomatic, this is not so for all. In a significant number of cases, the alteration in the normal physiology of the Eustachian tube and middle ear system results in frequent, recurrent ear infections. This can lead to frequent episodes of pain and discharge (suppuration). The loss of any part of the tympanic membrane can lead to a conductive hearing loss, as can erosion of the long process of the incus, which often accompanies the disease. The odoriferous discharge that also often accompanies this pathology is probably the most unpleasant aspect of the condition for the patient and can lead to more social difficulties than the hearing loss. Although not as common as in atticoantral disease, intracranial complications can also occur.

The decision to treat this condition depends on the severity and frequency of symptoms. In many cases, the patient may be completely asymptomatic with a dry perforation of the tympanic membrane and minimal hearing impairment. In these cases, there is a strong argument to leave well enough alone and not to interfere. Although the surgery to repair an isolated perforation is relatively simple, as with any middle ear surgery, the risks of dizziness, facial palsy, and dead ear still exist and must always be borne in mind before any operation. In contrast, in those patients suffering repeated episodes of infection and marked hearing loss, usually the result of erosion of the long process of the incus, the benefits far outweigh the potential risks. In these cases, it is important to first settle any acute infection by the use of oral antibiotics, topical antibiotic-steroid eardrops, and most importantly, regular and thorough aural toilet. The surgical procedures used are called *tympanoplasty*. This term implies surgery of the middle ear to remove disease and subsequently to reconstruct the hearing mechanism. Traditionally there are five types of tympanoplasty described:

Type 1—Repair of a tympanic membrane perforation alone.

Type 2—Repair of a tympanic membrane perforation and the reconstruction of an ossicular chain by devising a strut bridging the malleus handle and stapes.

Type 3—After disease excision, the tympanic remnant is allowed to drape itself directly onto the stapes or its remnant to encourage direct transmission of sound to the oval window.

Type 4—Fenestration cavity (now rarely if ever performed).

Type 5—Stapedectomy.

In tubotympanic disease, the most common procedure is a Type 1 tympanoplasty, although Type 2 is used frequently. Most often the tympanic membrane is patched using a tissue graft harvested from the patient at the time of surgery. In Type 2, the strut is created by using the remnants of the patient's incus and reshaping it to create a bridge between the malleus handle and the stapes remnant. Type 5 or stapedectomy is used under other conditions far more often and is included in the discussion of otosclerosis.

L.R., a 27-year-old female seen in a local clinic, is a typical patient one might encounter. She had a long history of chronic otomastoiditis and had a myringoplasty done when she was ten years old. At the time of her first visit to the local clinic, she presented with a nonhealing perforation on the left side and reported several episodes of draining from the ear. Otologic examination revealed a 30 percent perforation of the left tympanic membrane. The physician recommended tympanoplasty. At surgery, a piece of temporalis fascia was taken for a graft. A tympanomeatal flap was created, the perforation trimmed, and the layers separated. Elevating the annulus revealed normal ossicles, but many middle ear adhesions. The adhesions were dissected free as much as possible, and the fascial graft was placed under the tympanic membrane and the mucosa of the middle ear. L.R. tolerated the surgery well and was discharged from the hospital on the next postoperative day. Pre- and postsurgical audiograms showed that surgery reduced a 25-dB air-bone gap to about 5 dB. Furthermore, the recurrent discharge present before surgical intervention was eliminated.

Atticoantral disease is seen in a significant minority of individuals with glue ear in childhood who develop what is called a retraction pocket, or layered fold of the epithelial lining of the tympanic membrane. If the pocket remains shallow and self-cleansing, allowing the superficial squamous epithelium to migrate laterally, there are relatively few problems. However, if the pocket becomes too deep, there is a failure of normal migration and the pocket fills with the shed superficial keratinized squamous epithelium. Once this has occurred, technically a cholesteatoma has formed. (Strictly speaking these "tumors" have no cholesterol in them and so should really be called keratomas but tradition is not easily overcome and so cholesteatoma as a title persists). Retraction pockets usually develop in the posterosuperior part of the tympanic membrane, hence the atticoantral title.

With the constant shedding of squames, the cholesteatoma slowly enlarges and typically grows into the attic, antrum, and on into the mastoid system. Frequently, there is also spread into the middle ear. Unfortunately, the lining epithelium exhibits a number of interesting properties, the most important of which is its ability to erode bone. This ability is more pronounced when the cholesteatoma is infected, and thus it is bone erosion (with secondary infection) that leads to most of the complications and problems associated with this condition. For the typical patient, the main complaint is hearing loss. This is because the long process of the malleus is usually eroded early in the course of the disease. Recurrent infections may lead to otalgia and the associated and characteristic unpleasant discharge.

The amount of any auditory impairment is related to the size and position of a cholesteatoma and whether it has become secondarily infected. Sometimes a cholesteatoma will conduct sound. Therefore, sometimes audiometry does not accurately reflect the pathology, and the amount of hearing loss accompanying a cholesteatoma may not be a true indicator of the actual damage to the middle ear. If the cholesteatoma does not impede movement of the ossicular chain, there should be no hearing loss. If the ossicles are involved, erosion of the incus is common. As with other conditions interfering with the sound transducing properties of the middle ear conducting mechanism, a cholesteatoma can be expected to produce a flat audiogram with accompanying hearing loss ranging anywhere from 35 to 55 dB. Speech reception threshold is normally congruous with the pure tone audiogram, and given adequate loudness, the speech discrimination scores are usually normal.

Almost without exception, this is a disease requiring surgical treatment. The severity of potential complications demands attention to this condition. Only in the very elderly and infirm with a small and relatively asymptomatic cholesteatoma can conservative treatment be considered. These patients should be kept under regular review and have regular aural toilet to try to remove any keratin debris and to avoid further buildup. Surgical treatment requires complete removal of the cholesteatoma and its sac (Figure 6-5). The operation most

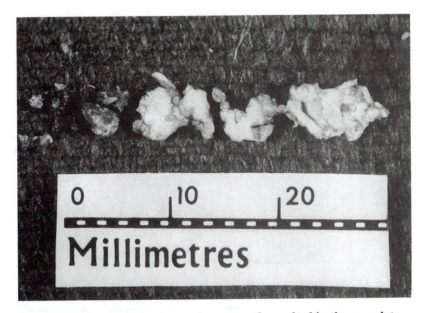

**FIGURE 6-5    Cholesteatoma whose growth resulted in the complete destruction of the middle ear of a teen-aged female.**

often performed has been in existence for many years and is called a *modified radical mas-toidectomy*. The procedure involves drilling out the infected mastoid air cells and the con-tained cholesteatoma, removing the incus and the malleus head, and excising any involved tympanic membrane. A tissue graft is then placed under the tympanic remnant and over the stapes remnant to create a Type 3 tympanoplasty. An essential part of this operation is the widening of the external auditory meatus (meatoplasty) to allow adequate aeration of the newly created cavity. Unfortunately, although this procedure is effective for disease con-trol, even with a perfect Type 3 tympanoplasty, the patient will be left with a significant con-ductive hearing loss. Consequently, other techniques have been developed to try to avoid that complication.

One technique, called the "combined approach" or "canal wall up tympanoplasty" is designed to preserve the anatomy of the ear to as close to normal as possible. Unfortunately, it is really suitable only for small and relatively localized cholesteatomas. Furthermore, the poorer exposure of the cholesteatoma with this technique sometimes results in an incom-plete removal and leads to higher rates of recurrence and multiple subsequent operations.

A long-standing cholesteatoma may result in damage such that hearing cannot be com-pletely restored except by surgical means. In the event surgery is not possible, Shambaugh (1967) reminds us that tympanoplasty is contraindicated if there is no air-bone gap or fails to restore hearing completely (as is often the case with mastoid surgery). Rehabilitative audiol-ogy becomes primary. The hearing loss may be alleviated by amplification, sometimes via a bone conduction hearing aid, and sometimes by more conventional models. Auditory train-ing and speech reading instruction may also be desirable. Continuous monitoring for recur-rence of middle ear pathology is essential.

## Complications of Middle Ear Disease

Throughout this discussion there have been references to complications associated with var-ious middle ear conditions. Generally, these are grouped into two categories:

### Localized Complications

- Erosion of the long process of the incus.
- Erosion into the labyrinth leading to either a perilymph fistula with consequent distur-bance of balance or more seriously suppurative labyrinthitis. A fistula is a connection between two epithelial lined cavities or structures. The presence of a fistula can lead to an internal hollow space subject to infection.
- Mastoiditis.
- Erosion and exposure of the facial nerve. The surrounding infection and inflammatory response may lead to a facial palsy.

### Intracranial Complications

- Erosion superiorly or backwards into the cranial cavity leading to meningitis, enceph-alitis, or intracranial abscess formation. Acute suppurative and chronic tubotympanic otitis media may cause this by direct spread through bone or through a congenital de-hiscence.

Hypothetically, almost any of these complications can occur from any middle ear condition, but in reality, they are almost never found in acute serous or chronic secretory otitis media. Intracranial complications are occasionally seen with both acute suppurative and chronic tubo-tympanic otitis media. Although generally intracranial abscesses are an extremely uncommon complication of ear disease, otologic causes are still their most common etiology, thus middle ear disease, and cholesteatoma in particular, should be taken seriously. In fact, all the complications are most frequently seen with cholesteatoma.

## *Audiological Considerations*

In the early stages of otomastoiditis there may be no measurable hearing loss for pure tones and no accompanying loss of sensitivity for speech, although tympanometry may be abnormal (usually tympanogram types B and C). In other words, the patient may not complain of an inability to hear. Instead, the complaint may center on pain or a sensation of fullness and the underlying illness that has produced the condition. As the disease progresses, of course, there are obvious audiometric signs. As with most conductive hearing impairments, the audiogram is expected to be flat or rising; that is, loss of auditory sensitivity should be about the same for all frequencies or a greater loss for lower frequencies than for higher frequencies.

Audiometric results usually display the most outstanding characteristic of any conductive hearing impairment, one that was discussed in Chapter 3—that is, an air-bone gap. Remember that the difference between an air conduction audiogram and the bone conduction audiogram is called the air-bone gap, and its extent is a measure of conductive hearing impairment. Because otomastoiditis is a condition of the middle ear, and there is no loss of sensitivity at the level of the cochlea, the inner ear is unaffected. Hence, if a signal were delivered directly to the inner ear so that it would bypass the middle ear conductive mechanism, an audiogram taken in this way would be normal. That type of measurement is done, of course, by applying a bone conduction vibrator to the mastoid. As a result, the middle ear conducting mechanism is removed from the test situation and the cochlea is assessed directly. In a patient with otitis media, an audiogram obtained through bone conduction will be normal, illustrating that there is normal cochlear function. If the test is via air conduction, that is, by placing an earphone over the external ear and passing the signal through the affected middle ear cavity, the result will indicate a hearing loss. Usually, in otomastoiditis, because there is normal cochlear reserve, and therefore no loss evident by bone conduction testing, the air-bone gap is identical in size to the loss of sensitivity by air conduction.

Not to complicate matters, but rather to alert the reader to other contingencies, it is important to point out that one can have a conductive hearing loss and a sensorineural loss at the same time. Consequently, in such a *mixed* loss, the audiogram would reflect both a loss in cochlear reserve up to the level of that deficit and an air-bone gap. There is further discussion of this concept later, but what is important here is to recognize that an ear may have several types of pathology simultaneously.

A tympanogram is a measurement of middle ear pressure and the compliance of the eardrum and is interpreted by the location of the peak pressure of the curve (positive, negative, or normal), the amplitude of the curve (high, low, or normal), and the shape of the curve (sloped, rounded, or peaked). Changes in a tympanogram are produced by alterations of the stiffness or the mass of the middle ear transduction system. Most middle ear pathologies have their own peculiar effects upon the tympanogram. For example, Figure 6-6 includes the audiogram and tympanogram of a child with chronic secretory otitis media. The presence of fluid in the middle ear cavity has increased both the mass and the stiffness. The result is a tympanogram showing negative pressures in the ear canal as indicated by the peak of the curves being below zero. Similarly, the amplitude of the tympanogram is reduced. In contrast, Figure 6-7 is from an ear with a cholesteatoma and ossicular destruction. Note how the absence of an intact ossicular chain has reduced the stiffness and mass associated with the tympanic membrane and created a somewhat flaccid drum.

What has been illustrated here are the typical and expected patterns associated with these pathologies. It should be appreciated that individual patients with individual pathologies may display individual variations of the expected patterns. Tympanometry is an essential diagnostic tool, but it should be used with other audiological procedures such as acoustic reflex measurements, speech audiometry, and, of course, with otoscopic examination.

**PURE TONE AUDIOGRAM**

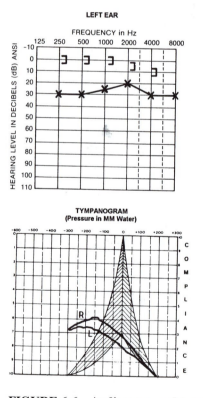

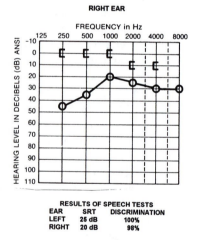

**FIGURE 6-6** **Audiogram and tympanogram of a child with chronic bilateral secretory otitis media.**

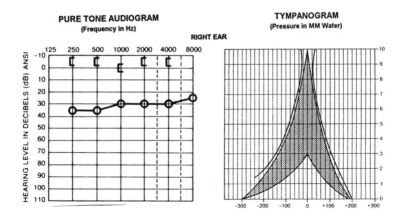

**FIGURE 6-7** **Audiogram and tympanogram of an adult ear with cholesteatoma and ossicular destruction.**

The patient with otitis media will have no difficulty understanding speech if it is sufficiently audible. That is to say, conductive hearing losses result in the same perceptual effect as a loss of loudness. Consequently, the patient with otitis media will display a loss of sensitivity for normal speech (i.e., depressed speech reception threshold) equal to the loss of sensitivity for air conducted tones. Speech discrimination scores will be close to 100 percent because they are measured at an intensity well above the speech reception threshold. The patient will have no difficulty understanding speech if it is of sufficient intensity to overcome any loss of hearing by air conduction.

## Comment

There is some evidence that most children outgrow these types of middle ear infections when their facial–skull structure elongates with age. Elongation of the face is accompanied by a downward slope of the Eustachian tube, which seems to facilitate drainage and reduce infections. Thus, there are far more of these infections seen in two- to five-year-olds than in five- to eight-year-olds. Nevertheless, outgrowing it later on in life does not negate the deleterious effects associated with the disease in the younger child. There are reports that indicate that children with chronic or recurrent ear disease appear to have somewhat lower IQs than matched controls as measured by standard tests (Howie, 1978). That is not to say that ear disease itself lowers one's intelligence. What it suggests is that frequent or chronic ear disease may deprive a developing child of information essential for successful learning and for the development of normal spoken language. It appears from the work of both Howie (1978) and Kramer (1978) that early and repeated ear disease may constitute the basis of a child's later behavioral and educational problems. Simply stated, a persistent hearing impairment may interfere with a child's ability to learn, due perhaps only to an inability to attend and to know what is going on all the time (Downs, 1978). Battin (1979) has cautioned that mild conductive problems may constitute "additive stress factors" for children otherwise at risk. The same conductive problem in a non-risk child will not result in behavioral and educational problems. Hence, recurrent otomastoiditis could be the source of the problem for some children. Potsic (1978) has noted motor and affective changes in children with chronic otomastoiditis. Downs (1984) has proposed the fitting of very low-powered hearing aids for children with mild, conductive, long-standing hearing losses. It remains, of course, a debatable approach to management, but one that certainly merits serious consideration in view of the potentially marked educational implications for the very young child.

The early detection of all forms of otomastoiditis is essential. There are many individuals and groups (nurses, office personnel, industrial technicians, service clubs, volunteers, etc.) ready to do screening. Unfortunately, the failure to apply rigid test standards and protocols often renders their efforts ineffective. The establishment and maintenance of adequate standards for detection and the development of new procedures and instrumentation for testing are imperative. The process must be improved and monitored so that screening can be done more often, more effectively, and less expensively. Audiologists must assume the major responsibility as the advocates, designers, and supervisors of audiometric screening programs at all levels from infancy to industry.

# Chapter 7

# *Bony Abnormalities of the Middle Ear*

Among other things, hearing depends upon the normal mechanical properties of the middle ear system. The middle ear is an impedance matching device allowing a reasonable amount of sound energy to be passed from the air to the cochlear fluids. This results from two mechanical factors, the lever ratio and the areal ratio.

The lever ratio is a mechanical advantage resulting from movement of the ossicular chain (Figure 7-1). The ossicular chain is not a piston; it does not go in a straight line from the tympanic membrane to the oval window. Rather, it rises into the attic of the middle ear and falls again across the relatively massive incus, thereby providing considerable increase of force at the incudostapedial joint. This increase of force is the lever ratio of the middle ear system. The area of the tympanic membrane is substantially larger than the area of the oval window. Consequently, the effect of the larger membrane acting upon a small membrane is that of an amplifier; that is called the areal ratio. It has been estimated that the ratio between the two areas ranges in different individuals from $14:1$ to $21:1$, the average at about $18:1$ (Bluestone,1991). No matter what the exact ratio, however, the effect is the same—that is, increasing the force of the signal at the oval window and facilitating movement of fluids into the cochlea.

Middle ear bony abnormalities interfere with that process. They do so by destroying the function of the ossicular chain, but that can be achieved by one of two opposite effects. First, they can result in insufficient bone structure or an inappropriate bone relationship within the ossicular chain itself. Second, they can result in too much bone or increased mass of the ossicular chain. Whether the problem is too much or too little bone, or a disrupted structural relationship, the ultimate effect is the same. That is, the lever and areal ratios are disturbed and middle ear mechanical function is interrupted.

Middle ear bony abnormalities may be of two distinct etiological types: (1) congenital malformations or (2) the result of a disease process. Although each is distinct from the other, congenital malformations may be considered as a group primarily because their medical-otologic and auditory considerations are so similar. Abnormalities resulting from

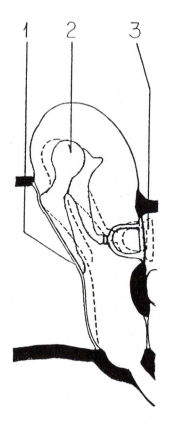

**FIGURE 7-1.    The lever action of the ossicular chain.** Note how the tympanic membrane is pulled into the middle ear space, forcing the head of the malleus to draw back, thus changing the angle of the incus and affecting the stapes. Note also how the footplate of the stapes moves in a rocking pattern in response to sound stimuli. The picture also illustrates the areal and lever ratios. The areal ratio is produced by the fact that (1) the area of the tympanic membrane is much greater than the area of the oval window membrane, while the lever ratio is created by the rising of the ossicular lever (2) and then (3) its fall.

disease processes, including ossicular erosion and ossicular fixation associated with tympanosclerosis as discussed earlier, may also be considered as a cluster. However, one disorder, otosclerosis, is so common and so typical in its patterns that it offers a clear example of the effects and treatment of all forms of bony middle ear disorders. For that reason, it has been singled out for detailed discussion below.

## Congenital Malformations of the Middle Ear

### Pathology and Etiology

There are well over fifty different syndromes associated with middle ear bony anomaly. There is no single etiology. The malformation may be genetic in origin, due to prenatal disease, the result of a toxin, the product of a developmental interruption related to a regional defect, or simply a slight variant on a normal theme. The various conditions described in Chapter 5 (Anomalies of the External Ear) may be expected to have concomitant middle ear anomalies. Embryologic development is such that anomalies of the external ear should cause the diagnostician to look for and expect anomalies of at least part of the middle ear as well. The pinna need not be severely anomalous in that respect. If a pinna is too low, or is in the wrong position, or is at the wrong angle, or if the two pinnae do not match perfectly, then there is reason to suspect a middle ear anomaly. Jaffe (1978) reported large numbers of surgically confirmed middle ear anomalies in which the first sign was the unusual position or appearance of the auricles. What form may an anomaly take? One possibility is a simple malformation of the malleus or incus as seen in Figure 7-2. Another is a fusion of the two into one large ossicle rather than two. In such a case, of course, the advantage of the lever ratio that normally accrues from the joint action of the malleus and the incus is diminished or lost. In extreme cases, the middle ear cavity is absent or even may be slitlike (Nager, 1973). Most often, however, middle ear anomalies are limited to malformed or fused ossicles.

If the middle ear is anomalous, surgical intervention is usually preferred. At one extreme would be a situation in which the middle ear cavity is absent and the solution is a complete middle ear construction or, in a severe dysplasia, use of a bone conduction hearing aid. At the opposite extreme would be an ear with moderately malformed ossicles that can

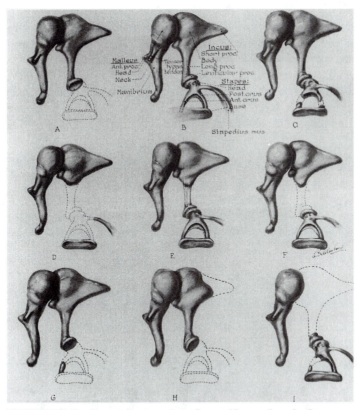

**FIGURE 7-2    Several examples of a malformed ossicular chain. There are many other variations possible, and examples A-I should be considered only illustrative. (From Papparella and Schachern, *Otolaryngology*, p. 1402, third edition. Courtesy of W.B. Saunders)**

be removed, reshaped, and replaced. This is called an autograft, or literally, to use the same tissue. Between these extremes lies a broad range of combinations of anomalous or fused ossicles and just as many solutions. For example, another alternative is replacement of the ossicles with ossicular homografts. In such cases, ossicles are removed from a cadaver and preserved for that purpose. The subject of tympanic homografts has been described in considerable detail by Perkins (1975). Admittedly, there is something more surgically aesthetic, and perhaps psychologically preferable, about the use of an autograft over a homograft, but it is not necessarily preferable acoustically.

Sometimes, an artificial prosthesis is a better choice. Such a device may be a piston attached at one end to the tympanic membrane and at the other end to the neck of the stapes; or a piston that attaches the tympanic membrane directly to the oval window; or a simple strut. Examples of these are shown in Figure 7-3. Prostheses usually restore hearing to as full an extent as do homografts or autografts.

## Audiological Considerations

If the middle ear system is not intact, the normal mechanical advantages of the ossicular chain obviously are not obtained. The associated hearing loss may be as high as 55 dB by air conduction. Bone conduction testing will usually reveal that a normal cochlea is present, and a significant air-bone gap will be present. Results of speech testing will be similar to that seen in patients with middle ear disease. That is, if the sound is loud enough, the patient will understand virtually 100 percent of what is presented. Once again, because the middle ear serves as a transducer and mechanical amplifier, bypassing it will reflect normal cochlear reserve.

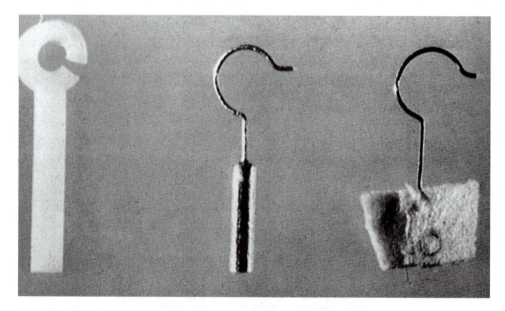

**FIGURE 7-3    Various prosthetic devices used in ossicular chain reconstructive surgery.**

Occasionally, a patient will be seen for audiological assessment who previously had normal hearing, but having suffered a blow to the head or trauma to the mastoid or temporal bone, has suddenly lost hearing. Tympanometry may reveal an extremely flaccid drum membrane. An air-bone gap of 50 dB or more may be present, and otoscopically the ear may look normal. If the test is presented at a comfortable loudness level, the problem may be compounded further by an elevated speech reception threshold but normal speech discrimination. A disarticulation of the ossicular chain—a break in the physical continuity of the ossicles—may be responsible. The total audiometric picture, except the case history, may be the same as that seen in a patient with a bony malformation of the middle ear. The audiogram will not provide sufficient information to make an audiological diagnostic judgment between the two possible diagnoses. However, tympanometry will provide information that the normal stiffness of the middle ear is markedly reduced, thus providing a clue to the etiology of the disorder.

Sometimes surgery is not the treatment of choice for a congenital malformation, or, because these types of anomalies are congenital, surgery may be postponed until head growth has nearly reached maximum. In such a case, just as in bone conduction audiometric testing, the middle ear can be bypassed and the cochlea stimulated directly by applying a vibratory-type hearing aid to the mastoid. Such a solution is called simply a bone-conduction hearing aid. The procedure may be satisfactory, but it is certainly less than perfect. Held on by a headband that is easily stretched, the vibrator may become so loosely held to the head that its effectiveness is diminished. Cosmetically, this type of hearing aid is marginally successful. The headband may disturb the hair or make the user self-conscious. The recent introduction of bone-anchored hearing aids is a much more satisfactory option (Figure 7-4). The quality of sound produced is much clearer, and they do not require a cumbersome and uncomfortable headband, and so they are much less externally intrusive. Their use does involve a surgical procedure to implant, and all which that implies, but it is a reasonably nonthreatening procedure, and the results have been reported to be excellent. Alternatively, a regular air conduction hearing aid may be a better choice, even though, for some of the reasons cited earlier, a bone conduction hearing aid may offer greater amplification. It is important that these issues be discussed thoroughly with the patient.

# Otosclerosis

## Pathology and Etiology

Otosclerosis literally means "hard ears." Simply, *oto-* refers to an ear while *sclerosis* is a hardening (e.g., arteriosclerosis: hardening of the arteries). The term otospongiosis has also been used to describe this disease (Goin, 1976). First described by Valsalva in 1735, otosclerosis is characterized by a growth of new bone, most often developing anterior to the oval window (Lindsay, 1973). Typically, the lesion is manifested by an irregular growth of new bone that is interspersed with many vascular spaces. It sometimes replaces the dense bone of the labyrinth. When it is active and growing, the new bone is spongy and loose (thus the term otospongiosis). When the growth stops, the new bone appears as a dense, mature, recalcified focus whose margins tend to be rather sharply defined. Initially, it is usually (but

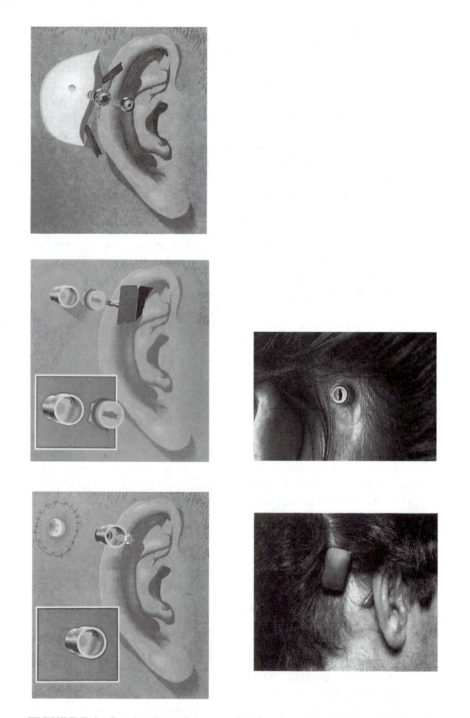

**FIGURE 7-4    Implanting a bone conduction hearing aid. (Reprinted with permission of Nobelpharma, manufacturers of the implanting device)**

by no means always) confined to the place where the anterior crus of the stapes attaches to the footplate and grows around the annular ligament of the stapes and oval window. If the disease progresses, it incorporates more and more of the stapes, inhibiting its movement. Sometimes the new bone also grows medial to the window, reaching into the cochlear vestibule. This leads to a condition that has sometimes been described as "inner ear conductive impairment" (Derlacki, 1976) or cochlear otosclerosis. This far more debilitating form of otosclerosis may be complicated by other symptoms, primarily vertigo and nausea.

A disease more prevalent in white women than in any other group, it has been estimated to occur in one of every five to ten (Goin, 1976). It occurs half as often in white males as in white females, but it occurs in only one in a hundred black people, and virtually not at all in other races. Fortunately, the effects of the disease are quite minor in most patients. Only about 10 percent of persons with histologic otosclerosis complain of hearing impairment; nevertheless, otosclerosis is the single most common cause of serious hearing loss in young adulthood.

Otosclerosis is a hereditary, degenerative disease apparently produced by an autosomal dominant gene with variable penetrance (Konigsmark, 1972). Because it is genetic and not congenital, it is an example of those kinds of diseases called familial degenerative or latent onset. Because otosclerosis is dominantly inherited—hence, it runs in families—and, because it occurs more frequently in women than in men, the probability of the disease appearing in the daughter of a woman who has had it is fairly high. A logical question often heard, then, is, "If it is not a sex-linked trait, how does it happen that the disease occurs more frequently in females than males?" The question is properly raised. The answer seems that, although the disease may be present in equal numbers in both sexes, it is aggravated and activated by certain metabolic and chemical changes that accompany pregnancy and menstruation. The disease rarely manifests itself before the third decade of life (although it has occasionally been reported in children), and it is in that decade (20 to 30 years of age) that most women bear children and undergo the associated biochemical changes. No special mechanism for this change has been isolated.

The patient will invariably present with a conductive hearing loss. Tinnitus is commonly associated, and as indicated earlier, there are patients who may also complain of vertigo and nausea. In about 10 percent of cases, otoscopic examination will reveal that the tympanic membrane exhibits a pinkish or rosy tint or even a reddish hue. This is called the Schwartze sign and reflects the increased blood supply of active new bone formation from dilated blood vessels in the mucosa of the promontory. It is one of the positive diagnostic indicators of otosclerosis. Thus, the audiologist or other clinician examining an ear with an otoscope before a hearing test should be alert to such a sign. Another physical sign is a bluish color to the sclera or covering of the eye. This is not seen in all cases, but should be recognized as unusual when present.

After determination that the hearing difficulty is the result of otosclerosis by various techniques, including audiometric and medical procedures, the physician is faced with either surgical or nonsurgical management. That decision is directly related to the extent of the patient's complaints and symptoms. The decision must always be made by balancing the potential benefit against the potential risk. While surgery can be very successful, as described below, it carries with it a real risk of producing a dead ear or a perilymphatic fistula. These will make the patient either deaf or dizzy, respectively. Consequently, if the hearing loss is mild or if the patient is elderly or infirm, medical treatment to attempt to reduce further growth and the recommendation of a hearing aid, rather than a surgical procedure to remove the disease process, might well be the best management option.

## *Medical and Surgical Management*

Medical (nonsurgical) treatment of otosclerosis has been attempted, but success has been minimal. Shambaugh and Causse (1974) treated their patients with large doses of sodium fluoride. The idea was to harden the bone, much as sodium fluoride hardens teeth. Just as softer teeth are more susceptible to cavity growth, softer bone continues to grow. By hardening the bone, theoretically, the growth would be restricted. Unfortunately, most of Shambaugh's patients showed no change, although one displayed a return to normal on radiologic examination. There are still many physicians today who use sodium fluoride treatments with their otosclerotic patients as a prophylactic measure.

Fortunately, otosclerosis does present one of the most dramatic and appealing examples of successful surgical intervention in terms of restoration of normal hearing. Historically, there have been three surgeries employed to correct the disease. These are called fenestration, stapedolysis, and stapedectomy. Only one, the stapedectomy, is truly successful and used extensively today. However, a review of the development of all three procedures provides an interesting insight into the treatment of conductive hearing loss. Further, an audiologist may occasionally encounter a patient who has undergone one of the earlier surgeries, and the clinician must be aware of what has happened to that patient and what to expect.

### *Fenestration*

Fenestration was developed by Lempert (1938). While conceptually a simple procedure, surgically it is not. The idea of the operation is that since the oval window is obliterated by bony growth, a new window (fenestra) needs to be made. Usually this window is drilled into the lateral semicircular canal at the level of the promontory. A successful fenestration operation cannot lead to a complete restoration of normal hearing. When the surgery is complete, there is a new window, but it is located in the vestibular region of the cochlea, and the ossicles are missing. The tympanic membrane has its medial attachment at the promontory between the oval and round windows, and the new oval window is exposed to outside air. As a result, fenestration fails more often than it succeeds, and thus is rarely done today.

### *Stapedolysis*

Stapedolysis, the second of the surgical procedures came about in 1953, when Rosen rediscovered a procedure called stapes mobilization or stapedolysis. That procedure had been done first by Kessel in 1878, but had fallen into disuse. As with the fenestration, the idea of the surgery is quite simple: if the stapes is stuck, free it. The procedure involves raising the tympanic membrane, exposing the contents of the middle ear, attaching a hook-like instrument to a crus of the stapes, and by jerking it, freeing the footplate from the otosclerotic growth. Frequently, the results of this procedure can be quite dramatic with the patient on the operating table suddenly hearing. Rosen's rediscovery of stapedolysis reestablished otology as a surgical specialty. However, it was eventually determined that the long-term effects of stapedolysis were not successful. The disease that captured the stapes in the first place, and that was not removed by the surgical procedure, continued. As a result, far too many stapes became involved a second time and had to be operated on again.

### *Stapedectomy*

Stapedectomy was the next logical step in the evolution of a satisfactory surgical approach to otosclerosis. An *-ectomy* is a removal. Stapedectomy, then, means to remove the stapes. In contrast to tonsillectomy or appendectomy, however, in which something is removed without replacement, a stapedectomy includes the replacement of the stapes with some kind of prosthesis. Although a homograft has been used, a typical prosthetic device is not a simulation or a copy of the normal stapes. It is usually a simple wire crimped around the lenticular process of the incus and inserted into the oval window. The point inserted into the oval window is packed with a material (e.g., Gelfoam) that retains it in place while normal tissue growth occurs. Eventually, the packing is absorbed into the surrounding mucosa. There is a 97 to 99 percent success rate for this procedure in expert hands (Meyerhoff and Papparella, 1991). A failure rate of only three percent for stapedectomy is excellent, especially when compared to the much larger percentages of failures associated with the stapedolysis and fenestration procedures.

On rare occasions, otosclerosis recurs in the same ear. Thus, most surgeons will operate on only one ear at a time, the poorer one, as they are unwilling to assume even the 3 percent risk of failure and the consequent deafness suffered by the patient. If the operated ear is successful, and it will be most of the time, some patients will request that the other ear be operated on as well. Although two ears are not necessary for normal hearing in the customary acoustic environment to which we are all exposed, a unilateral hearing loss, however moderate, is a nuisance, and for some it is a disability. Thus, the successful stapedectomy patient may often have the second ear done.

The procedure has been enhanced by several other recent developments. One of the most important has been the development of the operating microscope that permits accurate otic microsurgery with great success. In addition, improvements in pharmaceuticals, as well as development of new drugs, have significantly diminished the incidence of postoperative infection. Amoxicillin is the most commonly used prophylactic antibiotic and has been most successful against the threat of labyrinthitis. Nevertheless, there are instances of post-stapedectomy sequelae leading to an inner ear infection (endolabyrinthitis), eventually leading to destruction of the cochlear end organ and a resultant dead ear. Fortunately, that situation is extremely rare. More often, but still rarely, the otosclerotic growth continues and the neoplastic bone eventually captures the prosthesis. In such a situation, many surgeons would prefer not to attempt to operate a second time, either on the same ear or on the other ear. For these types of patients, amplification usually offers an adequate solution.

The value of stapedectomy cannot be overstated. Remember that otosclerosis is a disease that affects vast numbers of people. About 97 percent of those people can have their hearing restored to normal by a rather simple surgical procedure using a local anesthetic and requiring only one or two night's sleep in a hospital. Consequently, literally hundreds of stapedectomies are performed daily. Hence, although otosclerosis is a very common disease, its resultant hearing loss is rather easily corrected and with dramatic effects. The development of both the stapedectomy procedure and the simple prosthesis to restore hearing has combined to form a major landmark in otological science and is one of the great achievements of the surgeon's art.

## *Audiological Management*

As with other diseases and disorders primarily involving the middle ear, the impairment that accompanies otosclerosis is conductive in nature, and therefore, not likely to exceed 50 to 55 dB. That is to say, no one will become deaf from this disease. The exception occurs when advanced otosclerosis reaches into the cochlear vestibule causing a sensorineural hearing loss and produces a hearing loss as great as 90 dB or more. That is quite rare.

Otosclerosis has a characteristic audiometric pattern. Generally, in early otosclerosis, there will be a normal bone conduction audiogram and a mild hearing loss by air conduction, limited primarily to the lower frequencies. In other words, the loss appears the same as all other conductive losses and tends to have a rising audiometric contour. As the disease progresses, the hearing loss for the higher frequencies becomes as great as the hearing loss at lower frequencies and the contour of the air conduction audiogram will become flatter. Furthermore, the air-bone gap increases at *most* frequencies. However, there is an audiometric peculiarity to otosclerosis that sets it apart from other conductive hearing disorders. In most otosclerotic patients, the air-bone gap is diminished at 2000 Hz. That is, there is a "notch" or apparent sensorineural hearing loss reflected in the bone conduction audiogram at 2000 Hz (Carhart, 1950). This pattern, the closing of the air-bone gap at 2000 Hz, is called Carhart's notch. It rarely occurs at frequencies other than 2000 Hz and is common and specifically diagnostic of otosclerosis (Figure 7-5). It is important that Carhart's notch not be confused with notches occurring in the audiogram for other reasons (e.g., acoustic trauma). Carhart's notch is limited to the bone conduction audiogram; it does not appear in the air conduction audiogram.

Tympanometry is quite helpful in diagnosing this disease. Otosclerosis may be the best example of increased resistance due to increases of stiffness. Clearly, if the movement of the stapes is limited, then the entire ossicular chain is restricted in its range of motion. Hence, otosclerosis produces a characteristic tympanogram with decreased amplitude and a flattened slope as can also be seen in Figure 7-5.

Results of speech audiometric tests vary with the stage of the disease and the exact site of the conductive mechanism involved. A patient with an early, uncomplicated otosclerosis will generally display an elevated speech reception threshold in direct accord with the pure tone audiogram. Speech discrimination will be excellent, usually normal, if the signal is presented at a comfortable loudness level.

Patients with an advanced otosclerosis that has entered the cochlear vestibule do not fare so well. The audiogram reflects a decreased air-bone gap and an increasing sensorineural hearing loss as more and more of the cochlear structures are affected by the disease. The results of speech reception threshold tests and speech discrimination testing will mirror a corresponding difference in understanding. As long as it is only the conductive mechanism that is involved, speech tests are affected only by loudness changes. When there is a concurrent cochlear involvement, the value of loudness in increasing understanding is markedly decreased. In severe cases, speech discrimination scores may drop significantly below normal, reaching below 50 percent.

Perhaps otosclerosis is best understood when all the elements are together and described in a single case study. D.M., a 34-year-old male, had noticed some difficulty in hearing, a difficulty that had progressed over two years. He is a teacher and reported having trouble hearing in class. While he reported no history of ear disease or hearing loss, he stated

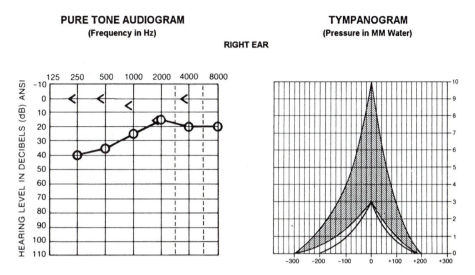

**PURE TONE AUDIOGRAM**
(Frequency in Hz)

RIGHT EAR

**TYMPANOGRAM**
(Pressure in MM Water)

**FIGURE 7-5    Typical audiogram and tympanogram from otosclerosis. Note Carhart's notch at 2000 Hz. The tympanogram shows a reduced mobility of the middle ear structures, as would be expected when the stapes in encased in otosclerotic growth.**

that his mother had a severe hearing impairment of unknown origin. Otoscopic findings revealed normal tympanic membranes bilaterally, although a slight reddish hue resembling Schwarze's sign was noted. A Rinne tuning fork test by the physician indicated a mild conductive loss. Pure tone audiometry confirmed an air-bone gap with an average loss of 35 dB in the right ear and somewhat more than 25 dB in the left. The contour of the bone conduction audiogram dropped bilaterally in the region of 2000 Hz, suggesting Carhart's notch. There was a Type C tympanogram. The speech reception threshold was consistent with the audiogram, and speech discrimination was normal. The family history, otoscopic signs, and the audiometric data suggested a diagnosis of otosclerosis. DM was initially observed for signs of hearing loss progression before surgical intervention was attempted. When progression was confirmed, it was decided to proceed with surgery. A stapedectomy was performed and a wire prosthesis placed. The patient tolerated the procedure well and has recovered. He has had no further difficulty and has returned to teaching.

## Comment

There are other pathologies affecting the middle ear that imitate otosclerosis. One, syphilis, is called "the great imitator." In its early stages it produces audiometric effects that can be confused with those of otosclerosis. Another disease with a similar pattern is osteogenesis imperfecta. Although its external signs are usually obvious, it also results in audiograms similar to those of otosclerosis. In addition, the blue sclera occasionally seen in otosclerosis may also appear in osteogenesis imperfecta.

The audiologist's role in otosclerosis is quite important for diagnosis. The combined audiogram, tympanogram, case history, and physical signs seen in the clinic are quite definitive. The audiologist may be the first person to see the patient and must respond accordingly and properly. This is clearly a medical and surgical problem initially and referral to the otologist is essential. A presurgical audiogram to help in the diagnosis and to establish a baseline of hearing, and a postsurgical audiogram to confirm the success of the operation, are important aspects of audiological care and management. If the patient has a problem that is inoperable or the surgery fails, the audiologist must assume the primary auditory rehabilitative responsibility for amplification, training, and counseling. At one time, the most successful hearing aid fittings were those done on otosclerotic patients. Today, those cases receive surgery and hearing aids are fit on only the more difficult ears. That means the success rate for hearing aid fittings is less than before and the effort far more challenging.

# Chapter 8

# Congenital Hearing Impairment

The word "congenital" means present at birth. It does not signify any particular cause, meaning only that the patient was born with the disorder. The term "genetic" refers to those disorders, whether or not congenital, carried by the genes. Since nearly half of all congenital hearing impairments are genetic, and the balance are not, it is easy for there to be confusion. Fraser (1976) summarized the problem succinctly when he said:

> *It is a paradox that underlies the distinction between congenital and genetically determined disease that genetic types of childhood deafness may frequently not be congenital, whereas acquired types due to causes acting in the prenatal period may often be truly congenital. This is one reason why diagnostic confusion may occur between these two types of deafness, in that congenital hearing losses that are acquired in fetal life due to infection or other cause may be falsely attributed to genetic determination.*

There is a certain amount of difficulty in addressing an issue as ultimately complex as congenital deafness. Consideration must be given, for example, to how great a loss is required for it to be considered "deafness." If discussion is limited to that small portion of the hearing-impaired population that suffers from a truly profound (by anyone's definition) hearing loss at birth, then the best available statistics indicate that about one child among 1000 born in the United States or Canada today will be in that category (Mencher, 1976). Roughly the same proportion is evident in other Western countries, although Barr (1965) reported only one profoundly hearing-impaired child in 2000 births in Sweden. In other parts of the world, the incidence is substantially greater. In the Middle East, for example, it is about double the incidence rate in the United States (Feinmesser and Tell, 1976), while in some parts of Latin America it is even greater (WHO, 1967).

When attempting to determine the incidence of congenital deafness, the problem is knowing that the impairment was, in fact, present at birth. There are at least two very good reasons why this is a problem. First, most children who are born in hospitals are not screened for hearing loss until they are nine to twelve months of age or even older. This is a particular tragedy since accurate screening methods do exist, and they are not being used. As a result, and aside from the educational and moral issues of not screening in the nursery, no one knows which children have hearing impairment at birth. Second, large numbers of children are not born in hospitals. In the United States today only about 75 percent of births occur in hospitals. It has been suggested by Gerber (1977) that the incidence of birth defects, including hearing impairment, is likely to be greater in the unexamined 25 percent than in the 75 percent available for an examination. This is because the nonhospital population is likely to have a larger proportion of children born in remote areas, or born to families of poverty or considerable ignorance to whom the kinds of medical and hospital services that the middle class is accustomed to either are not available or are not utilized.

In summary, if there is to be universal agreement as to what "profound" hearing loss means and how many cases there are in any given community, there needs to be a clear definition of the term. Furthermore, there needs to be a comprehensive analysis of the incidence of hearing loss at birth. Because neither of these is a reality, a clear and accurate reporting of the incidence of congenital deafness is a very difficult thing to do. However, the 1994 recommendations of NIH may improve the situation.

## Etiology and Pathology

The etiology of congenital deafness may be considered in terms of two main categories: genetic and nongenetic. Some forms of genetic deafness have associated abnormalities; most do not (Konigsmark, 1971). Those deafnesses that are nongenetic in origin may be due to infection, trauma, maldevelopment, and metabolic or toxic disorders.

### Congenital Genetic Deafness

About half of all cases of congenital deafness are inherited (Fraser, 1971; Mencher and Mencher, 1995). The form of genetic inheritance or what are called the forms of transmission may be autosomal recessive, autosomal dominant, or x-linked recessive.

#### Autosomal Recessive

Autosomal recessive genes are the basis of the vast majority (approximately two-thirds) of the cases of congenital deafness. According to Carrel (1977), there are at least five abnormal genes in each person that do not appear as distinct entities. When one of these genes is on a nonsex chromosome (i.e., autosomal) and is matched with another autosomal recessive abnormal gene mate, the risk for producing a deaf child is one in four. Since the risk is but one in four, there are three chances in four that a normal hearing child would be produced by such a mating. Figure 8-1 displays a typical pedigree for recessive deafness. If no hearing-impaired child has been produced for several generations, it is likely that the carrier of such a gene structure would be unaware of the potential of its presence. Consequently, there are many cases in which normally hearing parents produce a hearing-impaired child and honestly deny knowledge of any family history of deafness. Furthermore, if the baby was a first child, it would not have been automatically considered at risk. Therefore, the child would

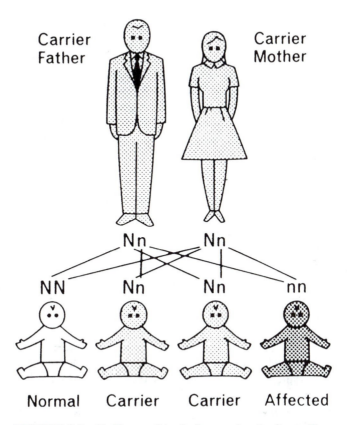

Carrier Father

Carrier Mother

Nn          Nn

NN      Nn      Nn      nn

Normal    Carrier    Carrier    Affected

**FIGURE 8-1    Pedigree of typical recessive deafness. For
each baby born to a recessive gene mating, there is a 50
percent probability of being a carrier of the gene, a 25
percent probability of not carrying it, and a 25 percent
chance of actually expressing the disorder. Each baby
should be considered separately, and the presence or
absence of these factors in other children resulting from
the mating has no effect on other progency. (Courtesy of
Pro-Ed, Inc., from Krajicek and Tearney, 1977)**

most likely not have been evaluated by a neonatal hearing screening program that was based
solely on the high risk register.

Bergstrom (1984) studied 427 patients who were hearing impaired at a very early age.
She found that somewhat more than 40 percent of the patients could ascribe their hearing
impairments to heredity, while slightly more than 31 percent related causation to factors
other than those that are inherited. Furthermore, and perhaps most interestingly, Bergstrom
found that 28 percent of the patients did not know the cause of their hearing losses. It is
probable that many among that 28 percent whose etiology was unknown were the first born

to normal-hearing parents who were carrying matched autosomal recessive genes. Konigsmark (1971) estimated that this phenomenon could account for as many as 35 percent of those who are congenitally deaf. If such a set of parents had the same autosomal recessive genes, rather than any other one of the available five or ten, then their risk for producing deaf children would be 100 percent (Carrel, 1977). Such a family is one in which a normal-hearing couple has produced three severely hearing-impaired children. There is no evidence that anything could have occurred within that family except for consanguinity or that "throw of the dice" that results in a matching of the same autosomal recessive genes for deafness.

### Autosomal Dominant

Autosomal dominant gene matings are normally at greater risk for producing an affected offspring than autosomal recessive gene matings. In dominantly inherited deafness, the genetic programming from only one parent is sufficient to produce the disorder. The risk of having a hearing-impaired child due to an autosomal dominant condition is 50 percent. In other words, if one parent carries the gene, each child has a 50 percent risk of being hearing-impaired. If both parents carry the same autosomal dominant disorder, the risk is 75 percent.

In some autosomal dominant conditions, the hearing disorder may not manifest itself, even though the child may receive the abnormal gene. An excellent example of such a variable expression is the Waardenburg syndrome (see below). Some people born with Waardenburg syndrome lack hearing impairment, some have a moderate hearing impairment, and some have a unilateral hearing impairment. Yet, all the people in each group carry the gene for the syndrome. Figure 8-2 displays a typical pedigree for dominant deafness.

### X-linked Recessive

X-linked recessive gene matings are not a frequent causative factor for hearing loss. In only slightly more than 3 percent of the cases of congenital deafness is this form of inheritance identified. That means that the gene locus that determines the condition is on the X chromosome, a sex chromosome. Females have two X chromosomes and males have one X and one Y. Because the male has only one X chromosome, if he carries the deafness gene on that chromosome, it is necessary for him to mate with a female who also carries the gene on only one of her two X chromosomes in order for them to produce an affected child. In such a case, there is a 50 percent chance of producing a son with a hearing loss or a daughter who will be a carrier of the trait, but without a hearing loss herself. Transmission is always from mother to son as shown in Figure 8-3. The mother does not have the hearing loss, the son does. When the son has children, his daughters may be carriers and their sons may have hearing losses, and so on. The pattern is quite similar to hemophilia.

## Forms of Pathology

All modes of transmission produce deafness with or without associated abnormalities of the outer, middle, and/or inner ears. Most often they do not. Anomalies associated with pathologies of the external and middle ear have already been discussed in Chapters 4 and 5, and need not be reviewed here. Nevertheless, they could quite properly fit into this discussion as well. Inner ear anomalies are generally rare, but occur often enough that they deserve men-

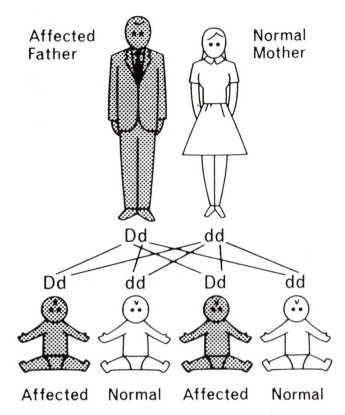

**Affected Father**

**Normal Mother**

Dd     dd

Dd     dd     Dd     dd

Affected   Normal   Affected   Normal

**FIGURE 8-2   Pedigree of a typical dominant deafness, where one parent does not carry the gene. For each baby born to such a dominant gene mating, there is a 50 percent probability of being affected and an equal probability of being normal. Should both parents be carriers of the dominant gene, probability of expression of the phenotype increases dramatically. (Courtesy of Pro-Ed, Inc., from Krajicek and Tearney, 1977)**

tion. The most extreme and rare form of an inner ear anomaly is called Michel anomaly. In such a case, there is no inner ear, and, in some cases, the entire auditory nerve may be absent. The disorder occurs in only about 1 percent of the profoundly deaf population. By contrast, according to Bergstrom (1984), about 70 percent of the congenital inner ear anomalies are of the Scheibe type. These usually are seen with an intact bony labyrinth, but with the loss of some of the vestibular and metabolic organs of the inner ear lost, and atrophy of the organ of Corti. The third major inner ear anomaly is called the Mondini anomaly. In the Mondini anomaly, the tissue of the cochlear duct and its contents is altered. For example, the first 1.5 turns of the cochlea may be normal, and the remaining turn absent or markedly mal-

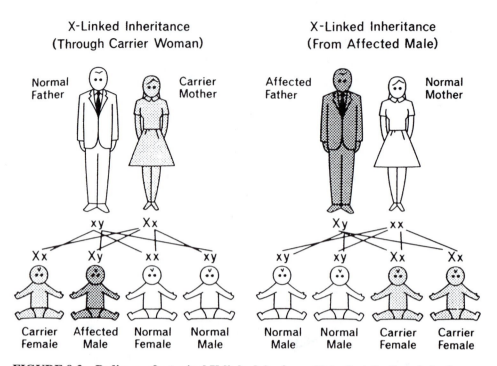

**FIGURE 8-3    Pedigree of a typical X-linked deafness. Note that the female is always the carrier and the male is always affected. This type of transmission is from mother to affected son to carrier daughter to affected son, and so on. Those familiar with hemophilia will notice an identical pattern of transmission and expression. (Courtesy of Pro-Ed, Inc., from Krajicek and Tearney, 1977)**

formed. Finally, a fourth anomaly may also occur. The bony anatomy may be completely normal but there may be various degrees of damage to the neuro-sensory epithelium. There is no specific name for that occurrence. There are other anomalies of the inner ear (e.g., Alexander and Bing-Siebenmann), but they are rare.

## Associated Anomalies

Congenital or genetic disorders with associated anomalies are usually called syndromes, that is, a collection of associated abnormalities and symptoms. For purposes of convenience, associated anomalies are classed as: (1) integumentary (pertaining to the skin); (2) skeletal; (3) ocular; and (4) other.

Perhaps one of the most inclusive examples of a congenital familial disorder with overt abnormalities in the four categories listed is the Waardenburg syndrome. Undoubtedly, that is because it characterizes many of the inheritable abnormalities that may occur. It is a dominant genetic disorder with variable expression. Since it is dominant, it will be passed to offspring with the frequency and in the manner described earlier. However, it is characterized, as are many dominant disorders, by the variable expressivity of its stigmata. That means that the collection of symptoms constituting the syndrome described by Waardenburg (1951) appears with all degrees of severity (including not appearing), from one patient to another. Waardenburg syndrome (Figure 8-4) is classified by Konigsmark's (1971) nosology as a congenital deafness with integumentary system disease. That is because its signs are primarily in the realm of pigmentary disorders, although a careful analysis reflects involvement of the ocular and skeletal systems as well. For example, a patient may present with heterochromia iridis (an alteration of eye color) in which the eyes are of different colors or more than one color may appear in the iris of each eye. Patients often have an alteration of hair color that is revealed by an unpigmented streak. The medial canthi of the eyes may be widely separated. The separation may be exaggerated by a characteristic flattening of the bridge of the nose. In some patients there is a typical heart-shaped mouth. Due to the variable expression of symptoms, some of these signs may not appear at all. Similarly, hearing loss may not appear, or it may present from mild to profound in one or both ears.

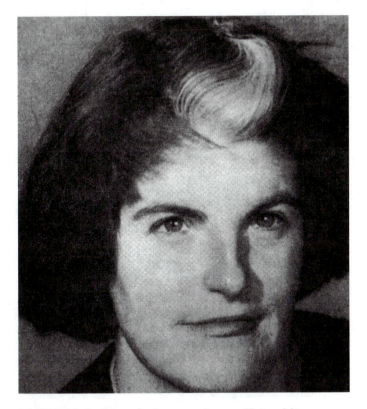

**FIGURE 8-4   Waardenburg syndrome. Note white forelock, hypertelorism, and other typical features. (From M.W. Partington,** *Arch Dis Child* **34:154–157, 1959)**

### Integumentary Anomalies

Integumentary anomalies (skin abnormalities) and congenital sensorineural hearing loss are the chief sequelae in many syndromes. Perhaps the best known is albinism. Tietz (1963) reported an extended family in which fourteen members showed the disorder. The hearing loss was severe. Besides albinism, or absence of the coloring pigmentation to the skin, integumentary anomalies may involve abnormal patterns of pigmentation. For example, hereditary piebaldism (strips of hyper- and hypopigmentation) and lentigines (leopard-like spots) may accompany severe congenital sensorineural hearing loss. These disorders tend to favor males.

### Skeletal Anomalies

Skeletal anomalies are less common than integumentary anomalies, but they certainly do occur with significant frequency. Perhaps the most often seen example of a genetic congenital hearing loss with associated skeletal defect is Klippel-Feil syndrome. Called an otocervical disorder, it involves the ear and the cervical vertebrae. The patient seems to have a shortness or absence of neck. Along with that, there is limited mobility of the head and what appears to be a lowered hair line in the back. The syndrome does tend to run in families, but, because its appearance is not so frequent or easily predicted, the disorder is said to be of "autosomal dominance with poor penetrance." As with Waardenburg syndrome, the disorder, and most of the others like it, has variable expressivity (Figure 8-5, *A* and *B*). That is, there is no consistent audiological pattern associated with it. Again, as with most other disorders in this category, it usually does involve some middle ear malformation (e.g., misshapen stapes, absence of oval window, etc.), and thus conductive losses occur often. However, sensorineural hearing losses occur more often, while mixed losses occur most often.

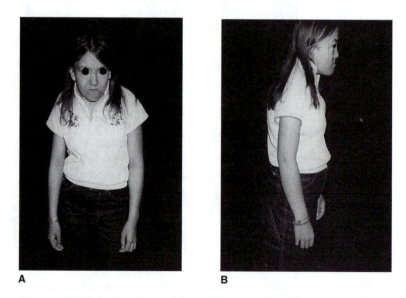

A    B

**FIGURE 8-5(*A*, *B*)    Klippel-Feil syndrome. Note the apparent absence of a neck, and shortened and rounded shoulders.**

### Ocular Anomalies

Ocular anomalies are commonly associated with hearing loss. Eye anomalies, extending as far as total absence of eyes (anophthalmos), occur with hearing disorders. In the European study of deafness (Martin et al., 1979; Martin, 1982), visual impairment was one of the three most common disorders associated with hearing loss. Physical and mental disorders were the other two primary categories. Rapin and Ruben (1979) reported eye anomalies in twelve of sixteen children with ear anomalies. Markedly bulging eyes, exophthalmos, is characteristic of Crouzon syndrome, and widely separated eyes, hypertelorism, accompanies several congenital deafness syndromes.

Usher syndrome, which appears in 3 to 10 percent of profoundly deaf children, offers the best example of a recessive genetic condition with hearing loss and associated ocular abnormalities. The first signs the patient notices are a narrowing field of vision and defective night vision. This usually occurs in early adulthood. The syndrome is specifically characterized by retinitis pigmentosa, a slowly progressive, bilateral, tapetoretinal degeneration. Eventually, total blindness can occur. The disorder may also be accompanied by mental retardation, epilepsy, psychological abnormalities, physical anomalies, and vertigo. The hearing loss is usually in the moderate to severe range, sensorineural, and frequently involves the high frequencies (Northern and Downs, 1991). Because the visual problem is progressive, the earlier the diagnosis, the more intensive and effective counseling can be. Family members should also receive genetic counseling.

### Other Anomalies

Other anomalies may also accompany congenital genetic syndromes with hearing loss. Two excellent examples loosely called "other" are actually of great significance and should not be treated so off-handedly. The first of these is called mucopolysaccharidosis, a group of disorders best illustrated by Hurler syndrome and Hunter syndrome. The second is commonly called Down syndrome although it is also known as trisomy 21 syndrome and mongolism.

There are actually seven disorders in the mucopolysaccharidosis (MPS) group, all of which are characterized by increased urinary mucopolysaccharide excretion. While all may present with hearing loss, only MPS I (Hurler syndrome) and MPS II (Hunter syndrome) count hearing impairment among their major stigmata. It has also been shown that chronic ear disease may be a characteristic of MPS VII (Wallace, Prutting, and Gerber, 1990). Hurler syndrome (Figure 8-6, *A* and *B*) is often reflected in mental deficiency and a specific constellation of deformities including reduced stature, osseous and articular (bone and joint) deficits, large heart, widely spaced eyes, and flattened nasal bridge. In contrast, Hunter syndrome (Figure 8-7, *A* and *B*) is less severe. Both disorders are considered an inborn error of metabolism (Northern and Downs, 1991). Most patients appear normal at birth, features gradually becoming coarse as the degeneration proceeds. In addition to the typical failure to grow, children with both these disorders usually suffer from chronic nasal problems, mental retardation, and stiffness of the joints. Patients with Hurler syndrome usually die by the age of ten years. Hunter syndrome patients usually live longer, but an early death is expected.

Patients with Hurler syndrome usually have some progressive hearing loss. Similarly, about half of the Hunter syndrome patients have a moderate hearing loss, primarily sensorineural. Because these disorders are also characterized by bone and joint malformations, middle ear and cochlear anomalies are common. A mixed conductive and sensorineural

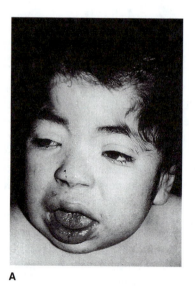 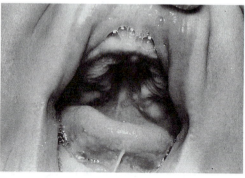

**A**                              **B**

**FIGURE 8-6    Hurler syndrome:** (*A*) **Note coarseness of features, large head, and flatted bridge of nose.** (*B*) **Note high palatal vault, oversized tongue and unusual shape of the gums and alveolar ridge.**

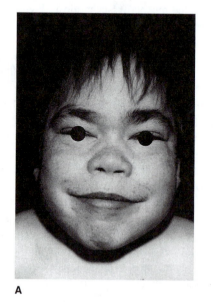 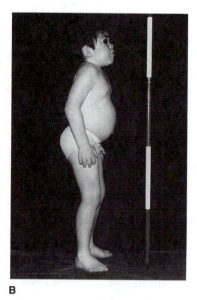

**A**                              **B**

**FIGURE 8-7** (*A, B*)    **Hunter syndrome. Note reduced growth, joint abnormalities, and malproportioned facial features.**

hearing loss may be present as a result of ossicular chain malformation and an inner ear anomaly (Kelemen, 1977; Konigsmark and Gorlin, 1976; Leroy and Crocker, 1966).

Down syndrome is, perhaps, the best known of all congenital disorders. Once known as mongolism because of a characteristic antimongoloid slant of the eyes, this disorder is the result of an extra chromosome at position number 21. This has led to it also being called the trisomy 21 syndrome. Incidentally, other major chromosomal disorders (trisomy 13-15 and trisomy 18) also result in severely involved children with marked degeneration of the organ of Corti. In those cases, however, most die in the first year of life. Estimates of occurrence suggest that trisomy 21 appears in one in 600 to 770 live births (Northern and Downs, 1991). The children may exhibit any combination of over fifty different anomalies. No single sign is considered diagnostic, and some of the characteristics appear in some normal persons. The most commonly associated stigmata include retarded growth, a flat hypoplastic face with short nose, prominent epicanthic skin folds, a protruding lower lip, small rounded ears with a prominent antihelix, a fissured and thickened tongue, stubby fingers usually without the middle section of the fifth finger, and a transverse palmar crease. Of all the characteristics, however, mental retardation, short fingers (especially the fifth), simian folds across the palms of the hands, and a flattened facial expression with the characteristic antimongoloid slant of the eyes are present in most patients (Figure 8-8).

Audiograms obtained from patients with Down syndrome may vary dramatically from person to person. Generally, because of the frequent presence of anomalies of the pinnae and ear canals, it is reasonable to expect, at worst, middle ear anomalies, and at best, a long series of middle ear infections. Most studies report the presence of middle ear problems in 50 to 80 percent of the cases. Gerber (1977b) has indicated that deafness, per se, is rare in the Down group. On the other hand, most authors agree that mild to moderate sensorineural hearing loss is present in many cases, with mixed sensorineural and conductive hearing loss

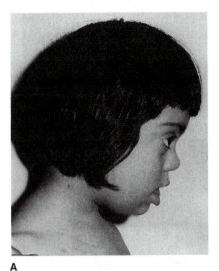

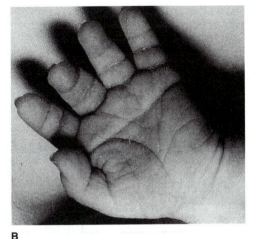

**A**                          **B**

**FIGURE 8-8    Down syndrome.**

present most often. The degree of mental retardation may influence the audiometric results obtained, and consequently, sensorineural hearing loss may appear to be far more severe than it really is. Play audiometry is usually very successful with these patients even at full adult chronological age.

## Congenital Nongenetic Deafness

Although nearly 50 percent of the children who are born deaf have a known genetic etiology, the information for the other 50 percent is not quite so well-defined. Certainly, a significant number within that second 50 percent fall into the "etiology unknown" classification. There is strong reason to suppose that many of those children are actually members of a latent onset group whose etiology is an autosomal recessive gene (Mencher and Mencher, 1995). However, firm evidence to support that notion is not easy to find. In any case, the remaining children—that is, those whose etiology is not genetic and is clearly known—constitute the *congenital nongenetic deafness* category. They constitute between 35 and 45 percent of the hearing-impaired pediatric population. Significant among causes of nongenetic congenital deafness are prenatal infections. Any viral infection can damage the central nervous system prenatally and, therefore, can cause congenital deafness. Generally, bacterial infections during pregnancy do not cross the placental barrier. Thus, although bacterial disease may cause a hearing loss in a child, it is unlikely to affect a fetus.

### Viral Deafness

The word "virus" is derived from a Latin word meaning poison, the same root as virulent, and implies a potent, destructive agent (Bergstrom, 1977). Some viruses may cause devastating effects on the fetal ear when they produce intrauterine infections that may be innocuous or even asymptomatic in the mother. There is reason to suppose that any viral disease that occurs prenatally may lead to congenital deafness. For example, one center reported a severely hearing-impaired girl born to a mother who had contracted viral influenza in the seventh month of her pregnancy. Granted, the cause–effect relationship is based on supposition; nevertheless, the principle is correct and should not be ignored. Viral disease may also result in severe inner ear or systemic effects when contracted in postnatal life. Notable among these diseases are measles, mumps, and meningitis.

Two of the most common viruses associated with congenital hearing loss are rubella and cytomegalovirus. Except for rubella and cytomegalovirus, no other viruses have been clearly documented as playing a major role in the causation of congenital deafness, although, as already indicated, viruses have been implicated in acquired postnatal losses. Today, at least in most nations in the Americas, children are immunized against rubella. This means the disease is rarely seen, and not that it has been eradicated. Consequently, children still appear in clinics with a hearing loss directly attributable to rubella during pregnancy. The issue here, however, is not rubella as a disease or whether it is slowly being erased as a public health menace. What is critical here is that rubella, as a disease process, behaves typically like a virus. Therefore, by a careful study of all we know of that disease, its effects upon the human body, its manifestations, and its treatments, the more we can generalize to other similar diseases. It is presented here as an example, one to be generalized and one to think of as a model for a host of other similar pathologies.

### Rubella

Rubella (German measles) is the best known of all the viral diseases associated with damage to a growing fetus. Similarly, historically, of all the viral diseases known to cause congenital hearing loss, the world at large has been most concerned about rubella occurring any time during the pregnancy and resulting in a baby with hearing impairment, visual impairment, cardiac defect, or mental retardation. In times of rubella epidemics, such as the epidemic of 1964–1965 in North America, as many as 25 percent of births with congenital hearing impairment can trace their deafness to this disease. It is a myth that rubella is dangerous only during the first trimester of pregnancy. According to the longitudinal studies of Bordley and colleagues (1967) and Baldursson and colleagues (1972), over 23 percent of the children with a hearing loss were born to mothers who contracted rubella during the second or third trimesters of the pregnancy.

The causal relationship between maternal rubella in pregnancy and congenital defects was first recognized by Sir Norman Gregg in 1941 (Brookhauser and Bordley, 1973; Hanshaw and Dudgeon, 1978; Hardy, 1973; Monif and Jordon, 1977). It was nearly 20 years after Gregg's discovery before progress was made either in an understanding of the pathogenesis of rubella, including the mechanisms of fetal damage, or in the development of a means of prevention. Before the isolation of the rubella virus, it was necessary to depend on clinical symptoms as the criteria for the diagnosis of the viral infection. Even now, the diagnosis of rubella is very often difficult and must be based on virological confirmation.

Fetal infection by the rubella virus generally occurs by one of the following routes: (1) the transplacental passage of virus; (2) spreading up birth canal with infection of the membranes; or (3) as a result of direct contact or contamination during the birth process. Neonatal infection may be acquired from the mother or the nursery attendants (Bergstrom, 1977; Hardy, 1973). Prenatal rubella infection differs in several important aspects from postnatally acquired rubella. Rather than being a mild, self-limiting disease, intrauterine rubella is often associated with a severe disseminated infection and a chronic infectious state that persists throughout fetal life. Sometimes infection may be incompatible with life and fetal death follows. The symptoms in those who survive depends on the organs involved and the degree of the damage.

The overall problem of rubella is further compounded by the fact that the virus has a very long life. Bordley and colleagues (1967) reported two hearing-impaired children born to mothers who had contracted rubella before conception. They also reported one hearing-impaired child in whom they could culture a live rubella virus at a postpartum age of fifteen months. The disease is insidious, and caution is required as infants may be severely damaged by prenatal rubella in cases in which the mother is free of symptoms.

Maternal rubella acquired in the first trimester of pregnancy usually results in fetal malformations: congenital cataracts, congenital heart disease, microcephaly, or mental retardation (Top and Wehrle, 1976). Hanshaw and Dudgeon also indicated that, in all the prospective studies that have been reported, the risk to the fetus is greater in the first eight weeks of pregnancy than in the second. Although the first trimester is the period of major risk, there is no distinct dividing line limiting risk after the thirteenth week of gestation. Hanshaw and Dudgeon also reported that malformations of heart and eye are uncommon after the twelfth week, but many cases of hearing loss, delayed development, and neurologic deficits have been noted if exposure occurs before the sixteenth week (fourth month), but those disorders are less frequent with exposure after that time. Information on the risk of fetal damage from maternal rubella after the fourth month of gestation is sparse.

Hardy, Sever, and Gilkeson (1969) reported that fifteen of twenty-two infants born to mothers who had clinical rubella sometime between the thirteenth and thirty-first weeks of gestation had evidence of fetal damage. The defects noted consisted mainly of poor delayed development and speech disorders (Bordley et al., 1967). Kohji and colleagues (1979) conducted a correlational study of the relationship between gestational age at the time of prenatal rubella and the type of congenital anomaly. They analyzed instances of congenital rubella syndrome for which the last menstrual period and the date of appearance of rubella rash were known. The history of prenatal rubella in these cases was from 16 to 131 days (approximately 2 to 19 weeks) of gestation. Kohji and colleagues found 46 cases of deafness out of 55 such patients. They also found that there was no special relationship between the time of prenatal rubella and the degree of hearing loss. Thus, despite the paucity of documented evidence on the incidence of defects associated with rubella contracted beyond the twentieth week of pregnancy, it can be concluded that the risk of incurring hearing loss diminishes after the twentieth week.

One aspect affecting the reported incidence of defects due to prenatal rubella is the age at which the children are assessed for evidence of damage. Hanshaw and Dudgeon (1978) cite several studies that indicate the progressive nature of hearing loss as a result of prenatal rubella. Studies reported by Manson, Logan, and Loy (1960) of children born in England and Wales (1950–1951) following prenatal rubella indicated that the incidence of sensorineural hearing loss detected at age two years was 2 percent and that of suspected sensorineural loss was 6 percent. When the same group of children was reassessed at four to five years of age, 12.8 percent were found to have sensory deafness. A third follow-up of this group of children at age eight to eleven years showed that the incidence of sensory deafness was 16 percent. Bearing in mind that, as children get older they respond better to audiometric testing and further that the incidence of sensorineural hearing loss in a population of normal eight- to eleven-year-olds is markedly less than 16 percent, this information suggests that there is progressive hearing loss due to prenatal rubella. Anvar, Mencher and Keet (1984) reported similar findings, as did Bordley and Brookhouser (1973), Downs (1984), and Tell (1976). These observations stress the importance of continued assessment of children known to or thought to have been exposed prenatally to rubella.

The histopathology of prenatal viral disease is often identical to that of an acquired endolabyrinthitis and is structurally the same as some of the congenital anomalies of the inner ear. Bordley and colleagues (1967) described the pathology as that of the Scheibe type. A most interesting observation was reported by Lindsay and Matz (1966). They had acquired the temporal bones of a child with a well-documented congenital hearing impairment who subsequently had mumps that caused an additional hearing loss. Studies of the temporal bones revealed that the cochleae were abnormal indeed, but there was no way to tell which abnormality was congenital and which was acquired.

Temporal bone studies of children congenitally deafened by rubella have revealed localized lesions in the inner ear. These are mainly confined to the stria vascularis, Reissner's membrane, and the tectorial membrane (Bergstrom, 1977; Hanshaw and Dudgeon, 1978). Necrosis of the epithelium of the cochlea with damage resulting from small hemorrhages and inflammatory cells in the stria vascularis are common findings. The main histopathologic changes observed by Friedman and Prier (1973) consisted of inflammation and necrosis, with adhesions between Reissner's membrane and the tectorial membrane. The latter may be found retracted away from the organ of Corti and covered by inflamed cells. The degenerative and inflammatory processes are often ongoing, leading to profound deafness, and offering an explanation for the late onset of hearing loss in some children. Another problem encountered in rubella is related to a lesion in the brain resulting in a form of central auditory imperception.

Sometimes hearing loss is the only defect associated with congenital rubella. Severe deafness was a prominent feature following a rubella epidemic in Iceland in 1963–1964 (Baldursson et al., 1972). Thirty-seven children with rubella syndrome were detected, none had cardiac or ocular defects, but there were various degrees of hearing loss among them. Many of the children had behavioral disorders but normal intelligence. Another similar type of epidemic was seen in Trinidad between 1960–1961 (Karmody, 1969). Serologic tests for rubella on children with deafness of unknown etiology indicated that maternal rubella in subclinical form probably caused many of these cases.

The pattern of hearing loss associated with maternal rubella was reported in a study by Brookhouser and Bordley (1973). They found that the hearing loss was sensorineural in character with a mild conductive component present in few cases. Severity of the loss varied from patient to patient and between the ears of the same patient. Audiometric patterns varied among individual patients and between the ears of the same patient. Some patients showed no response at any frequency in either ear, while others responded to most frequencies but with a distinct asymmetry between ears. Audiograms most frequently associated with rubella showed a curve with greatest loss in the middle frequencies between 500 and 2000 Hz. Poor speech discrimination was seen often. A subsequent follow-up study of rubella infants reported a decrease in auditory acuity from the initial hearing tests in about 25 percent of the cases.

Some studies suggest that there is a high coincidence of conductive hearing loss related to otitis media in children with rubella-associated hearing losses (Bordley et al., 1967). Hardy and Bordley (1973) report that, although the primary hearing loss is sensorineural, all rubella-affected children may have concurrent middle ear difficulty. This suggests that the host for the rubella virus in cases of progressive hearing loss may lie in the middle ear disease. The report of Mencher and colleagues (1978) seems to support that notion. They noted several cases of progressive sensory hearing loss in rubella-affected children with a full history of middle ear disease. There was a contrasting absence of sensorineural hearing loss in children from the same epidemic with a negative history of middle ear disease. It appeared, therefore, that the rubella virus may have survived in the diseased middle ear tissue and reentered the inner ear, producing additional sensorineural hearing loss. The implications for other viral-based congenital sensorineural hearing losses and their relationship to ongoing middle ear pathology are obvious and need to be included in future planning.

Anderson, Barr, and Wedenberg (1970), in reviewing twenty children with hearing loss due to prenatal rubella, found that thirteen of nineteen parental pairs had hereditary abnormalities of hearing. From this, Proctor (1977), like Anderson, Barr, and Wedenberg, concluded that genetic disposition to hearing impairment appears to be a prerequisite for rubella deafness. This seems to be a fairly broad generalization, especially in consideration of the other defects resulting from rubella in the first trimester of pregnancy. Clearly this hypothesis requires further investigation.

Figure 8-9 illustrates three typical children, all the result of the same rubella epidemic. All were born within a few weeks of each other, all within the same general geographic region of Nova Scotia. All are now in their late teens, and a significant amount of information has been gathered about them. The first is considered deaf and blind. He has totally lost all his vision and hearing and is responsive to sign language via his hands. He retained some vision until just after puberty. He now resides in a specialized home designed to teach him self-help skills and independent living. The second boy is physically involved, but has vision. He has had difficulty with leg muscles and walking and would be considered cerebral palsied as well as hearing-impaired. In spite of these disabilities, he was mainstreamed in school and with significant help from his family and by his own efforts, he graduated from high school and is now entering Gallaudet University. He has a moderate to severe sensorineural hearing loss and is entirely dependent upon hearing aids, sign language (total communication), and auditory training systems for communication. However, he is quite independent and has a solid future before him. The third child has a severe hearing loss and no other obvious disabilities. He has been enrolled at the special school for the hearing impaired in the Atlantic Provinces of Canada and has just graduated. He is now enrolled in a technical–trade program with excellent prospects for a job in the mechanical field. His speech is excellent and is quite intelligible. These are special boys whose only misfortune

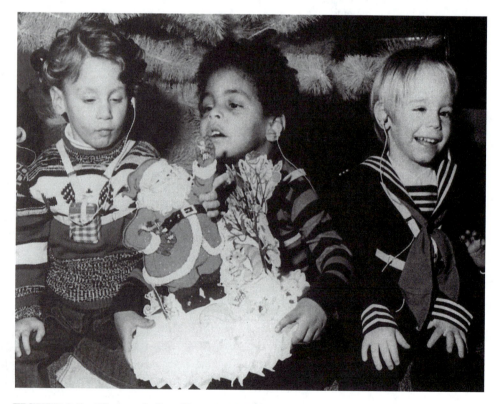

**FIGURE 8-9    Three rubella-affected children.**

was to be born at the same time in the same place in the middle of a vicious epidemic. Today, they would all have been born normal because their mothers would have had the opportunity to be immunized against rubella.

Rubella embryopathy was numerically the single most important known prenatally acquired cause of congenital childhood deafness, and the highlighting of such an avoidable cause of deafness clearly shows the urgent need for an effective immunization program. The total number of cases of rubella deafness has been substantial in any year, and in epidemic years has risen to catastrophic figures. Fortunately, today, rubella is on the wane. Rapid progress has occurred in the development and testing of rubella virus vaccines (Sever and Bethesda, 1973). The criteria for an ideal vaccine include: (1) safety and no untoward reactions; (2) no adverse effects on the fetus; (3) not transmissible from vaccinees to women of childbearing age; and finally, (4) long-lasting immunity. Several strains of rubella vaccine have been tested. Results indicate that not all are satisfactory for mass immunization programs, but local health authorities are aware of limitations and have developed programs accordingly. As a result, and despite problems still faced, immunization has rendered rubella a preventable disease and its incidence has markedly decreased. It has been a number of years since we have seen a rubella deaf infant. However, we must not become sanguine about this fact. Carrel (1977) expressed concern that our decreasing attention to prenatal rubella may lead to increasing numbers of children who are not immunized against this potentially devastating disease.

Ultimately, if the vaccines used to prevent rubella are effective there will be a further gradual decline in the incidence of the disease. This will not only prevent unnecessary suffering for individual children and their families, but will also reduce the number of children requiring special education for deafness and partial hearing. The resultant economic saving will be remarkable, it will more than offset the actual cost of the immunization programs and greatly exceed the cost in terms of human suffering.

### Cytomegalovirus

Concern cannot, and should not, be limited to rubella. Cytomegalovirus (CMV) is far more common today than prenatal rubella. It is estimated that 2 to 3 percent of pregnant women excrete this virus and that it may be found in 1 to 1.5 percent of newborns. The disease resulting from cytomegalovirus is silent (i.e., asymptomatic) in as many as 98 percent of the infants who have it (Marx, 1975). Furthermore, Marx estimated that by the age of thirty years, fully 80 percent of the population of the United States at some time will have carried a live cytomegalovirus. Thus, the disease is extremely common and apparently easily transmitted. In the 1960s, scattered reports of congenital deafness resulting from CMV infection began to appear. CMV was first isolated in 1956, although it had been suspected as a cause of cytomegalic inclusion disease for the greater part of this century (Amstey, 1977). Ten times as many infants are infected by CMV at birth as by rubella. The infection is asymptomatic in the mother, who may shed organisms for weeks or months in saliva, urine, breast milk, feces, or tears (Bergstrom, 1977). Transmission may occur during pregnancy by the transplacental route. Intrapartum infection is possible during the passage of the fetus through the birth canal in women with cervical CMV, but this is usually not associated with disease. The infant who may be ill one month after birth is asymptomatic otherwise. In postnatal life, CMV is transmitted only by intimate contact in adults, frequently by sexual contact and by fresh blood transfusion. Although, theoretically, babies with congenital CMV may be infectious, there is little evidence that CMV is readily disseminated to other patients or personnel in a hospital setting (Affias and Embil, 1978).

When CMV contacts the unborn infant, the infection may be contained by the several host defense mechanisms of the fetus, or there may be disease ranging from subtle abnormalities not detectable at birth to severe generalized disease in the newborn period. The latter, more recognizable form of the disease has been far better documented than the milder manifestations. Classically, cytomegalic inclusion disease is characterized by enlarged liver and spleen (hepatosplenomegaly), jaundice (hyperbilirubinemia), blood and skin abnormalities (thrombocytopenia with petechiae or purpura), a variable involvement of the central nervous system, including cerebral calcifications, microcephaly, chorioretinitis, deafness, and psychomotor retardation (Weller and Hanshaw, 1962). There are several variations and combinations of these findings (Figure 8-10). Overt congenital CMV, which occurs in 2 percent of the cases, is usually fatal (Aballi and Korones, 1963). Hyperbilirubinemia is a common manifestation of congenital infection occurring in more than half of symptomatic infants in the first week of life. Hyperbilirubinemia is one of the high risk factors for sensorineural hearing loss. Since it is a common symptom of congenital CMV, monitoring the bilirubin level is one way to be alert to the hearing status of newborns who might develop a hearing loss associated with CMV.

There is growing evidence that most infants with congenital CMV infection have little or no outward clinical manifestations of the disease, but develop subtle neurologic deformities that become apparent in the late preschool and early school years. Hanshaw and colleagues (1976) sought to determine if CMV-infected asymptomatic children were developmentally different from uninfected controls as they approached the demands of elementary school education. Of the fifty-three children who were seropositive for CMV at birth, forty-four had psychometric and pediatric evaluations at three and a half to seven years of age. The group's mean I.Q. was nine points below that of a group of matched controls. Bilateral hearing loss was present in five of forty children with antibodies against CMV and in only one of forty-four matched controls without antibodies. The predicted school failure rate, based on I.Q., behavioral, neurologic, and auditory test data was 2.7 times that of matched socioeconomic controls and 8 times that of randomly selected controls. In one particularly severe case, the child did not have symptoms of CMV in the newborn period, and the possibility of congenital infection was not considered by his physicians. He was microcephalic, hypotonic, and had a profound bilateral, sensory hearing loss. His I.Q. was below thirty at seven years of age, and he continued to excrete CMV in his urine. Hanshaw and colleagues (1976) concluded, from their study, that clinically inapparent congenital CMV infection definitely could have an adverse effect on central nervous system development.

The first CMV case report involving pathology of the cochlear end organ was described by Myers and Stool (1968). However, the infant died in the first month of life and hearing had not been evaluated. Cytomegalic inclusion-bearing cells were found in epithelial cells of the saccule, utricle, and semicircular canals and on the epithelial cell layer (endolymphatic side) of Reissner's membrane and the stria vascularis. Hydrops of the saccule of both ears, of one utricle, and of the scala media of both ears was present. The stria vascularis was degenerated and contained a cystic structure in one ear.

According to Dahle and colleagues (1974), a severe-profound, high-frequency, progressive sensory hearing loss is often associated with congenital CMV infection. The hearing

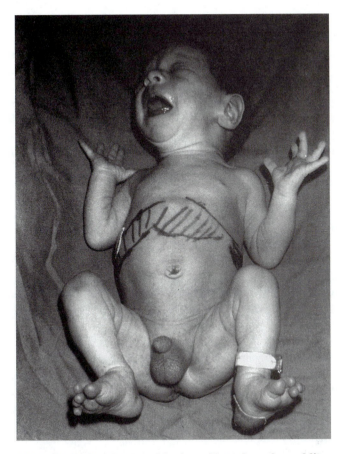

**FIGURE 8-10    Cytomegalovirus. Note the enlarged liver
and spleen. This child is also quite jaundiced.**

sensitivity of eighteen children with subclinical CMV infection was studied. Nine of the eighteen children had some hearing loss ranging from slight high-frequency impairment to a severe–profound unilateral loss. Indirect evidence for a progressive disease process was discovered by analyzing the number of cases with a hearing loss compared with the age at time of testing. It was found that only two of eighteen children under thirty months had a hearing loss, whereas seven of eighteen children over thirty months had a hearing loss. The most severe hearing losses were seen in children over forty months. Later, Dahle and colleagues (1979) presented four case studies in which CMV may have been the cause of progressive hearing loss. The subjects were part of a longitudinal study involving 182 children seen for audiologic evaluation and serologic studies. All four cases had progressive hearing loss and a history of chronic middle ear disease since early infancy. This suggests that, as with rubella, there is a need for close monitoring for progressive hearing loss.

Gerber, Mendel, and Goller (1979) reported a case study of a female child with congenital CMV whom they monitored audiometrically over a long period. Although examination at birth was unremarkable, it was reported that at four weeks of age, she was not responding to events occurring in her acoustic environment. At the age of two months, an audiological diagnosis revealed no responses to speech or narrow band noise at 90 dB in the sound field, but normal tympanometric measures. At ten weeks she was seen for electric response audiometry and responses were obtained at levels indicating a moderate flat hearing loss in the left ear and an upward sloping audiogram for the right ear. Again, impedance results were normal. A pediatric examination revealed a positive titer for cytomegalovirus. At twenty-two weeks, auditory brain stem responses were found at 95 and 103 dB HL. On her last visit, at the age of thirty-one weeks, auditory brain stem responses were obtained at the limits of the system, 103 dB bilaterally. The authors concluded that, in this case, it appears that CMV led to a degenerative sensory hearing impairment, and it is therefore possible that pattern is a natural sequela of CMV infection. Although not confirmed by other reports in the literature, clearly, such a situation and interpretation are possible and plausible. Thus, as with the relationship between ongoing middle ear pathology and rubella discussed earlier, these elements must be included in planning patient care.

Attention has turned to the possible development of a vaccine to prevent CMV. If 1 percent of all infants excrete CMV at birth, then out of 3,000,000 infants in the United States, 30,000 were born with infection in 1975 (Amstey, 1977). The numbers in Canada represent about 10 percent of the U.S. totals. In California, the most populous of the United States, 600,000 infants are born each year. Hence, 6,000 of them can be expected to be born with and shedding CMV. This is an extremely large number of children and should encourage the development of some type of preventive measure. Given the absence of a primary care preventive vaccine against CMV, the next (but less satisfactory) step is secondary care or the earliest possible identification and institution of a treatment program to prevent further disability from occurring. Unfortunately, not only is there no vaccine to prevent the disease, there is no medical therapy for treatment of congenital CMV infection. Severe congenital anomalies are not usually produced by CMV; however, intrauterine infection produces an inflammatory reaction in fetal tissues leading to the observed changes at birth. It is the child with mild disease or the asymptomatic virus excreter who may benefit from therapy. It would be hoped that a medical therapy might prevent subclinical disease, mild handicaps, mental retardation, or deafness. According to Hanshaw (1979), many antiviral agents have been used in the treatment of congenital and acquired CMV infections. Although virus excretion has been temporarily halted in some instances, no role in the treatment of these infections has been established for these agents. Further, Hanshaw states that the use of these agents is potentially toxic and has not been adequately studied. The final stage is, of course, tertiary care or treatment of the active disease process and rehabilitation. Treatment of the disease is based on symptom management. Rehabilitation is based on identification, diagnosis, amplification, aural habilitation, speech–language development, special education, and all the other factors seen with hearing-impaired children.

## Protozoal Infections

The most dramatic example of congenital nongenetic deafness caused by protozoal infection is toxoplasmosis. Children affected by Toxoplasma gondii, which is acquired transplacentally, are usually multiply involved. The mother may acquire the protozoan by eating uncooked or partially cooked meat that contains the infection. It is also transmitted via the feces of certain animals, most notably in North America the domestic house cat. It is strongly recommended that pregnant women avoid contact with pet cats and their litter boxes. The disease, generally, tends to be more prevalent in communities in which animals are less contained and cleanliness is secondary. It has even been said that 10 to 20 percent of profound childhood deafness is caused by this infection (Theissing and Kittel, 1962). Stein and Boyer (1994) suggested the number may be even higher than that. However, Mencher and Mencher (1995) reported only one case in ten years in Nova Scotia, Canada. The disease may occur more often than recognized, but the number and extent of hearing losses associated with it has yet to be confirmed. Suffice it to say, toxoplasmosis does cause hearing loss and other neonatal disorders. Hydrocephalus, seizures, mental retardation, visual impairment, and neuromuscular deficit are frequent sequelae in addition to the hearing loss. The disease apparently develops as calcium deposits on the stria vascularis and the spiral ligament. The resultant hearing loss is therefore slowly progressive. The hearing impairment may begin in early childhood as a mild loss and will advance toward profound deafness with time. The disease does not respond well to drug therapy, and, because of the multiple involvements, prognosis is poor. Audiologic differential diagnosis is extremely difficult; nevertheless, habilitative efforts can be quite rewarding.

## TORCHS Syndromes

TORCHS is an acronym for TOxoplasmosis, Rubella, Cytomegalovirus and Herpes and Syphilis. These represent the major nongenetic congenital causes of sensorineural hearing loss in neonates. Although the discussion in this chapter has followed a slightly different order, the first three of these diseases have been discussed in detail. Herpes (a virus) and syphilis (a bacterium) represent diseases that not only attack the newborn and cause congenital hearing loss, but also can attack an adult or manifest themselves in the adult (even though they have been present since birth) and result in an acquired hearing loss. Consequently, they are discussed in brief detail here and again in Chapter 9.

### Congenital Syphilis

Congenital syphilis (lues disease) can be prevented. With proper blood tests before pregnancy (the test is called the VDRL), the mother can know she is a carrier of the disease. Given those circumstances, proper antibiotic management throughout the pregnancy can ensure that both she and her baby remain symptom-free. Failure to recognize the presence of the disease can lead to spontaneous abortion in a high percentage of cases, or failing that natural solution, a seriously involved neonate with a rash over the entire body, anemia, dental anomalies, central nervous system deficits, cardiac anomalies, and hearing loss (Figure 8-11). In most of these cases, the baby will not survive. In a large number of cases, the baby may be symptom-free at birth, but the disease will express itself in the second decade of life, usually around puberty. About one-third of those cases will have a hearing loss.

A typical case involved a brother and sister aged thirteen and fifteen. Both had been symptom-free and neither they nor their parents admitted knowledge of congenital lues. The fifteen-year-old girl came to the clinic complaining of dizziness, tinnitus, and difficulty understanding conversation in noise. Audiometric results indicated mild sensorineural loss, normal speech reception threshold, but poor speech discrimination in one ear at 60 percent. The other ear was slightly better at 86 percent. At first, the otologist tried to rule out the pres-

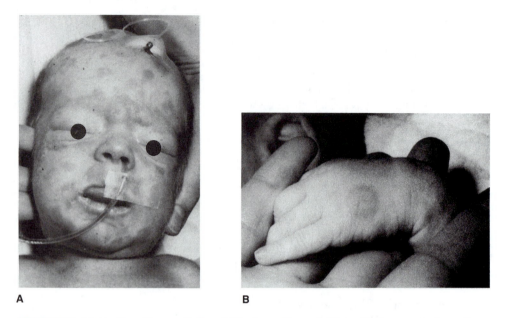

**A**                                **B**

**FIGURE 8-11** (*A, B*)    **Congenital syphilis (lues disease). Note the large number of vesicles covering the child's body. This child also suffered from severe central nervous system damage and other associated pathologies.**

ence of a variety of pathologies, including Ménière disease, eighth cranial nerve tumor, labyrinthitis, and so forth. The girl was scheduled for a complete evaluation and an appointment scheduled in two weeks. Within that short period of time, the patient developed visual difficulties, primarily blurred vision. She was admitted to hospital and a complete program was instituted. Blood serology tests confirmed the presence of lues. Medical treatment by antibiotic therapy was instituted, but the young woman continued to fail. Within six months she was almost totally deafened in one ear, had a severe loss in the other, and was essentially blind. At that point, her brother, who had also undergone medical analysis and testing with similar results, began to show identical symptoms. This story does not have a happy ending. Both patients died within two years. Temporal bone analysis confirmed total destruction of the cochlear structures and the organ of Corti. In addition, at autopsy it was noted that the cortical structures of the temporal and occipital lobes were severely damaged by the disease. The really sad part of this story is that it could have been prevented if the proper testing procedures had been followed at the time of the marriage or the pregnancy.

*Herpes Simplex Virus*
Herpes simplex virus (HSV) is one of the most commonly transmitted sexual diseases. According to Northern and Downs (1991), HSV infects the genital tracts of an estimated 20 to 25 percent of the world's population. If the mother is infected, the disease will be transmitted to the baby during the birth process, and it has been suggested that as many as 50 percent of those infected will die. Consequently, in most cases when HSV is present, the delivery will be

by caesarean section. If, by chance, the disease crosses the placental barrier prior to delivery, as with lues disease, this too will often result in a spontaneous abortion or severe malformations of the child. Hearing loss is usually present at birth for those who are infected. Because most cases of congenital HSV are also symptomatic of the entire disease process at birth (including rash and other associated sequelae) it is not hard to recognize. Immediate referral to audiology for examination and follow-up is essential. Audiological treatment follows the same lines as all congenital infections including diagnosis, amplification, speech and language development, special education, and so forth. There is no cure for HSV. As a virus, it remains one of the more difficult disease processes for medical science to conquer.

## Medical Considerations

To provide the maximum in educational and audiological programming, and thus, presumably, the maximum opportunity for normal development, the congenitally deaf or hard-of-hearing child must be identified at the earliest possible time in life. The recommended procedures for screening newborns are in print and are presumably well known to physicians and others engaged in early identification efforts (National Institutes of Health, 1994) Predicated on longitudinal research data, recommendations were refined at the 1974 Nova Scotia Conference on Early Identification of Hearing Loss (Mencher, 1976) and adopted and subsequently modified several times by the Joint Committee on Infant Hearing until the most recent statement (Joint Comm. on Infant Hearing, 1994). They have also been adopted by the Canadian Advisory Coalition on Childhood Hearing Impairment (CACCHI), the Canadian equivalent organization (Kassirer, 1984). A core element in the early identification process is something called the High Risk Register for Hearing Loss (Table 8-1).

Originally based on a concept outlined by Downs and Silver (1972), the register is a series of the most common causes of congenital sensorineural hearing loss in newborns. If possible, all children are to be screened for hearing loss at birth by either auditory brain stem response audiometry or otoacoustic emissions. However, failing that capability, a center may use an alternative model in which only those children found to be on the high-risk register for hearing loss may be screened by use of these electrophysiologic approaches. When a child has been identified as at risk for hearing loss and has failed a preliminary hearing screening, procedures to confirm or deny the presence of hearing impairment should be implemented immediately and with the utmost care. Children failing the screening examination or those referred directly to diagnostic centers are to be evaluated by both audiological and medical techniques that follow a specific sequential procedure and, consequently, most family physicians or pediatricians will refer to otological and or audiological centers.

Medical approaches are aimed at two definitive purposes: (1) identification of a hearing loss and (2) identification of the etiology of any hearing loss. Procedures such as pneumatic otoscopy are aimed at separating sensorineural from conductive problems. Fundoscopic examination is germane to relating etiology to rubella or retinitis pigmentosa (although that is not likely to be spotted in a newborn). Urinalysis may identify kidney disease or one of the mucopolysaccharidoses. An examination of thyroid function may reveal Pendred syndrome, while chromosomal studies may specify several different etiologies. Chromosomal examinations may also lead to genetic counseling and possibly to the prevention of future children

**TABLE 8-1    High risk register for early identification of hearing loss.**

*Indicators Associated with Sensorineural and/or Conductive Hearing Loss*

For use with neonates (birth through age 28 days) when universal screening is not available.

1. Family history of hereditary childhood sensorineural hearing loss.
2. In utero infection, such as cytomegalovirus, rubella, syphilis, herpes, and toxoplasmosis.
3. Craniofacial anomalies, including those with morphological abnormalities of the pinna and ear canal.
4. Birth weight less than 1500 grams (3.3 lbs.)
5. Hyperbilirubinemia at a serum level requiring exchange transfusion.
6. Ototoxic medications, including but not limited to the aminoglycosides, used in multiple courses or in combination with loop diuretics.
7. Bacterial meningitis.
8. Apgar scores of 0–4 at 1 minute or 0–6 at 5 minutes.
9. Mechanical ventilation lasting 5 days or longer.
10. Stigmata or other findings associated with a syndrome known to include a sensorineural and/or conductive hearing loss.

In addition to the above items, head trauma, recurrent or persistent otitis media with effusion for at least 3 months, neurofibromatosis Type II, neurodegenerative disorders, and anatomical deformities and other disorders that affect Eustachian tube function are considered significant indicators of an at risk child.

From the Joint Committee on Infant Hearing (JCIH) (1994) Position Statement, Asha, 36:38–41.

with hearing loss. A systematic approach to diagnosis requires that a specific and sequential procedure be followed. One such sequence in seen in Table 8-2 (Mencher and Gerber, 1981). Ruben (1996) has developed a detailed list of necessary procedures.

It is important that all the disciplines concerned with identification of deafness in children, specifically audiology, otology, and pediatrics, be familiar with and understand the procedures reviewed here, the limitations of their usage, and the rationale for the priorities specified. Only through a clear understanding by all involved of the what, why, and how of sister disciplines can the team approach be developed and the best interests of the patient be served. Finally, the general otologic considerations for a patient with congenital sensorineural hearing loss are no different from what they would be in any normal-hearing person, except perhaps, that greater caution is required. Identification of middle ear disease in a patient with a congenital sensorineural hearing loss is far more difficult. That is, the sensory loss may hide any change in middle ear function that would normally have been reflected in a conductive hearing loss. Furthermore, the significance of the development of ear disease in the one good ear is doubled when dealing with a patient having a unilateral hearing loss.

## *Audiological Considerations*

The disabling effects of congenital hearing impairment are extensive and variable. Genetic deafnesses range from mild to profound with audiometric contours from flat through odd-shaped, affecting one or both ears. Some genetically based hearing impairments are degen-

**TABLE 8-2    Sequence of procedures to follow for diagnosis of sensorineural hearing loss in newborns.**

1. Essential to the assessment
   a. Standard pediatric examination
   b. Pneumatic otoscopy and/or otomicroscopy
   c. Funduscopic examination
   d. Observations for specific physical abnormalities
2. Strongly recommended in the assessment
   a. General laboratory examinations
   b. Appropriate serology examinations for toxoplasmosis, rubella, cytomegalovirus, and herpes
   c. Urinalysis
   d. Family audiograms
3. Include when indicated
   a. Thyroid function
   b. Polytomography of middle and inner ear
   c. Electrocardiogram
   d. Chromosomal study
   e. Fluorescent treponemal antibody absorption test for syphilis
   f. Appropriate testing for mucopolysaccharidosis

From Mencher and Gerber (eds.) (1978). Early Diagnosis of Hearing Loss (NY: Grune and Stratton).

erative; some are not. Among those that are degenerative, some appear within the first weeks of life, and some not until much later. Some children with hereditary degenerative hearing losses appear, at first, to have no hearing loss, but become quite profoundly impaired.

Congenital hearing losses that are not genetically based are equally variable. Hearing impairment consequent to prenatal viral diseases is usually very severe. For example, audiograms associated with prenatal rubella have sometimes been called "corner audiograms" because the only responses are in the lowest frequencies and at the highest intensities. In comparison, hearing losses associated with some prenatal familial dispositions, such as diabetes or thyroid diseases, are not as severe. The point is that it is not easy to predict the severity or extent of a congenital hearing loss. To every rule, there is an exception. The only constant is that genetically based hearing losses appear with equal severity in both children and adults. Furthermore, in spite of, or perhaps because of, the variety of conditions, audiometric patterns, and causes for hearing losses within this group of disorders, there seems to be little, from an audiological view, to distinguish congenital from acquired hearing impairment.

There is a set of audiological diagnostic tests and procedures that, when used together, should result in a comprehensive auditory assessment of a suspect infant (Gerber and Mencher, 1978). Obviously, the age and physical condition of the patient, as well as the information available from and about the family, and the type and degree of any hearing loss, will influence which procedures will yield what information, and under which conditions. The results of the assorted special audiological tests should be consistent with each other and with the audiometric contour. As with other forms of cochlear pathology, a patient with a congenital hearing impairment may display the phenomenon known as recruitment (see Chapter 11) or abnormal sensitivity to changes in loudness, and therefore the examiner must be aware of its possible presence during testing procedures (and during rehabilitation, particularly if recommending amplification). Finally, audiological procedures must be considered simultaneously and in conjunction with the medical steps outlined earlier. An audiological battery should include the following:

1. An extensive behavioral history by parental report
2. Observations of behavioral responses to appropriate auditory stimuli
3. Visual reinforcement audiometry (where age appropriate)
4. Acoustic immitance measurements (including tympanometry, acoustic reflex, and static compliance)
5. Electric response audiometry (as indicated)
6. Otoacoustic emissions

## *Comment*

For most profound losses, test procedures will be at the limits of the clinical audiometer. However, some caution should be exercised in this regard. When dealing with a patient who cannot respond to any of the sounds an audiometer can generate, one cannot conclude that there are no sounds to which the patient responds. The only safe conclusion is that the equipment cannot generate sounds to which the patient can reply. Expectations that speech reception and speech discrimination scores be consistent with pure tone audiograms, to the same extent expected in an adult with an acquired hearing impairment, must also be tempered with reality. Audiometric data should not lead to the assumption that a profoundly hearing-impaired patient should not be provided with amplification. The fact that an audiogram is not acquired in the usual manner does not preclude a hearing aid evaluation. There is often great success in providing amplification to very, very young hearing-impaired infants who do not display auditory behavioral responses. Further, when examining and when providing rehabilitative programming, the audiologist must consider all the special problems of someone who has never had any hearing or never had sufficient hearing to communicate aurally.

Finally, when dealing with a child who is congenitally severely hearing-impaired, it is unfair and, perhaps, even unkind, to expect performance beyond capability. Granted, capability should change with habilitation, but there is no question but that spoken English is equivalent to a foreign language to such a child. The language of signs is the native language of most congenitally deaf. Total communication that incorporates signing and oral language represents a bridge between languages. It behooves the professional to deal with patients in the language of their choice, and not the clinician's. This should not be construed as argument for or against oral language, sign language, or total communication. It should serve only to remind the readers to start from the patient's perspective, skills, and experiences, not from their own.

*C h a p t e r* **9**

# Acquired Hearing Impairment

Consider again that 1 in 1000 to 1200 births results in an infant with a profound hearing impairment, and that 1 in 400 or fewer infants is born with some lesser degree of hearing impairment (Carrel, 1977). On the other hand, in the United States alone, there are about 10 million people of all ages with sufficient hearing impairment to cause some degree of disability. Clearly, the vast majority of hearing-impaired people became that way postnatally. The rate of increase throughout each decade of life in the number of people with hearing loss is really rather astounding.

First is a group of children with a hearing impairment that is apparently of latent onset, but occurs so early in life that it has the same effect as deafness at birth. Second, at any given moment, as many as 5 or 6 percent of the school age population have a hearing impairment, although usually conductive and therefore usually treatable medically. Third, and finally, is a vast group of children and adults with adventitious or acquired hearing impairment. Many impairments arise from the same kinds of things that cause congenital deafness. Still others are related to systemic disturbances, diseases (viral or bacterial), or degenerative disorders. Some of the losses are idiopathic, that is, they are said to cause themselves. That term usually is used because the problem has no clearly known or discoverable cause. On the other hand, some of the hearing losses have rather obvious causes including drugs (ototoxicity), noise (trauma), and age (presbycusis).

Of course, there are individuals who, in addition to the typical middle ear problems, also have an acquired sensorineural loss due to one of the various disease processes. The reader is reminded of the temporal bone study of Lindsay and Matz (1966) that describes a child who had fever and subsequent hearing impairment overlaid upon what may have been an existing congenital sensorineural hearing loss. She wore hearing aids and seemed to do quite well with them. Tragically, she was killed in an automobile accident. A local physician sent her temporal bones for investigation. The studies revealed that the child had abnormal cochleae and there was a "healed stage of degeneration . . ." In other words, it was not possible to separate congenital pathology present before her exposure to disease to what was a result of the disease.

The effects upon the cochleae were similar. From a clinical perspective, that can mean that the auditory behavior of an acquired loss is not very different from that of a congenital loss, and the audiological treatment thus may be similar. That concept is further exemplified in this chapter. It is important for the reader to understand that the overt results of systemic disturbances, diseases, and hereditary degenerative disorders, all acquired, are often quite similar and difficult to tell apart, and therefore lend themselves to combined study. Consequently, they are considered together in this chapter. On the other hand, ototoxicity, noise trauma, and presbycusis, each with its own special effect on hearing, are reviewed independently in following chapters.

## Tinnitus and Recruitment

The two most typical characteristics associated with all acquired sensorineural hearing losses are tinnitus and recruitment. Tinnitus is the sensation of noise or ringing in the ear. Recruitment is an abnormal sensitivity to loudness changes. Both require detailed explanations to understand their relationship to sensorineural pathology.

### Tinnitus

Tinnitus is a term commonly used to describe noise in the ear. Different people describe the sound differently; some patients describe ringing, some report noise, some report whistling, and some will say that it "Sounds like . . ." Tinnitus is a symptom that appears when internal sounds are subjectively louder than environmental or external noises. Tinnitus can interfere with pure tone audiometry, particularly when the patient cannot discriminate the sound of the audiometer from the sound of the tinnitus. Special precautions or instructions may be needed. The specific cause of tinnitus is unknown, but certain hypotheses are tenable under certain circumstances. For example, tinnitus following exposure to intense noise may be a sign of auditory fatigue, and tinnitus following a blow to the head may indicate compression of a blood vessel. If the tinnitus is the sign of a disease, it may disappear with cure or relief of the problem, although frequently it does not.

It has been suggested that tinnitus is of two general classes: vibratory and nonvibratory. The first, vibratory, appears when the underlying etiology originates from outside the patient. Noise is the obvious example; head trauma is another. On the other hand, nonvibratory tinnitus appears when the cause is due to disease, or drugs, or some other internal (e.g., metabolic) process. The distinction could be important for diagnosis. For example, if the patient reports a whistling sound, then one would lean toward an impression of nonvibratory tinnitus and seek diagnosis among disease or other toxic processes. The next chapter describes the tinnitus that is expected to be an adverse by-product of some medications. If, on the other hand, the patient reports noise that sounds like water running, one might look for pathology within the middle ear space. Why? If the patient has had a blow to the head, it is possible that a blood vessel passing through the middle ear has become constricted, or pinched, between the bones. Sometimes patients may correctly claim that they are able to hear their pulse. A constricted blood vessel might indeed be heard.

Tinnitus is said to be objective if people other than the patient also can hear it. That is a very rare phenomenon, indeed. Although recently, a case of objective tinnitus was referred by a neurosurgeon to a local clinic because of concern about the validity of the complaint. The patient had incurred a stenosis (narrowing) of the jugular vein on one side, and she (and the examiners) could hear her pulse at her ear on the affected side. A low-power hearing aid was recommended to serve as a masker, that is, to mask out the internal noise by amplifying external sounds. But it was not a satisfactory solution. The patient was not hearing impaired and did not need a hearing aid. The solution lay in the hands of the neurosurgeon who ligated the jugular vein and cut out the stenotic part. The tinnitus disappeared.

Everyone seems to experience tinnitus some time. It is common to hear someone say, "My ears are ringing; someone must be talking about me." Of course, gossip isn't the reason for tinnitus. However, persistent tinnitus should alert the examiner to look farther. Sometimes, tinnitus may be an indication of auditory fatigue; the hair cells responding to abuse. People who are exposed to high levels of noise, whether in noisy occupations or at rock concerts, frequently report the presence of tinnitus for some hours or even days afterward. They often experience a temporary threshold shift accompanied by tinnitus. This is an early warning sign that hearing is being lost by trauma to the ear. One is losing auditory sensitivity.

Noise exposure is not the only case in which tinnitus is an early warning sign. It may be a precursor to drug-induced hearing impairment, hearing loss caused by active disease processes or central pathology, an increase in tinnitus reflecting the metabolic processes associated with aging, or it may show a lifetime of noise exposure, or other difficulties. The point is, tinnitus occurs commonly; persistent tinnitus is not normal; and the astute diagnostician uses the patient's description of the tinnitus as a guide to further testing. The diagnostic clinician must not forget, however, that for many patients, tinnitus is severe and disabling. Management is also a critical element. Generally, it involves reassurance, an explanation as to the cause, and the use of behavioral therapies to control response. Hazell (1990) has had particular success with his patients by retraining them to perceive the tinnitus sound as nonthreatening. Other clinicians recommend their patients use a tinnitus masker, although the evidence on the overall success of that instrument is still pending.

## *Recruitment*

Recruitment is the abnormal growth of loudness such that when sound levels exceed the threshold of hearing, they abruptly become too loud. Recruitment of loudness refers to a condition of the cochlea that makes intense sounds abnormally loud to the patient who cannot hear sounds at moderate or lesser intensities. This can be an exceedingly annoying condition. The familiar story of the person who says, "Speak up, I can't hear you," and then says, "Don't shout at me" is an excellent example of the phenomenon. The sounds of the environment tend to be either not loud enough or too loud. Recruitment is a frequent concomitant of all sensorineural hearing losses, but especially ototoxic hearing impairment. What is the basis for the phenomenon of recruitment? The evidence is not entirely clear, but a physiologically based model of recruitment employs the notion of spread of excitation along the basilar membrane (Gulick, Gescheider, and Frisina, 1989; Ward, 1973). This notion suggests that, when intensity is sufficient to stimulate hair cells adjacent to the damaged area, neural excitation will be initiated because healthy hair cells in that adjacent area will fire. As the signal level continues to increase, more and more of the unaffected area's sensory units will be excited as the displacement of the basilar membrane gets broader and broader. DeBoer (1967) and Evans and Wilson (1977), among others, gave credence to this model of recruitment when they found no evidence under various conditions of lateral inhibition on the basilar membrane.

There is no concrete evidence linking recruitment with specific pathologic disorders, although the phenomenon is always associated with cochlear pathology. Management is quite difficult because the patient's tolerance for loudness changes is quite restricted. Patients suffering from recruitment typically are the most difficult to fit with a hearing aid and are the least satisfied hearing aid users. Devices with a limited dynamic range, clipping, and careful amplification settings for the various frequencies involved can be used. However, these patients require the most time and care during the fitting.

## Acquired Disease

### Viral Diseases

The relative significance and the danger to the hearing mechanism associated with the so-called diseases of childhood vary somewhat, and the effects of individual disease may differ prenatally from postnatally. For example, rubella is less significant as a cause of acquired deafness postnatally than prenatally. On the other hand, measles (rubeola) has a far greater significance postnatally. Many years ago, McCabe (1963) determined that measles was the most common cause of acquired hearing loss among children in residential schools for the deaf. Of course, this is no longer true, primarily because of immunization programs against viral diseases of childhood. Children are now routinely inoculated against rubella, rubeola, diphtheria, mumps, tetanus, pertussis, influenza, and poliomyelitis; and now varicella (chicken pox). Nevertheless, people still do develop these diseases and do incur hearing losses subsequent to them. No matter which viral disease is the cause of deafness, the mechanism, the destructive pattern, and the auditory consequences are essentially the same (Figure 9-1). The organ of Corti is affected primarily at the basal turn; individual hair cells are severely damaged or missing. The stria vascularis may become atrophied. The tectorial membrane appears shrivelled or rolls up. Finally, Reissner's membrane may completely collapse to the point that it attaches itself to the basilar membrane.

#### Cytomegalovirus

Cytomegalovirus was discussed in the previous chapter as a rather common cause of congenital deafness. It is the most common viral disease among the newborn (Sever, 1983) and the most common viral cause of mental retardation. It is, moreover, one of the most common viral diseases of the human species: eighty percent of the population of the United States carries cytomegalovirus antibodies by the age of thirty-five to forty years (Marx, 1975). However, in contrast to the other destructive viruses to be discussed in this section, cytomegalovirus is an excellent example of a virus that can be quite destructive to the fetal ear during formation, but has no effect upon the normal functioning ear after birth. Evidence shows that cytomegalovirus does not produce impaired hearing after the age of three weeks (Johnson, 1986). Apparently, there has not been a single reported case of cytomegalovirus deafness in a child past that age, even though the virus can be transmitted in breast milk.

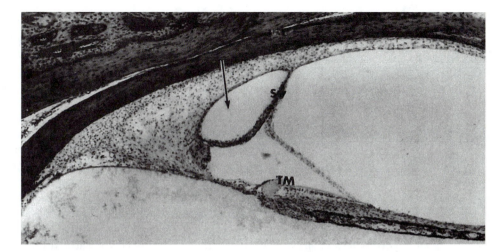

**FIGURE 9-1    Destruction of the cochlea resulting from a virus attack (rubella) during pregnancy. Note how the stria vascularis (SV) and tectorial membrane are misplaced. (Hemenway, Sando, and McChesney,** *Arch Klin Exp Ohren Nasen Kehlkopfheilkd* **193:287, 1969).**

### Mumps

Mumps (myxovirus parotidis) has been, historically, quite a common contagious disease. Transmitted by close contact with the patient, it is not as contagious as measles or rubella. The period of risk extends from a few days before the onset of the first symptoms until the swelling of the parotid gland has disappeared. Like cytomegalovirus, mumps may be silent, that is, without symptoms. In fact, only about two-thirds of the patients who become infected with mumps virus manifest the disease. The disease focuses on the parotid glands, structures located below and in front of each ear. These salivary glands were called "tumors near the ear" by the ancient Greeks. When the virus inflames the parotid gland, it may enter the inner ear by infiltrating through the internal auditory meatus. When it does, it can cause extensive damage to the organ of Corti and associated structures. Consequently, the mumps virus is a well-known cause of sensorineural hearing loss in childhood, although it can have the same effect in adults. Actually, any of the so-called diseases of childhood (which are not limited to children) may lead to a viral labyrinthitis. Chicken pox, the common cold, and such things as influenza and poliomyelitis, like mumps, are produced by viruses that may attack the inner ear. Measles was once the most frequent cause of virally produced severe hearing impairment (McCabe, 1963). Antibiotic drugs, in general, are ineffective against viruses. Consequently, there is little that can be done to cure the problem during the acute stage of these diseases, although drug therapy may be used to prevent further associated infections.

The phenomenon of severe to profound unilateral hearing loss is peculiar to mumps among all acquired hearing impairments associated with viral disease. That is because the focus of the disease is the parotid gland and not the entire body. Thus, it may limit its attack to one parotid gland rather than both. If it does, and it enters the ear on that side only, the result is a unilateral profound hearing impairment rather than a bilateral one (Ruben, 1972).

Conversely, even if both parotid glands are involved, the disease can lead to a unilateral profound loss if the course of the disease leads to that pattern. Consequently, when a clinician is faced with a patient who has an evident severe unilateral hearing loss, the question of mumps should be first to arise.

A typical example of mumps is a case of a young teacher who contracted from her pupils bilateral mumps that resulted in a mumps endolabyrinthitis. Ms. D., age twenty-seven, reported a severe hearing loss in her left ear following an illness she described as "swollen glands." This was medically diagnosed as mumps. She had no family history of hearing loss and was in otherwise good health. Both air and bone conduction thresholds in the right ear were within normal limits. Air conduction thresholds in the left ear ranged from normal at 250 Hz to a profound loss at 8000 Hz (Figure 9-2). Bone conduction thresholds followed the configuration of air conduction thresholds. Testing of the left ear was done with appropriate masking noise presented to the right ear.

Speech reception thresholds were consistent with pure tone averages: -5 dB on the right and 65 dB on the left. Speech discrimination scores were 98 percent at 40 dB SL on the right, but only 52 percent at the same sensation level on the left. A Type A tympanogram with stapedial reflex thresholds within normal limits was recorded from the right ear. A Type A tympanogram was also recorded from the left ear, but stapedial reflex thresholds appeared at lower sensation levels than expected (35 dB SL), suggesting the presence of recruitment.

Because the overall results suggested one perfectly normal ear and one ear with a permanent severe to profound sensorineural hearing loss, and the woman has just completed a confirmed case of mumps, the diagnosis was established as moderate to severe sensorineural

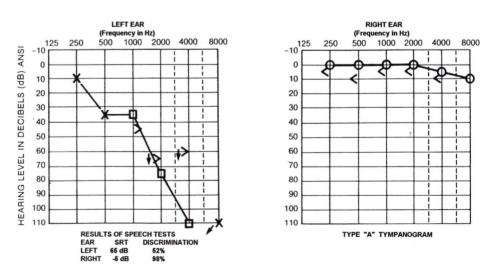

**FIGURE 9-2    Audiogram, left ear of post myxovirus parotidis (mumps) patient.**

hearing loss secondary to myxovirus parotidis. In cases of acquired loss, a course of monitoring audiometry is indicated to aid in the differential diagnosis, to track any progression, and, of course, to plan rehabilitation. Unilateral hearing losses, in which the other ear is normal, usually do not require intensive auditory rehabilitation. Therefore, it was recommended that Ms. D. return for a follow-up evaluation in six months to be certain that her hearing was not deteriorating.

The clinician should enquire about mumps in every patient who complains of a unilateral hearing loss. However, deafness of sudden onset due to vascular disease or accident may also be unilateral. In addition, some of the degenerative genetic disorders sometimes appear unilaterally. Syphilis, too, may present with a unilateral impairment, but the loss soon becomes bilateral. More on those phenomena as the disease processes are reviewed and considered elsewhere in the book.

### Acquired Immunodeficiency Syndrome

Acquired immunodeficiency syndrome* caused by the human immunodeficiency virus (HIV) threatens to produce the worst epidemic in the history of the human species. It must be clear that HIV and AIDS are not the same thing. HIV is the microbe that produces AIDS. A patient may carry the HIV, that is, be HIV+, and not have AIDS. Moreover, some people who are HIV+ never express AIDS, although most do.

Since the first description of the acquired immune deficiency syndrome in adults (Centers for Disease Control, 1981a, b; Gottlieb, Schroff, and Schanker, 1981), followed by initial reports of its appearance in children (Simonds and Rogers, 1992), AIDS has shown itself to be a disease with multifaceted clinical manifestations. Now approaching 2 million cases in the United States, the effect of the virus on the central nervous system (*neurotropism*) and in the immune system (*lymphotropism* and *immunodepression*) have challenged otorhinolaryngology, audiology, speech–language pathology and others concerned with hearing, voice, language, and communication. The problem recently has been compounded as we have begun documenting a growing pattern of otolaryngologic structure involvement.

The HIV, first identified by Luc Montagnier of the Pasteur Institute in May 1983, is a RNA retrovirus whose genome has been well characterized (Flower and Sooy, 1987). The viral particle includes regulatory genes for the replication and the pathogenic actions of the virus. HIV has a selective tropism for T4 cells—the helper–inducer subset of T-lymphocytes that express the CD4 phenotypic marker (Fauci, 1988) and are a critical inducer of most immunogenic functions. The resulting depletion causes a profound impairment in the individual's immune system. So far, the amazing genomic characteristics of the virus, its high mutability rate, and our lack of understanding of how it works and what cofactors trigger the replication phase, have frustrated efforts to produce a useful vaccine or to generate more antiviral effective agents.

Up to 20 percent of patients with AIDS have neurologic involvement as a presenting symptom (Berger, 1987). Because over 90 percent of autopsies in AIDS patients show central nervous system abnormalities (Koralnik, Beaumancir, and Hausler, 1990), a great deal has

---

*The authors gratefully acknowledge use of materials provided by Dr J.J. Madriz and Dra. G. Herrera, Ministry of Health, Costa Rica, which were included in an article printed in September 1995 in the Journal of the American Academy of Audiology.

been learned about the structural–functional correlation that results from cerebral damage due to polyneuropathy, vascular myelopathy, opportunistic infections, and AIDS encephalopathy. One of the most fearsome consequences of HIV is brain destruction and, at the end, dementia is a common outcome in adults (Ollo, Johnson, and Grafman, 1991). Estimates of the frequency and degree of motor, cognitive, and behavioral abnormalities in adults with AIDS vary widely in the literature (32–78 percent), while in asymptomatic HIV+ individuals, cognitive abnormalities tend to fall to 5 to 20 percent (Goethe, Mitchell, and Marshall, 1989).

AIDS is becoming a disease of children. Madriz and Herrera (1992) used the acronym PAIDS to indicate pediatric AIDS. The Centers for Disease Control (CDC) of the United States defined PAIDS as any incidence of AIDS appearing before thirteen years of age. However, the largest proportion of PAIDS patients expressed the disease at a much earlier age. The CDC reported that 1988 saw the smallest increase ever of new cases of AIDS (9 percent). However, that year also witnessed a 47 percent increase in the incidence of PAIDS. The actual number of cases remains small but continues to increase on an annual basis. Most of the children with PAIDS probably were born HIV+. About 80 percent of them have parents who are or were intravenous drug users. There is a slight preponderance of males and a large preponderance of black children. If a mother is HIV+, one cannot accurately determine if her child is HIV+. For at least the first three postpartum months, the baby could carry the mother's HIV antibodies. It seems that, after that time, some 30 to 50 percent of the children will display their own antibodies; that is, if they are HIV+, and most of them will eventually express PAIDS.

In children, although the fatal element is immunodeficiency, brain involvement continues to develop slowly. There is no latent or dormant period for the virus (Ho, 1992). HIV is working silently within the infected cells with a low rate of duplication. What is yet to be determined is what causes the phenotypic change and acceleration of the replication rate that leads to immunosuppression. It is now clear that AIDS is a primary viral phenomenon and only secondarily an immunologic event (Ho, 1992).

It is important to note that AIDS is neurotropic as well as immunotropic. The consequences of PAIDS to communicative behavior in general and auditory function in particular are massive. Although AIDS is a fatal disease, these children may live with the disease for some years. A congenital or early-appearing encephalopathy, with its expected consequences, is virtually universal. Kastner and Friedman (1988) predicted that PAIDS will eventually become as common a cause of mental retardation as Down syndrome and fetal alcohol syndrome. Apparently the encephalopathy has two forms, one static and one regressive. In the first case, the infected child fails to achieve expected developmental milestones; in the second case, the child seems to lose the milestones already achieved. Studies of neuropathology correlate with the behavioral findings (Epstein, 1986). The first group displays microcephaly; the second displays an apparent shrinking of cerebral tissue. In either case, however, the child will eventually have developmental delays or disabilities with obvious communicative consequences.

General otolaryngologic manifestations of HIV and AIDS in both children and adults are directly related to abnormal immune response and/or a central nervous system and auditory pathway disruption caused by the disease process. For example, patients are seen with neck masses, mucocutaneous candidiasis, epiglottal disease, parotid enlargement, and Kaposi sarcoma to name a few (Sooy, Oleske, and Williams, 1987; Williams, 1987). Cytomegalovirus infections involving the larynx and causing a voice disorder requiring a differential diagnosis have been reported (Marelli, Biddinger, and Gluckman, 1992).

Otologically, patients also complain of hearing loss, otalgia, otorrhea, vertigo, and tinnitus (Kohan, Hammerschlog, and Holliday, 1990). Common findings also include various forms of otitis media. Williams' (1987) reported that 90 percent of his patients were microsomic, while developmental delay occurred in 90 percent, and inflammatory ear disease occurred in 80 percent. Probably the most striking blueprint for HIV and AIDS is the presence of *Pneumocystis carinii* in middle ear infection, mastoiditis, cutaneous pneumocystosis, and aural polyps, among others (Coulman, Greene and Archibald, 1987; Gherman, Ward, and Bassis, 1988; Park et al., 1992). More and more frequently other opportunistic infections by unusual agents are described: malignant otitis by *Pseudomonas auriginosa* (Rene, Mas, and Villabona, 1990); necrotizing otitis externa (McElroy and Marks, 1991); otitis media by *Nocardia asteroides* (Forret-Kaminski et al., 1991); otomastoiditis by *Aspergillus fumigatus* (Strauss and Fine, 1991); malignant otitis externa (Rivas-Lacarte and Pumarola-Segura, 1990); otosinusitis by *Candida albicans* (Poole, Postma, and Cohen, 1984); Herpes zoster oticus (Mishell and Applebaum, 1990); and others that involve the nasal and laryngeal system.

HIV does not modify the general occurrence of acute otitis media in asymptomatic HIV+ children, compared with normal children (Principi, Marchisio, and Tornaghi, 1991). However, HIV/AIDS-infected children experienced significantly more episodes of acute otitis media than paired normal controls and asymptomatic HIV+ children. Principi and colleagues concluded that HIV infection does not seem to favor the occurrence of acute otitis media per se, but that it predisposes one to a higher recurrence and to a greater failure rate in response to treatment. The pathogenic reasons for these results remain to be investigated. AIDS-infected children with recurrent otitis media will undoubtedly come to our offices and soundproof chambers sooner or later. Key findings such as *P. carinii or C. albicans* have to be interpreted as diagnostic features in high risk patients. HIV must be suspected and the clinician vigilant. There is an old saying, "If you don't know what you're looking for, you probably won't understand what you're looking at."

One intriguing facet of HIV/AIDS, with only a limited number of formal reports in the literature, is sensorineural hearing loss. Due to its neurotropism, HIV has to affect the auditory and vestibular pathways. Nevertheless, there are substantially fewer reports of this than ones related to other neurologic complications. That may be because clinicians are not looking for it, or perhaps, by the time manifestations occur, the life-threatening condition of the patient doesn't allow for priority status to the symptoms and signs of hearing loss. The potential for ototoxic drug therapy should not be overlooked, particularly as more aggressive treatment thwarts a more aggressive disease process. Audiometric monitoring of AIDS and HIV patients should be part of routine care.

As practitioners, audiologists and speech–language clinicians (and all others as well) must be acutely sensitive both to the needs of the patient and to the risk of the spread of infection. HIV is not an airborne virus, and one cannot "catch" it simply by being in the presence of an AIDS-infected person. It is, however, fluid borne; and this fact demands that we take great care in handling materials that may have been in contact with AIDS-contaminated fluids. For example, what must we do with the earphone cushions that had been placed on that patient with otorrhea? The customary cleaning procedures—soap or ultraviolet light—will have no effect on HIV. A bleach solution works, but that process will destroy the cushions on the earphones. Infection control is essential with any disease, not just HIV or AIDS. Consultation with appropriate infection control centers in the departments of health, hospitals, community health centers, and so forth. will provide the most current and appropriate information to the clinician. This protects the institution, the clinician, and most important of all, the patients. Glutaraldehyde is now being recommended (Ballachanda, Roeser, and Kemp, 1996; Cohen and McCollough, 1996).

### *Herpes*

Herpes virus has several common forms: herpes simplex, herpes zoster, and varicella (chicken pox). In Chapter 4, we described the effects of herpes viruses on external auditory structures. In Chapter 8, it was indicated that the herpes simplex virus obeys the same rules as most other viruses; that is, the effects it can have in prenatal life range from fetal mortality to severe, multisystem involvement (including hearing loss) in a surviving newborn. Damage to the ear also mirrors damage associated with other viral diseases (Figure 9-3 *A* and *B*). Varicella may lead to irreversible sensory hearing impairment; it is uncommon, but it does occur (Lindsay, 1973).

There are, however, other sequelae of herpes viruses, particularly on cochlear and retrocochlear function. Herpes zoster, for example, is an infection of the primary sensory neurons and ganglionic cells. The patient initially feels an increased hypersensitivity and irritability associated with fever and other signs of a systemic disease. A rash or pattern of vesicles may appear. This is often diagnosed as shingles. As the disease progresses, visual tracts become

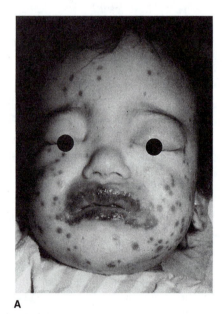 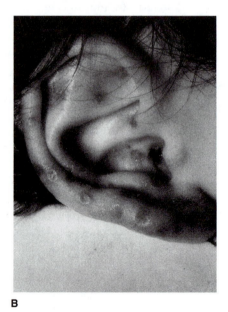

**A**                                             **B**

**FIGURE 9-3 (*A, B*)   Infant with herpes type 1. Note the vesicles around the lips and ears.**

involved and if the auditory system is affected, transmission of signals beyond the cochlea becomes difficult. Tests for central lesions will assist in diagnosis, and, of course, auditory brain stem testing may be affected. If the disease affects the trigeminal and facial nerves (fifth and seventh cranial nerves), an involvement that is common, the speech–language pathologist may see a patient with a motor paralysis of the mandible and masticatory musculature, a pseudobulbar palsy, and/or paralysis of some facial musculature.

## Bacterial Diseases

### Meningitis

Among the most significant diseases that can result in acquired sensory hearing loss is meningitis. But what is meningitis? The brain and spinal cord are surrounded by fairly rigid bone that protects them from injury. Within that bony housing there are three membranes that also encase the brain and cord. The outermost, a strong fibrous structure, is called the dura mater. The second layer, called the arachnoid, is also fibrous, but less so than the dura mater. The innermost structure, quite delicate and filmy, is called the pia mater. The three together form a covering over the brain and spinal cord called the meninges. An *itis* is an "inflammation." Therefore, meningitis is an inflammation of the lining that surrounds the brain and spinal cord. Clearly, any serious infection of the meninges can lead to serious damage to the central nervous system structures beneath. Consequently, the effects of a meningitis, among other things, include deafness, blindness, coma, and damage to motor centers of the brain.

The difficulty is further compounded by the fact that sometimes the expression of the disease is not obvious for several days after it has begun to ravage the body. Thus, it is possible to have suffered severe central nervous system damage even before it is recognized that the disease is present. The initial symptoms include high fever, malaise, vomiting, and in extreme cases, coma. Initially, the patient may appear to have a serious flu and be treated accordingly. If a cerebrospinal fluid culture is taken by spinal tap, the disease may have done its damage before the laboratory can process the results. Finally, since the disease can be either a viral or bacterial type, treatment may or may not be directly effective. Viral meningitis is more frequent than bacterial meningitis, but no matter what the pathogen, it is a very serious disease.

It is the leading postnatal cause of hearing loss among school-aged deaf children (Catlin, 1981). The incidence of profound hearing impairment after viral or bacterial meningitis has been increasing because of the greater number of people surviving the disease. Sometimes, especially in early infancy, the hearing impairment is accompanied by other severely disabling neurological disorders (Robertson and Whyte, 1983). Hence, while the incidence of meningitis may have remained constant or even decreased, the prevalence of sequelae has increased.

According to Hicks (1986), the underlying organism of the disease has a considerable influence on whether hearing impairment will follow meningitis. Of the twenty patients who had pneumococcus, eleven (55%) had sensorineural hearing impairment after recovery. However, hemophilus influenzae is the most common bacterial cause of meningitis, so that ratio is worth noting. Other bacteria causing meningitis had auditory sequelae much less frequently. However, virtually 20 percent of all patients who had meningitis had subsequent hearing impairment. Of course, not only the hearing mechanism can be involved. Sometimes, a purulent labyrinthitis is a consequence of bacterial meningitis; sometimes it is a precursor.

Vestibular difficulties and the severity of the hearing impairment are the most striking things about postmeningitic deafness. It is usually profound to the extreme. For example, the audiograms of twenty-eight children in special classes for the hearing impaired in California were examined and grouped according to severity. The purpose was to illustrate to parents what an audiogram shows and what is meant by such terms as profound, severe, and moderate hearing loss. All the children with profound hearing losses were those who had had meningitis, and all the children who had had meningitis were in the profound hearing loss group.

The disease processes that invade the human body rarely limit themselves to a single location or a single effect. Pneumococcus is one of the best examples of the interrelationship among disease processes. In Chapter 6, purulent otomastoiditis, a bacterial disease, was discussed at length. It differs from secretory otitis media by the presence of bacteria in the fluid rendering it purulent. According to Eichenwald (1979) and Howie (1975), the most frequently found pathogen (35%) is pneumococcus, followed by *Hemophilus influenzae* (29%). Besides the risk to the middle ear, when it is due to pneumococcus or other bacteria there is potential threat of mastoiditis and bacterial meningitis from a simple middle ear infection.

Meningitis acquired from a middle ear infection demands heroic treatment. Characterized by pain in the ear, high fever, and headache, the meningitis must be treated first. Bacterial diseases usually respond to antibiotic treatment if the spectrum of the antibiotic is appropriate and if the individual in treatment has not developed an immunity to the effects of the therapy through previous overuse of the drug. If the prescribed treatment is not effective, alternative programs will be prescribed. In the very rare extreme when the middle ear disease cannot be resolved, surgical intervention in the form of mastoidectomy may be indicated.

### Syphilis

Syphilis (lues) provides a good illustration of a condition that may produce sensory and/or neural hearing loss of delayed onset. Fortunately this disease is now treatable and preventable, and consequently, fewer cases are being seen in our modern, first world practice. Caused by a bacterium in spiral form called a spirochete, the disease can be treated and its spread prevented. Blood tests prior to pregnancy and/or marriage in most Western nations ensure that infected women are aware of their situation and are given appropriate antibiotic treatment during pregnancy to ensure a healthy baby. However, if preventive therapy fails and the disease is transmitted to the fetus, most will die as spontaneous abortions or shortly after birth. If the child survives, congenitally based degeneration of various systems typically begins in the second decade of life, although 37 percent of the cases have been reported to have otologic signs before the age of ten years (Shulman, 1979). There is also a form of congenital syphilis in which symptoms do not appear until later in life. Congenital syphilis may never result in hearing impairment; but, when it does, it is rapid in development. It often starts as a unilateral problem and becomes symmetrical and profound rather quickly. Some individuals, particularly females, and most particularly those who were pregnant, have reported fluctuation in the early stages of their hearing losses. Sometimes, loss of hearing and what appears to be eighth cranial nerve involvement are the first signs of the presence of the disease. The patients are almost always also troubled with vertigo and tinnitus. Therefore, all the signs of Ménière disease or eighth cranial nerve tumor are present. No wonder that this disease has been called "the great imitator." Diagnosis focuses on medical questions related to case history, physical examination, blood serology, and vestibular tests.

If the disease results in symptoms of a latent onset, the process is often degenerative and treatment is, at best, severely limited. One of the most serious cases involved a fourteen-year-old girl who came to a university center complaining of some visual field difficulty and tinnitus. Her audiograms indicated bilateral high-frequency hearing losses starting at approximately 2000 Hz, appropriate speech reception threshold levels, but speech discrimination scores at less than 50 percent. Ophthalmologic studies reported rapid destruction of the optic nerve and impending blindness. Blood tests confirmed the presence of lues disease, which was determined to be congenital. Within one year the young lady was virtually totally blind and her audiogram had slipped to a minimum 75 dB loss at all frequencies with speech discrimination reduced to nearly 10 percent. Note that these symptoms began as mild difficulties around the time of changes associated with puberty. The girl died before reaching her sixteenth birthday.

If syphilis is acquired, usually through sexual contact, symptoms may appear at any time and their rate of progression and severity are highly variable. Syphilis may manifest itself as a suppurative otitis media (otosyphilis), and the syphilis spirochete may find its way to the inner ear. The otitis media associated with syphilis would be treated as a purulent otomastoiditis, in addition to the general treatment for syphilis, which is usually penicillin. Sensorineural hearing loss is less frequent when the disease is acquired. If there is a hearing problem, it is often the product of an associated meningitis or secondary problem. This late stage is often called neurosyphilis.

## *Sudden Onset and Degenerative Disorders*

A significant group to be considered under the general heading of acquired hearing loss is sudden onset of hearing loss (usually for some undefined reason) and those whose losses are due to a degenerative disease that is also undefined. In reality, these are not disease-related pathologies, nor are they acquired in the same fashion as mumps or syphilis. Nevertheless, they do result in hearing loss later in life.

In the previous chapter, it was noted that some genetic disorders are congenital (present at birth), while some that appear later in life are not. The outstanding example is otosclerosis, which is dominantly inherited but does not usually appear until the third decade of life. Furthermore, some forms of so-called early presbycusis (a hearing loss due to aging) are likely to have a genetic component. Some genetically based hearing disorders not present at birth may appear early in life. These are collected under the general headings of early-onset recessive deafness and early-onset dominant deafness. There is some difficulty with the term "early" as it is used here, in that it is not really known at what age the hearing loss develops. Most authorities agree, however, that degeneration is well underway by the time the patient is three years of age and frequently even younger than that. The actual age of presentation then will obviously depend on the rate of progression, with a rapidly progressive condition presenting earlier and causing more problems.

Hearing loss of sudden onset with no known etiology is another of the more dramatic and interesting problems encountered by the audiologist. Goodhill and Harris (1979a) described the problem as an otologic emergency. It may occur as a result of lesions in the internal auditory meatus, cerebellopontine angle, or the central nervous system. Because outer and middle ear obstruction or damage are usually amenable to medical or surgical treatment, those types of lesions are not considered in this section. The discussion here focuses on sensorineural hearing loss of sudden onset (e.g., overnight or perhaps within a very few weeks) and with no apparent etiology.

The etiology of the problem has been variously attributed to viral disease, vascular insult, endocrine imbalance, and allergic reaction. No doubt individual cases result from each of those etiologies. The most prevalently listed etiologies are viral and vascular. In many histopathologic studies, the destruction seen within the cochlea is quite similar to that seen in mumps or meningitis. Mumps, discussed elsewhere in this chapter, is certainly a major contributor. There may be such things as atrophy of the stria vascularis, displacement of the tectorial membrane, or collapse of the cochlear duct (Papparella and Schachern, 1991). Often the disorder is diagnosed as a vascular accident, and the patient is led to believe there has been a small stroke. Although occlusion of a blood vessel of the inner ear by an embolus or thrombus has probably not occurred, the problem may be due to a vascular spasm, capillary sludging, hypercoagulation, or a host of other vascular system disorders. There has been some evidence to suggest that sudden severe hearing loss may be due to a rupture of the membranes within the labyrinth or to a labyrinthine fistula.

Rubin (1968) developed a classification system for categorizing the effects of the disorder based on severity of the hearing loss and audiometric configuration. These classifications range from Type I with a mild low frequency hearing loss, to Type II with a fairly flat 60-dB loss across all frequencies, to Type III that is typical of a severe hearing loss with markedly reduced speech discrimination. The tinnitus and vertigo that often accompany the onset of the disorder and that frequently lead to a tentative diagnosis of Ménière disease, will usually disappear after a week or two. Furthermore, as the disease abates, hearing will often return, sometimes to normal.

Because the etiologies of most of these disorders are unknown, they tend to be nonresponsive to medical intervention. Nevertheless, the audiologist and the otologist have a central role in such cases. If the disorder cannot be medically treated, these professionals must assume a role as advisor, counselor, and referral source. Referral for genetic counseling should be basic. In all cases of adventitious hearing loss, when the medical treatment is completed or not possible, the otologist has an absolute obligation to refer the patient to the audiologist for further case management.

## *Trauma*

Head trauma can result in a disarticulation of the ossicular chain (see Chapter 4). Head trauma that results in fracture of the temporal bone, however, sometimes leads to sensorineural hearing loss. Generally, the head trauma resulting in hearing impairment is due either to a direct blow to the head or to a penetrating wound such as that caused by a gunshot. Clearly, emergency medical procedures are required in either case, and auditory assessment and rehabilitation will be postponed. A common sequela of head injury is a serious dysfunction of language behavior (i.e., aphasia), properly the concern of the speech–language pathologist, but that can be a factor in hearing aid selection or auditory rehabilitation. There is a distinction between the effects of penetrating and nonpenetrating wounds. The distinction is significant not only for language dysfunction but also for auditory dysfunction because penetrating wounds destroy neural tissues whereas those that do not penetrate result in inhibition of function. Penetrating wounds result in language dysfunction more often than nonpenetrating wounds, but those that do not penetrate (such as blows to the head) are more likely to result in auditory dysfunction. Furthermore, nonpenetrating injuries to the head occur more frequently than those that do penetrate.

From an auditory point of view, the primary concern is with blows to the head that fracture the temporal bone (Abd Al-Hady et al., 1990; Ghorayeb and Yeakley, 1992; Liu-Shindo and Hawkins, 1989; Williams, Ghorayeb, and Yeakly, 1992). Approximately 80 percent of temporal bone fractures are longitudinal, and 20 percent are transverse, although they may occur together (Parisier, 1983). The distinction can be acoustically important. If a fracture of the temporal bone runs lengthwise through the petrous pyramid, it is described as a longitudinal fracture (Figure 9-4). Such fractures usually result from blows to the side of the head, or technically, from circumscribed blows to the temporoparietal area. Transverse fractures occur horizontally across the petrous pyramid and typically result from blows over the frontal or occipital areas, that is, blows to the front or the back of the head. A transverse fracture line may be extended through the otic capsule, resulting in injury to the inner ear.

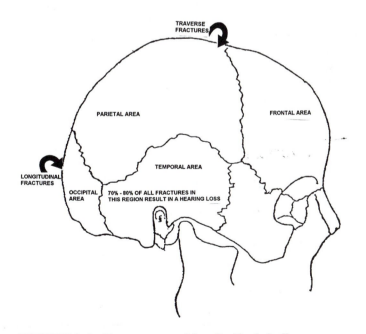

**FIGURE 9-4    Transverse and longitudinal skull fractures and their effects.**

Transverse fractures are more critical for hearing because they may result in profound sensorineural hearing losses and frequent severe vertigo. To be sure, these consequences may appear with longitudinal fractures but they are less common. Electronystagmographic disturbances have been reported to persist as long as eight years after blunt head injury in children (Vartianen, Karjalainen, and Karji, 1985). In addition, injuries to the facial nerve are both more common and more severe following transverse fractures, and such injuries may result in phonologic impairments.

Because head trauma, both penetrating and nonpenetrating, may occur to any part of the head and with any degree of severity, the auditory consequences are equally variable. Such a patient may have a conductive impairment, a sensorineural impairment, or a mixed impairment. A conductive component is found more often with longitudinal fractures, whereas transverse fractures seem to more frequently invoke sensory losses. Jerger and Jerger (1981) report that tinnitus occurs in at least 25 percent of patients with temporal bone fractures, and dizziness may be observed in 45 percent or more of them. Invariably, when cochlear damage occurs, a correspondingly severe sensory hearing impairment occurs.

Sometimes the blow does not result in a direct fracture, but rather what is called the contre coup effect, literally, to "blow across." That is, a blow to one side of the head creates a pressure wave inside the skull that forces the opposite side of the brain against the bone and damages it. This is much the same principle as pushing water on one side of a container and creating a wave that strikes the opposite wall. If the blow is to the left temperoparietal area, the right side may be more seriously affected, or if the blow is to the frontal lobe, the occipital lobe may take the force of the blow. In any case, the effect is just as serious and the consequences for the auditory system just as severe. The phenomenon of contre coup is an audiometric curiosity since it is the only instance in which a bone conduction audiogram can be poorer than an air conduction audiogram in the same ear. This results, presumably, from a failure of the bony labyrinth to vibrate and compress the labyrinthine fluids in a normal manner.

Management of the head injury is primarily neurosurgical. If a hearing loss is present, there is usually nothing that can be done. The otologist's role in these cases is usually confined to treating any coexistent facial nerve palsy or cerebrospinal fluid leak. A facial palsy is usually treated by exploring and decompressing the facial nerve. Surgical repair is required if the nerve has been divided. Cerebrospinal fluid leaks often settle spontaneously. If they do not, the otologist may be required to explore the mastoid and middle ear system to find the leak and plug it. This is most often done using temporalis fascia and local muscle flaps. It is important to keep in mind always that head trauma resulting in brain injury is more serious than just simply an injury to the temporal bone. It was a wise and thoughtful caution offered by Bordley, Brookhouser, and Tucker (1986) who reminded us that serious head injury can pose a threat to life and neurosurgical concerns on possible intracranial injury must take precedence over otologic considerations.

## Hearing Loss Associated with Systemic Disease

All those diseases, conditions, and pathologies affecting the general metabolic system or biochemical homeostasis have the potential to result in hearing impairment. Within this group are such diverse problems as thyroid disease, diabetes, kidney disease, and perhaps one of the best known hearing disorders, Ménière disease. It would be difficult to find a common medical or surgical treatment plan for systemic disorders, as each disease is unique. Diseases of the kidney would most certainly require different management from diseases of the thyroid or of other organs. Therefore, any discussion of medical considerations pertaining to systemic diseases must consider each of the symptoms.

## Thyroid Disease

Thyroid disease offers one of the more interesting and singular examples of an adventitious disorder. Perhaps the best known to be associated with auditory pathology is called Pendred syndrome. A recessive endocrine-metabolic disorder, Pendred syndrome is genetic, and usually appears with deafness and goiter (Figure 9-5). A unique member of the family of thyroid diseases, Pendred syndrome has been the focus of extensive research by Fraser (1976). The peculiarity is that deafness is present at birth or shortly thereafter, while the symptoms of the thyroid disease itself, including the goiter, appear later. Pendred syndrome produces 5 percent of all cases of deafness (Fraser, 1976), most cases with a bilateral loss. There is evidence of progressive hearing impairment in some, but this may be abated by appropriate thy-

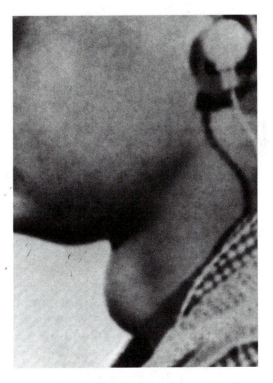

**FIGURE 9-5   Pendred syndrome showing
the goiterous enlargement of the thyroid
gland in a deaf patient.**

roid therapy. In addition to Pendred syndrome, cases of idiopathic hypothyroid disease with similar auditory symptoms and similar responses to thyroid therapy have also been reported (Cotton, 1977). Fraser advised that careful differential diagnosis is essential before confirming Pendred syndrome as the actual thyroid disease or disorder involved. This is very important for appropriate and successful genetic counseling.

## Diabetes Mellitus

Among the other systemic disorders that seem to contribute to or are associated with sensory hearing impairment, one will find diabetes mellitus. Diabetes mellitus is associated particularly with those sensory impairments in which the threshold of hearing seems to fluctuate. In fact, Meyerhoff and Liston (1991) reported that there are frequent findings of fluctuant hearing impairments among diabetic patients. The cause of this is not clear although glucose is required for normal neurologic function. Furthermore, in longstanding diabetes, a microangiopathy develops (disease of small blood vessels) that may also account for the impaired cochlear function.

## Kidney Disease

Another cause of severe adventitious hearing loss is kidney disease. Because the kidneys are required to remove naturally-occurring toxins from bodily systems, it follows that if they fail those toxins will also not be removed from the endolymphatic and perilymphatic spaces. Thus, due to the intimate association between kidney function and other bodily functions, fluctuations of auditory sensitivity frequently accompany kidney disorders. On the other hand, a study by Visencio and Gerber (1979) reported unexpected and unpredictable variations in pure tone thresholds among patients undergoing dialysis treatment for kidney failure. The study correlated auditory function with dialysis treatment and thirty different blood tests. Their expectation was that, as certain chemicals varied in levels present in the blood stream, so would auditory sensitivity. Sometimes it did, and sometimes it did not. Results suggested the function of the kidneys is so broad and so complex that no easy prediction can be made about the variability of auditory sensitivity. The only possible generalization is that hearing impairment should be expected to accompany kidney disease, but the severity of the impairment is not necessarily correlated with the severity of the disease, nor is recovery or relief from the disease necessarily correlated with recovery of hearing.

There is also a congenital disorder known as Alport disease (Alport, 1927), characterized by nephritis (infection of the kidneys) and congenital deafness. The hearing loss is progressive, males showing degeneration faster and more often than females. The disease is often fatal. Nevertheless, amplification and rehabilitation offer support. Constant monitoring of hearing is required as the disease reaches various stages of progression and stabilization.

## Multiple Sclerosis

Multiple sclerosis is an excellent example of a group of demyelinating diseases that may affect the auditory and vestibular pathways. The disease usually first appears in young people in their late teens or twenties or thirties. It is characterized by widespread patches of demyelination that seem to break off and destroy the integrity of the central nervous system.

It usually attacks the spinal cord first, resulting in a spastic paresis of the legs. As it progresses, the disease affects the brain stem and mid brain, resulting in dysarthric speech, hearing loss, and a host of other neurologic symptoms. Known to cause visual disturbances, poor coordination and control of muscle groups, and vestibular difficulties, the disease is characterized by periods of remission and exacerbation. Silman and Silverman (1991) suggested that hearing loss may be both profound and transient, with spontaneous remission accompanying a general improvement of the patient. The cochlear and vestibular nuclei are often the site of the primary lesion if the spinal cord is not attacked first. Consequently, audiometric studies indicate retrocochlear pathology. Speech discrimination scores are lower than would be predicted by pure tone thresholds, as seen in presbycusis, another disorder associated with disintegration of the central pathways. There is no single consistent audiometric pattern associated with multiple sclerosis. However, Strome (1977) cautioned that fluctuating sensorineural loss in a young adult with or without vertigo should suggest the possibility of multiple sclerosis. Conversely, in patients with multiple sclerosis, fluctuant hearing loss is often found.

## Connective Tissue Disease

There is a group of disorders and diseases called connective tissue disease that includes such things as rheumatoid arthritis, systemic lupus erythematosus, polyarteritis nodosa, dermatomyositis, and temporal arteritis, among others. The body essentially reacts with an autoimmune reaction against some of its own structures. Frequently, these patients also demonstrate some degree of hearing impairment that parallels the disease activity. It should be noted that there is a school of thought that suggests that Ménière disease may also have an autoimmune origin.

## Ménière Disease

Ménière disease is an outstanding example of acquired idiopathic hearing impairment limited to the auditory system. Idiopathic means self-originated or of a spontaneous nature coming from within itself. Ménière disease was first described in 1861 by Prosper Ménière, for whom it was named.

Ménière disease is characterized by a unique group of symptoms: hearing loss, tinnitus, and vertigo (a characteristic form of dizziness). Accordingly, the American Academy of Otolaryngology—Head and Neck Surgery (1985) defined Ménière disease as: "an idiopathic disease involving the inner ear as characterized by vertigo, hearing loss, and tinnitus. The hearing loss and vertigo are characteristic. The hearing loss is fluctuating, sensorineural in type, and associated with tinnitus. It is a low frequency, often flat, impairment." All three symptoms must be present to enable a diagnosis of Ménière disease. If all three are not present simultaneously, then the disorder may be something else; although, of course, Ménière disease cannot be completely ruled out. The Academy points out that "additional evaluation may serve to exclude other disorders and facilitate monitoring the course of the disease."

Pulec (1984) has argued that the etiology of Ménière disease is frequently allergic but that other kinds of systemic deficiencies may also cause the disorder. Pulec has also claimed that, in 45 percent of his patients with Ménière disease there was no known etiology (Table 9-1).

**TABLE 9-1   Causes of Ménière disease.**

| Cause | Percent |
|-------|---------|
| Idiopathic | 45 |
| Allergy | 14 |
| Adrenal–pituitary insufficiency | 7 |
| Congenital or acquired syphilis | 6 |
| Hypothyroidism | 2 |
| Vascular problems | 3 |
| Estrogen insufficiency | 2 |
| Combination of above | 12 |
| Internal auditory canal stenosis | 3 |
| Physical trauma | 3 |
| Acoustic trauma | 2 |
| Viral infection | 1 |

From: J.L. Pulec, Ménière disease. In J.L. Northern, ed. (1984). *Hearing Disorders*, 2nd ed. (Boston: Little, Brown).

Ménière disease is characterized by endolymphatic hydrops, a watery swelling of the cochlear duct and vestibular organs. Schuknecht (1975) listed a series of pathologies: enlargement of the cochlear duct, dilation of the saccule, rupture of the membranous labrynth, collapse of the membranous labyrinth, degeneration of neural elements in the apical cochlea, and proliferation of fibrous tissue in the vestibule. In summary, he concluded that Ménière disease is caused by dysfunction of the endolymphatic sac.

The disease may occur at any age but rarely appears before age forty, although it has been known to be present in children and may be considered genetic in some cases (Papparella, 1991). The disease is more likely to occur in males than females. It does not occur in black people. Over 75 percent of the cases are unilateral A most striking characteristic of Ménière disease is its cyclical nature. The report of a tendency to feel disoriented is often a sign of Ménière disease. Most patients who suffer from this disease are not affected all the time. They get attacks of hearing loss, tinnitus, and vertigo. The disabling effects of Ménière disease vary with the severity of the symptoms. Some patients are severely disabled; they are unable to walk, unable to hear, and suffer from frequent and violent attacks of nausea and vomiting. On the other hand, some patients have mild, rare attacks of fleeting dizziness, with some annoying tinnitus. Over a period of time, the hearing impairment and the tinnitus worsen, even though they may be relieved somewhat between attacks. Cody (1978) stated that perhaps the most characteristic feature of Ménière disease is a fluctuation of auditory acuity with a tendency for hearing ability to deteriorate. In the majority of cases, with the passage of time (often 10 to 15 years), the disease tends to "burn itself out" and the attacks of vertigo cease although the patient may be left with a marked sensorineural hearing loss.

For example, recently, a hospital clinic reported on one of their patients who had her first attack of Ménière disease in rather old age (over 80). She had no earlier problems of the kind and had no more hearing loss than one normally expects as a function of age. Suddenly one day, she was rendered quite ill with nausea and vomiting and very distressing ringing in the ears (tinnitus). She had frequent attacks of Ménière disease for several months. After that time, she had virtually no more attacks of vertigo and tinnitus, but her auditory sensitivity deteriorated rapidly. About five years after her first attack, she had regained her ability to walk steadily; but she heard very poorly, even with a properly fitted hearing aid. Five years later, she heard virtually nothing, even aided.

Ménière disease has associated audiometric characteristics. Patients with Ménière disease usually have a rising audiogram, that is, one with a more severe hearing loss for lower frequencies than for higher frequencies. In earlier discussions, it was indicated that a rising audiogram with an air-bone gap is a sign of middle ear disease. In patients with Ménière disease, the problem is cochlear (sensory), there is no air-bone gap. As the disease progresses, and the hearing deteriorates, the audiometric contour becomes flattened and then, eventually, falling with greater deficit in the high frequencies than in the lows. That is, after time, the audiometric contour assumes the shape customarily associated with sensorineural hearing impairment. During the early stages of the disease, when the hearing loss is limited primarily to the lower frequencies, the patient has very little loss for speech discrimination. As both the magnitude and configuration of the hearing loss change, so do the speech reception threshold and speech discrimination scores. Other audiological tests are usually consistent with the pure tone audiogram, and results of special tests (e.g., for recruitment) are characteristic of cochlear impairment.

Furthermore, remember that the presenting complaint of patients with Ménière disease is usually one of dizziness. The presence of vertigo is one distinguishing sign of this disorder. If the patient does complain of vertigo, then the vestibular system needs to be examined, and it is frequently the audiologist who does the test. The essential test is electronystagmography. Nystagmus is an oscillation of the eyes from side to side that occurs when a normal vestibular system is disturbed.

Abnormalities of the vestibular system may be reflected in this oculomotor activity and can be measured by electronystagmography. An electronystagmograph is a device that records even tiny nystagmic movements. Many things influence the electronystagmograph: it results from labyrinthine, proprioceptive, and exteroceptive inputs. Hence, the diagnosis of Ménière disease—or, for that matter, any other isolated clinical entity—cannot depend on a single test. Nevertheless, the electronystagmograph is essential as part of the diagnostic armamentarium for Ménière disease. Figure 9-6*A* illustrates how the electronystagmograph is done, while Figure 9-6*B* compares a normal electronystagmograph to one obtained from a confirmed Ménière disease patient.

Ménière disease responds well to any supportive and sympathetic therapeutic approach, regardless of which treatment modality is ultimately used (e.g., there is a strong placebo effect). Treatment can be either medical or surgical and can be regarded as a therapeutic ladder, climbing from the simple to the complicated. Utilizing that philosophy, Goodhill and Harris (1979b) developed a model program for the patient with Ménière disease. They argued that for these patients management is a far better term than treatment. Their management model is based on fluctuation of physiologic changes in the endolymphatic labyrinth, with osmotic, vascular, and endocrine interrelationships. This model of medical treatment leaves care for other physical problems (e.g., diabetes) to the family physician. Goodhill and Harris reported that most patients will respond, particularly as far as vertigo is concerned, to the therapy plan they outlined. They did suggest, however, that surgical management may be indicated if the patient is nonreponsive to treatment.

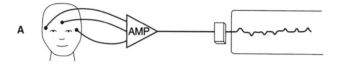

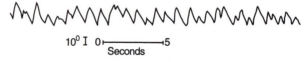

**Figure 9-6 (A) Recording electromystagmography (ENG). (B) The upper trace is a normal ENG; the lower trace displays a caloric response induced by putting warm water into the external auditory meatus.**

Medical management starts with the manipulation of diet in an effort to reduce salt and fluid intake, and strong psychological reassurance. Betahistine, a labyrinthine vasodilator, has been shown to give significant symptom control. Vestibular sedatives are useful for short-term symptom control and are best prescribed to be taken at the onset of any attack. Diuretics are frequently prescribed, but as yet there is no good study to demonstrate any greater efficacy than with a placebo. Initial medical treatment normally provides sufficient symptom control in about 80 percent of patients to avoid surgery.

If medical management fails, the simplest surgical procedure is the insertion of a grommet in the affected ear. This procedure is without logical or scientific support and probably works by placebo effect alone. However, the mainstay of surgery for Ménière disease is decompression of the endolymphatic sac with the aim of treating the underlying pathophysiologic abnormality without destroying the function of the ear, particularly hearing. Decompression is achieved by simply opening the sac or by the use of a shunt to provide prolonged drainage. Although 90 percent of patients report initial satisfactory symptom control, by five years this figure is down to 60 percent. There is some controversy concerning endolymphatic sac surgery. This concerns the Danish sham study in 1981 in which sac surgery was compared to simple cortical mastoidectomy. The study was blind and demonstrated no significant differences between the two surgical options.

More radical surgery for Ménière disease involves vestibular nerve section, which abolishes signals from the troublesome labyrinth while still preserving hearing. Control rates of 90 percent, maintained for up to ten years have been reported, although morbidity is higher because a neurosurgical approach is required. The vestibular labyrinth may be selectively destroyed by the use of ultrasound, but this technique does also risk cochlear damage.

Finally, in those ears with poor hearing, a total labyrinthectomy may be the procedure of choice. This is usually achieved by opening the labyrinth surgically or by direct local application of gentamicin, a highly ototoxic drug.

All of these procedures are unilateral, and thus, the patient usually still has essentially normal hearing in the sound field through the other ear, but has lost localization ability. One can adjust to the loss of that ability and skillfully use the remaining ear. These patients have an excellent potential for normal living.

## *Comment*

Adventitious hearing impairments are as different otologically as they are etiologically. Usually, but not necessarily, postnatal viral or bacterial disease does not lead to as severe a hearing impairment as when the disease occurs prenatally. The major exception, of course, is meningitis, which does not occur prenatally at all, and can result in the most severely disabling hearing disorder. Hearing impairment after viral or bacterial disease is usually unchanging, that is, the hearing loss should not get worse. On the other hand, metabolic disorders (which may also be acquired) often display fluctuant hearing losses. There is also the question of unilateral versus bilateral losses. Most adventitious hearing impairments are bilateral and often severe. Consequently, more than just monitoring audiometry is needed.

The audiometric configuration should be similar in all sensory hearing losses; that is, there is usually a greater loss for the higher frequencies than for the lower frequencies. Speech reception thresholds are usually consistent with the pure tone audiogram. Speech discrimination usually is as good as, or as poor as, the audiogram suggests. In spite of these broad generalizations, however, it must be understood that each disease entity may have its own characteristic patterns. For example, hearing losses associated with thyroid disease may be profound. On the other hand, those associated with kidney disease are as diverse as the patients and as Visencio and Gerber (1979) found, pure tone thresholds in the same ear were sometimes improved by dialysis and sometimes not, and sometimes fluctuated and sometimes did not. More often than thyroid or kidney disease, the most profound hearing impairments arise from viral or bacterial endolabyrinthitis. Sometimes it is impossible to obtain a response from the ear, and sometimes only a corner audiogram may be obtained. A corner audiogram is one in which the only responses are to extreme intensities, usually only to sounds in the low frequency range. Of course, speech audiometry is out of the question in such a case.

Except for Ménière disease there is little that can be done surgically specifically for acquired sensory hearing impairments. They are not subject to surgical intervention, nor are they usually amenable to medical–otologic treatment. Of course, the underlying disease is a medical problem that needs to be treated, and that treatment may have a beneficial effect vis-a-vis the hearing impairment (e.g., as in hypothyroidism). In short, the entire medical, audiological, and psychoeducational armamentaria may be called upon to treat those with adventitious hearing losses. In addition to the specialists needed to deal with the disease processes, amplification, auditory training, speech reading, and personal and family counseling may all be essential. Special education may be required for children, as well as the services of the school audiologist and speech–language pathologist, and related psychoeducational experts should be consulted.

# Chapter *10*

# *Ototoxicity*

The word "ototoxicity" means literally ear poisoning. More specifically, it is defined as the partial or total reduction of cochleovestibular function as a result of chemical interaction with drugs (commonly therapeutic agents) or other toxic substances or procedures. Excluded from this discussion are ototoxic losses in which the toxin itself is part of the disease process (e.g., as in kidney disease). Although over 200 ototoxic substances have been described, there is a small group of regularly used agents consistently associated with toxicity. If a hearing loss has resulted from a drug therapy regime, that loss is said to be *iatrogenic*. This literally means doctor caused (from the Greek *iatros* or physician). The reader should not conclude that a physician would intentionally cause deafness. Unfortunately, often the drugs of choice—almost always in critical situations—are among those that count hearing impairment among their side effects. It is usually a question of saving a life and suffering the consequences.

## *Pathology*

Most of the iatrogenic ototoxins are specifically cochleotoxic, although some are vestibulotoxic and some are also nephrotoxic (dangerous to kidney function). Many are neurotoxic. The severity of any hearing impairment varies from patient to patient depending upon the sensitivity or predisposition of the individual, the size of the dosage and the size of the individual, the method of drug administration, the length of time the drug has been taken, and finally, any previous damage to the auditory system.

The sensitivity or predisposition of the individual is affected by the metabolic rate, previous damage to the renal system, genetic makeup, previous drug exposure, and various biochemical factors too numerous to name. There is strong evidence that the body accumulates drugs of this nature, and it is the total accumulation that is the critical variable. In other cases it may be that when the drug exceeds a certain concentration in the blood stream, effects will occur. To avoid overaccumulation and associated ototoxicity, many patients are given blood tests regularly to monitor the serum level of the drug. If the serum level is low enough, the drug may be reintroduced or continued.

The size of the dose is normally based on the size of the patient. This is predicated on the assumption that a body of a specific size will tolerate a dosage of a certain size. Sometimes, however, a physician may call for an excessive dose in order to counteract a serious threat to life. This is sometimes seen with meningitis in which case the disease can cause far more serious damage to the entire central nervous system than an ototoxic drug can cause to one system. The method of drug administration is also a factor. Intramuscular injections act more slowly than intravenous solutions placed directly into the blood system. Pills and capsules act more slowly than intramuscular injections. Thus, the physician can regulate the dosage by strength (dosage) or time (method of delivery). This combination can help to avoid ototoxic side effects.

Previous exposure to the drug of choice and previous damage to the auditory system by ototoxic substances have been shown to predispose a patient to greater damage. It is usual for the second dose to result in far greater damage than the first, and a third to be far more traumatic than a second, and so on. There are some drugs that act synergistically to produce adverse effects at a much lower dose than either drug alone. One of the best examples of this is the combination of an aminoglycoside with a loop diuretic. The actual mechanism of action of the toxins varies with different agents and is not always clearly understood. Figure 10-1 shows the audiogram and cochlea of a patient who had suffered ototoxicity compared to normal.

## *Drugs and Chemicals That Affect Hearing*

There are seven groups of substances and chemicals that are known to affect hearing and/or the vestibular system:

1. Antibiotics
2. Loop diuretics
3. Analgesics and antipyretics
4. Antimalarial agents
5. Antineoplastic or chemotherapeutic agents
6. Miscellaneous drugs
   a. Antiheparinizing agents
   b. Anticonvulsive drugs
   c. Beta-blocking agents
7. Chemicals and general toxins (mercury, lead, alcohol, etc.)

### *Antibiotics*

Among the currently used ototoxic drugs are the aminoglycoside antibiotics such as amikacin, gentamicin, kanamycin, neomycin, netilmicin, streptomycin, and tobramycin. Note that all these drugs end in "mycin." It is easy to conclude, therefore, that they are all related and of the same general family. That is not the case. The mycin ending merely establishes that these drugs are drawn from a fungus. (Remember, the fungus in the ear canal was called an otomycosis.) Consequently, the reader should not assume that these pharmaceutical products are related in any chemical way. Moreover, there are many -mycin drugs that are not ototoxic.

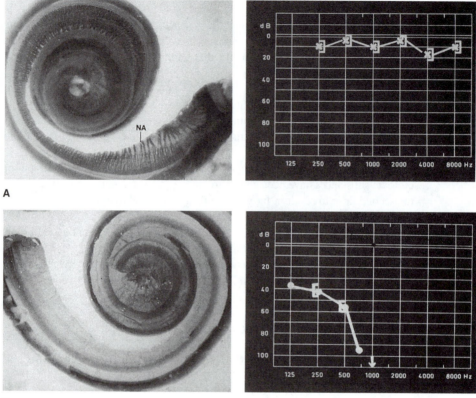

**FIGURE 10-1**   (*A*) **Normal human cochlea compared to a cochlea (*B*) damaged by ototoxic drugs. Note the regular rows of hair cells and the normal audiogram in the normal ear compared to the missing rows of hair cells, primarily in the higher frequencies and how that is mirrored in the accompanying audiogram of the ear exposed to ototoxicity. (Permission by Dr. R. A. Tange; published in *The Inner Ear*, Duphar, 1984)**

Cochleotoxicity seems to be related to the number of free amino groups (-NH$_2$) on the molecule. These are more common in neomycin and kanamycin. Vestibulotoxicity relates to the number of free methylamine groups (-NHCH$_3$), which are more common with gentamicin and tobramycin. However, a report by Jung and Nissen (1991) noted cochlear damage to be greatest with amikacin and gentamicin, with an incidence of about 10 percent, followed by tobramycin and netilmicin (2 percent). Vestibulotoxicity is less common with an incidence of about 3.5 percent for amikacin and gentamicin and 1.5 percent for netilmicin. Ototoxicity may occur as long as 6–12 months after aminoglycoside usage. Secretion and resorption are performed by the stria vascularis. Damage occurs to the cells of the cochlea, in particular the outer hair cells, and to the ampullary cristae and macculae of the utricle and saccule. The degree of damage can be related to the concentration of the drug in the peri-lymph and endolymph. These drugs are excreted by the kidney, and their dose is usually markedly reduced in the presence of renal failure. This process of excretion explains the synergy between aminoglycosides and loop diuretics.

Probably the best known of all ototoxic drugs, or at least the one that has been studied the longest, is streptomycin. It was the first aminoglycoside to be discovered. Strepto-mycin has been, and still is, a drug of choice for the treatment of tuberculosis. Tuberculo-sis, still a common life-threatening disease, can occur in any part of the body (including the ear) except the teeth and nails. Streptomycin, besides being cochleotoxic, is vestibulo-toxic. Consequently, the tubercular patient may report a sensation of mild vertigo, proba-bly with tinnitus, before complaining of hearing loss. Bergstrom and Thompson (1984) observed that vestibular damage due to streptomycin is more frequent than hearing loss. Some years ago, to avoid the vestibulotoxic effects of streptomycin, a drug called dihy-drostreptomycin was developed. It is just as cochleotoxic as streptomycin, but does not produce vertigo. As it turned out, this was not a good idea at all. By removing the vestibu-lotoxic effects, one of the early warning signs of ototoxicity was also removed. Many peo-ple were thereby deafened; and, consequently, dihydrostreptomycin has not been used for many years.

Essentially all ototoxic drugs, including streptomycin, produce tinnitus. The patient is warned to be especially alert to the onset of tinnitus. When tinnitus occurs, and if the patient's life is no longer at stake, the dose is reduced or the drug is removed entirely for a period. The presence of tinnitus and the use of monitoring audiometry influence the extent and degree to which all drugs are used. That is the proper procedure for administration of any known oto-toxic substance. However, as tuberculosis is a life-threatening disease, patients with it and other diseases for which streptomycin is most effective, and patients with severe burns, are still treated with it. A program of monitoring audiometry is essential even after the drug has been withdrawn. It is likely that there will be a latent onset of hearing loss due to the persis-tence of the drug in the cochlear fluids.

Gentamicin is the most widely used aminoglycoside antibiotic and seems to be less ototoxic than streptomycin (Shulman, 1979). However, it is both ototoxic and vestibulo-toxic. Gentamicin and kanamycin are commonly used in pediatric practice as part of the treatment of seriously ill newborn infants. Again, it should be understood that the pediatric community knows that these drugs are potentially harmful; their use is judicious and only when necessary. Consequently, confirmed deafness from kanamycin or gentamicin when the drug was given in early life has been observed only very rarely (Abrams, 1977). The low incidence figures may be related to the possibility that sensitivity to the ototoxic effects of these drugs is something that develops later in infancy (Hawkins, 1975). Although kanamycin crosses the placental barrier, it affects auditory function only after development is complete (Uziel, Romand, and Marot, 1979). Moreover, kanamycin has been known to lead to unilateral hearing impairment. In contrast to their somewhat mild negative effects on children, when used with adults, the ototoxic effects of these drugs are quite striking. In fact, their ototoxicity is so well-established and so well-understood that they are given to experimental animals as part of ongoing investigations of the pathologic effects of ototoxic drugs.

## Loop Diuretics

Loop diuretics are in common use for patients with heart failure and peripheral or pulmonary edema. They inhibit reabsorption of sodium and water in the loop of Henle, one of the important tubular structures of the kidney, and improve diuresis (the flow of urine). Because of that action, they derive the name loop diuretics. Three of these drugs—furosemide, bumetanide, and ethacrynic acid (in high doses)—may produce a reversible high-frequency hearing loss. They appear to act by producing edema and damage to the stria vascularis. This impairs its function and probably upsets the metabolism of the hair cells, although the organ of Corti remains macroscopically normal. Generally, these effects are reversible upon withdrawal of the drug. However, there is enhanced permanent toxicity if these drugs are in simultaneous usage with aminoglycoside antibiotics. The dispenser of any of these medications is made aware by the manufacturer of their potentially adverse side effects. The drugs are used cautiously and appropriately. Nevertheless, as new drugs are developed, new problems can appear. Caution and audiometric monitoring are usually indicated.

## Analgesics and Antipyretics

Aspirin is a common name for a form of salicylic acid and is the analgesic and antipyretic in most extensive use today. An analgesic is a pain reliever, while an antipyretic fights fever. Aspirin appears under many well-known brand names such as Alka Seltzer, Anacin, and Bufferin. Salicylic acid is an ototoxic drug that causes a hearing loss and tinnitus. It appears to be purely cochleotoxic, and recent evidence suggests a direct effect on the outer hair cells. There is no known consistent change within the hair cells or the cochlear end organ associated with salicylate ototoxicity. The effect may be produced by vasoconstriction of the small vessels or microvasculature of the cochlea. Shulman (1979) ventured that the mechanism of the hearing disorder is related to a reversible alteration in biochemical or enzymatic function. This surmise is consistent with vasoconstriction.

Aspirin is rapidly cleared by the kidney, and the adverse effects appear to be invariably completely reversible. After stopping the drug, hearing may improve within 72 hours (Shulman, 1979). It has been reported, on the other hand, that the drug disappears rather slowly from cochlear fluids following withdrawal (Goin, 1976). It appears to take a great deal of salicylic acid to impair hearing, but once again, that is a function of body size, age, and so forth. An excellent example of this is arthritis, a disease for which aspirin had been the drug of choice because of its anti-inflammatory effects and its low risk factor. Arthritics who take aspirin therapeutically consume much larger quantities of salicylic acid than those of us who take two aspirins for a headache. Dosage may equal 2 tablets every 4 hours. Few of them will suffer from ototoxicity, but a relatively high number do report tinnitus.

If a hearing loss does occur, it is usually mild to moderate, rarely exceeding 40 dB. There may be some decrease of speech discrimination ability at the peak of the toxic cycle, but this too will improve upon withdrawal. There are no vestibular consequences. It should be noted that there is the rare possibility of a permanent cochlear effect in the patient who has had salicylate poisoning.

## *Antimalarial Agents*

Quinine was used for many years in the treatment of malaria and is still used today also for the treatment of nocturnal leg cramps. It appears to have cochleotoxic effects very similar to aspirin, except that the hearing loss may progress despite withdrawing treatment and may be permanent. It was thought for many years that hearing loss was a necessary result of malaria. The fact is, though, that hearing loss did not result from the malaria, but from treatment of the disease with quinine and other antiprotozoal agents. Degeneration of the stria vascularis, cochlear neurons, and hair cells has been associated with long-term quinine use. A patient treated with quinine may develop a steep hearing loss with severe impairment limited to the high frequencies (Figure 10-2).

A greater danger is not to the malaria patient, but to the fetus of a pregnant patient given that quinine has been known to cross the placental barrier and to result in severe congenital deafness (Jaffe, 1977). Fortunately, the drug is not in common use today because substitutes have been developed. Nonetheless, the reader should be warned that Quick (1973) reported that small doses of quinine, even in a "palatable gin and tonic" can cause tinnitus in susceptible individuals. Chloroquine, also used for the treatment of malaria, has caused permanent sensorineural deafness. The typical symptoms include tinnitus, ataxia, hearing loss, and blurred vision. Fortunately, malaria is no longer seen to the degree it was just a few years ago, but, by the same token, it is by no means eradicated. The same care and monitoring associated with other diseases are essential.

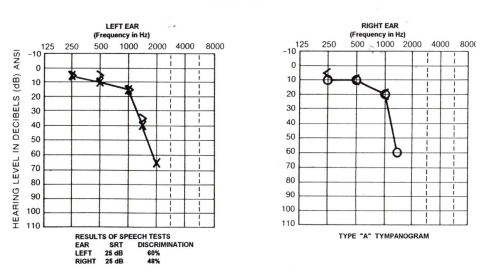

**FIGURE 10-2** **Audiogram of patient with malaria. Patient had been taking heavy dosage of quinine and other medicines for the disease.**

## *Antineoplastic or Chemotherapeutic Agents*

A number of toxic agents are used in the treatment of cancer. By their very nature they are highly toxic to living tissues. If they reach a sufficient concentration in the fluids of the labyrinth, an irreversible hearing loss will result. One of these drugs, cisplatin (cisplatinum) is in common use and its description offers a model of most of the others while simultaneously allowing us to review one of the most potentially ototoxic drugs in current use (Mencher et al., 1995). Chemotherapy regimens using cisplatin have been reported to cure 60 to 100 percent of patients with advanced germ cell tumors affecting the head and neck, ovaries, and other soft tissue areas. The ear appears to be most affected by single, high-dose injections, but the cumulative effect of repeated low-dose treatments has also been noted (Blakley and Myers, 1993).

Van der Hulst and colleagues (1988) reported incidence rates for hearing loss ranging from 4 to 91 percent, but noted that variability is a function of the definition used to define ototoxic change. The hearing loss is usually bilateral and permanent, primarily affecting 4000 Hz and above, although lower frequencies have been affected in some patients. It has also been suggested that patients might develop a base amount of hearing loss, which is unspecified, and which remains constant no matter what the dosage or how long it is prolonged. There are also reports of partial recovery of hearing following termination of drug therapy.

Typically the damage resulting from ototoxicity is to the outer hair cells. However, cisplatin is an exception to that pattern in that it seems to cause exclusive damage to the inner hair cells, leaving the outer hair cells almost completely undamaged. The importance of this finding has not been lost on cochlear physiologists who have developed an animal model to look at the phenomenon and to further investigate the function of the separate inner and outer hair cell systems.

Individual susceptibility to ototoxicity is an ongoing area of detailed study. Preexisting hearing loss, age, and kidney function have been shown to be significant factors in cisplatin ototoxicity. Further, Schwan and colleagues (1992) found statistically significant differences between those resistant and those susceptible to hearing loss for the factors albumin, hemoglobin, red blood cell count, and hematocrit. These results suggest that a patient's poor nutritional and physical condition (something known to occur in head and neck cancer patients) might be associated with greater risk for cisplatin-induced hearing loss. These authors suggest that lower plasma albumin levels may have resulted in higher levels of active cisplatin in plasma, because only that fraction of the cisplatin not bound by plasma proteins is considered to be active in toxicity. They also conclude that red blood cell count, hemoglobin, and hematocrit results in the susceptible group suggest relatively poorer oxygen transport capabilities. This could mean that intervention by blood transfusion, nutritional support, and supplemental oxygen could reduce the risk of cisplatin-induced hearing loss. Clearly, if this susceptibility model is accurate, and was applied to other ototoxic drugs, it could be a valuable tool in preventing hearing loss.

Focal irradiation is a treatment for patients with carcinoma as a supplement to or alternative for chemotherapy, Adverse effects depend upon the amount of radiation absorbed and the quantity delivered. The basic reaction to radiation is inflammation of the endothelium of the blood vessels leading to vasodilation and then destruction of the vascular lumen, resulting in soft tissue that is injured or prone to injury and highly susceptible to infection. It is common for the effects of radiation treatment to be delayed for months or years after exposure. In the ear, radiation may result in inflammatory changes in the skin of the auricle and external auditory canal and in the mucosal membrane of the middle ear, atrophy of the organ of Corti, destruction of hair cells, and atrophy of the basilar membrane, spiral ligament, and stria vascularis (Schuknecht and Karmody, 1965). If bony structures are affected, a necrosis of the outer and middle ear structures including the ossicles is common. Because the focus of the radiation and the dosage level can vary significantly, there is no specifically defined hearing loss associated with these cases (Talmi, Finkelstein, and Zohar, 1989).

Obviously, if the choice is hearing loss or death, use of therapeutic techniques that may result in hearing loss is more understandable. A keen awareness of acceptable levels of exposure is necessary to reduce risk, to limit actual loss, and to facilitate management of the patient whose hearing is affected. Given that there is careful monitoring of those exposed to toxic drugs and radiation therapy, it follows that there must be some control over the number of persons developing hearing loss. However, because treatments such as cisplatin and radiation are so effective in limiting the growth and spread of carcinomas, those techniques are in greater use and consequently more patients are living longer. This suggests that it is quite likely that more patients are encountering hearing loss. Unfortunately, prevalence figures are unknown because ototoxicity and radiation statistics on hearing loss are not well kept and cause–effect factors are difficult to interpret. Further, many patients do not survive, and consequently, their hearing losses are unrecorded. Nevertheless, it is clear that ototoxicity and radiation therapy are much larger etiological factors in acquired hearing loss than had been suspected and clearly should be recognized as such. It is vital that these patients be routinely monitored for hearing loss, and that every step be taken to ensure that their prolonged lives have richness and quality as well as quantity.

## Miscellaneous Drugs

There are three general categories of drugs that have been known, on rare occasions, to be ototoxic or vestibulotoxic. Antiheparinizing agents are used as anticoagulants. In particular, they have been used with patients being treated for renal failure, although they can be used in many situations calling for a decrease in the clotting time. Beta-blocking agents are used to block beta-1 and beta-2 receptors that function at the synaptic level. These drugs are used by a variety of medical specialties including cardiology and ophthalmology. Both types of agents have been known to cause hearing loss, but rarely, and only with long-term usage. Another group of drugs, called the anticonvulsant drugs, tend to be more vestibulotoxic, although that is also rare. There is evidence that withdrawal of these drugs will return the patient's hearing to normal (Health and Welfare Canada, 1988).

## Chemicals and General Toxins

Any poisonous or noxious substance is a toxin. So the term "toxin" includes substances occurring in the environment, drugs used voluntarily to alter behavior, and even radiation. Viruses and bacteria are naturally occurring toxins. Other toxins also appear in the environment and find their way into the food or water. These include some metals, airborne allergens, food additives, and environmental chemicals (e.g., herbicides and pesticides). The group also includes industrial toxins such as carbon disulfide, benzene, carbon tetrachloride, and others. Many such substances are neurotoxic, whether or not they have ototoxic effects, and many of them are teratogenic (may cause birth defects). Christian (1983) noted that these toxins place us at risk long before birth and the risk persists long after birth.

Significant among environmental toxins are metals, especially lead, but also cadmium, gold, iron, and mercury. Excessive exposure to lead can result in changes of red blood cells and chronic kidney damage in addition to its well-known effect on the central nervous system. The indirect potential for ototoxicity via kidney damage should be evident. Lead can disrupt renal function and that can impair hearing. Lead is also vestibulotoxic. Furthermore, it has been observed that children unduly exposed to lead are disorganized, distractible, hyperactive, and impulsive (Brackbill, 1987). Lead is ubiquitous: in 1984, 120 million pounds of lead were discharged into the atmosphere in the United States. Most of it comes from automobile exhaust and industrial emissions. These discharges also include other ototoxins such as carbon monoxide. The Environmental Protection Agency, therefore, continues to endeavor to lower lead in exhaust. In California, for example, one can no longer buy leaded automobile gasoline. An American Academy of Pediatrics (1987) policy statement observes that the proper level of lead in blood is zero, none at all. Cadmium has effects similar to those of lead. Used in a variety of manufacturing processes, cadmium finds its way into the air, into the water, and into the food chain. It also appears in cigarette smoke. In addition to the cadmium effects that are the same as lead's, that is, kidney damage and an ensuing otopathology, Padmanabhan (1987) found that prenatal exposure to cadmium produced congenital defects of the outer, middle, and inner ears.

Mercury ranks highest among environmental toxins released into the air by human activity versus that which occurs naturally. It is used in a variety of manufacturing processes, particularly in smelting operations, and finds its way into the soil from the air. In this way, it enters the food chain. Historically, of course, people were known to die of mercury poisoning. Mercury has the same effects as other metals. It is known to lead to hearing loss and to disrupted speech and language function. Moreover, environmental mercury has been a significant cause of birth defects. The mercury in paint is toxic if eaten, and so is the mercury in some species of fish.

Petroleum and petroleum products act in the environment in much the same way as metals: They enter the food chain. Ingestion of petroleum has yet to be reported as fatal, but there are permanent sequelae including effects of neurotoxicity. One study described this group as having "significant CNS depression" (Fazen, Lovejoy, and Crone, 1986). Recently, certain groups have taken to inhaling petroleum fumes for recreational purposes. The effects on the central nervous system are well documented, but there is no report of permanent hearing loss associated with this dangerous and foolish activity.

## Behavioral Toxins

We have coined the term "behavioral toxins" to embrace drugs people choose to take. The group excludes, therefore, those substances taken without choice, that is, prescribed medicines and environmental toxins. In reality, some of the behavioral toxins are medications that are abused: the so-called uppers (amphetamines) and downers (barbiturates). Both amphetamines and barbiturates can be vestibulotoxic, although this occurs far more often with barbiturates.

A greater number of people are affected by alcohol than by the other drugs. Consumption of alcohol, even to excess, can be socially acceptable by certain groups, at least in certain times and places (e.g., twenty-first birthday with the gang at the local pub!). Alcohol is a neurotoxin. It is also an ototoxin and produces vertigo during periods of intoxication. While this may abate with the onset of sobriety, among chronic alcoholics, nystagmus may persist (Jung and Nissen, 1991; Kassirer, 1988). Fetal alcohol syndrome (Figure 10-3) is a term used to describe a baby who has suffered significant congenital malformations and disorders as the result of alcohol abuse during the pregnancy. Counted among the symptoms are low birthweight, failure to thrive, mental retardation, central nervous system dysfunctions, and anomalies of the skeleton and internal organs. Micrognathia, cleft palate, abnormal pinnae, and both conductive and sensorineural hearing loss may also be present (Church and Gerkin, 1987). Thus, alcohol is not only vestibulotoxic to the user, but is life-threatening to the unborn fetus.

Cocaine is fast becoming one of the most serious drug issues in the world today. There is no evidence that cocaine is ototoxic, except as a teratogen. Even in that case, there is no

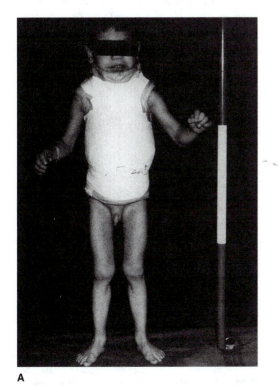 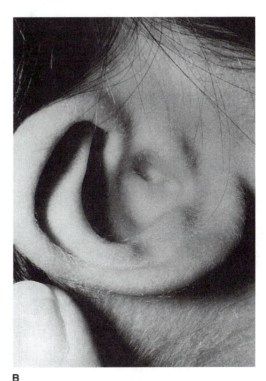

**A**    **B**

**FIGURE 10-3** (*A, B*)    **Child with fetal alcohol syndrome.**

indication that the teratogenic effects of cocaine are necessarily lasting in every patient. We do know, however, that auditory brain stem responses are abnormal in virtually every baby born to cocaine-abusing mothers (Salamy et al., 1990; Shih, Cone-Wesson, and Reddix, 1988). The nature of the abnormality suggests neurotoxicity, but ototoxicity does seem to appear in a small number of these infants. To date the data on incidence are contradictory. However, because there seems to be an increasing number of these children produced, and because they continue to develop and eventually come to school, we should get an opportunity to learn if there are lasting communicative effects. The difficulty with confirming the etiology of any disorders seen with these children is that people who use illicit drugs typically use more than one. In addition, they usually use alcohol, smoke (nicotine may be ototoxic), have poor diets, are not healthy, do not have good prenatal care, and live in poor conditions. Further, these folks are not likely to open up and disclose how much they have taken of what drug and when . . . if they can even remember. For that reason, it is nearly impossible to relate a particular disorder to a particular etiology.

## *Comment*

When it is necessary for a physician to prescribe a life-saving drug whose use could lead to a severe hearing impairment, it is important that the patient have some form of monitoring. In some cases, such as with aminoglycoside antibiotics whose adverse effects are related to the concentration of the medication in the blood stream, this will take the form of monitoring serum levels of the drug. In most other cases, some form of auditory or vestibular monitoring is appropriate. Unfortunately, even a relatively simple pure tone audiogram becomes a major undertaking in a seriously ill patient. It is not always possible to move the patient to the audiology department, nor will the ward environment provide the ideal background noise levels for the performance of a meaningful audiogram. Obviously, the problems are even more complicated for monitoring vestibular function. In the worst situation, common sense and caution are about the best that can be offered.

Hearing impairments arising from ototoxicity are variable in severity but are frequently characterized by tinnitus and recruitment. Withdrawal of the drug may limit the degree of hearing loss. These patients require extensive counseling and support and much patience on everybody's part. That is true at the onset of their hearing loss, during the adjustment to that loss, and finally, during rehabilitation. Without that combination, success will be marginal at best. Audiological intervention includes use of hearing aids that compress or eliminate sound at very high intensities, but provide enough amplification through the normal range of hearing to permit communication. Thus, some rehabilitative relief is offered the patient.

A hearing and speech clinic reported a case of a twenty-two-year-old male enrolled in the second year of the medical school at their affiliated university. The young man developed a bilateral nephrosis, a disease process attacking both kidneys. He became toxic and entered a coma. In order to save his life, his physician recommended a drug known to cause ototoxicity. The options were discussed with the family before administration, and the decision was simply one of survival versus possible deafness. A medical colleague confirmed the diagnosis and the limited options available under the circumstances. The family approved administration of the drug. The patient responded immediately to treatment and was stable and well on the road to recovery within two weeks. Unfortunately, his hearing did not fare so well. He developed a bilateral profound sensorineural hearing loss, responses no better than 95 dB at any frequency. Speech responses were consistent with the pure tone audiogram.

The initial problem faced by this young man was psychological. He could hear perfectly when he entered the coma, and he was effectively deaf when he awoke. He still had all his mental faculties and ambitions, but his goal of continuing in medical school was shattered. He was worried about his potential for a family and for life in general. He became quite depressed and admitted to considering suicide. Initial efforts focused on psychological counseling. In addition, he was enrolled in a group auditory rehabilitation program at the hearing and speech clinic. It was important to work with him to ensure that he did not lose his speech abilities now that his auditory feedback was so severely limited. Fortunately, he also demonstrated excellent speech reading abilities. When he was ready for it, the idea of a hearing aid was introduced and he was appropriately fit. Approximately seven years after the insult, he was an active participant in the hard-of-hearing community and working as a computer programmer for a national corporation. It has taken time, counseling, empathy, a supportive family, and a self-motivated individual to reach this point.

Generally, ototoxic losses are not subject to medical intervention except in those cases in which a cochlear implant is an option. That would be in cases in which essentially all residual hearing was gone from the ear. Deafness caused by such drugs as kanamycin, neomycin, or cisplatin is characteristically profound; therefore, too little residual hearing is available for amplification. The use of a cochlear implant for such patients has been a considerable boon. No claim is made that these implants restore hearing in the usual sense. However, they do allow patients to reestablish contact with the acoustic world. For example, a cochlear implant may allow the ototoxic deaf patient to know if the phone rings, even though that patient cannot use it. An implant may restore the early warning function of hearing. That is, it could allow a patient to hear the siren of a fire engine or the blast of a car horn. Moreover, cochlear implants have been found to be significant aids to speech reading (Rose, 1994). Although there has been occasional controversy over the benefits of cochlear implants, ototoxicity is not part of that controversy. The ototoxic deaf patient is often the ideal candidate for a cochlear implant, and if the success of that implant is measured in terms of awareness of the environment, then the success rate for these patients is very high.

# Chapter *11*

# *Noise Exposure and Hearing Loss*

What is noise? To some it is the sound of a lead guitar. To others it is the whine of a cranky child. To some, the guitar is playing music and the child's cry a pleasant opportunity to express love and affection. In other words, for most of us, the definition of noise depends on our mood, the situation we are in, and the need we have to concentrate on a specific activity without interruption or distraction. But that definition is a psychological one. It is limited to what we think and to what we feel. When we speak of noise and noise-induced hearing loss, however, we go beyond the psychological and move into the physiological. We mean an acoustic stimulus of such intensity and duration that it can do more than create a psychological reaction, it can actually affect the physical structures of the ear. There is little room for subjective interpretation in this definition. The auditory structures are fatigued or damaged or they are not damaged. It does not matter if we like the noise that has caused the damage, such as a rock band using highly amplified instrumentation, or we dislike the noise, even if it is as good for us as an alarm warning signal.

## *Epidemiology*

Noise is undoubtedly one of the world's great health problems and the single most common form of environmental pollution. Today in our industrialized Western civilization, no one is free from the effects of high level noise. That is unfortunate, because noise exposure is as accepted as it is unavoidable, a risk taken for living in a modern mechanized world (even though it is not true!). The problem is further compounded in that there are those who are willing to experience more noise exposure than they should or need to accept. In our society, noise is everywhere. Automobile horns toot at 110 dB SPL. Jet engines scream at us at 120 to 140 dB. Even household appliances (80 dB), road traffic (70 to 100 dB), and our home lawn-mowers (92 dB) reach levels that can be dangerous to the delicate mechanisms of the ear

(Figure 11-1). The irony is that for thousands of years humans lived in an environment that, except for gunpowder and war, was quiet and harmless to our ears. Pliny the Elder, who lived from about the year 23 to about 79 CE, thought it unusual enough to suffer industrial hearing loss that he described a village near one of the cataracts of the Nile in which artisans (probably coppersmiths) became deafened as they plied their trade. Noise-induced hearing loss is a relatively new phenomenon. It is strictly a human-made pathology, and one that can be easily overcome with forethought, planning, and simple care and protection of ourselves and those around us. Audiology as a profession can trace its origins to the effects of the noise of war and its interference with communication. Thus, it is appropriate that it is the audiologist who plays the major role in the diagnosis of the problem, its prevention, and its treatment.

Community noise is a major problem, whether at home or out on the street, and thus there is much to consider when discussing community noise controls that will affect our daily living and the good health of our citizens. Noise pervades our homes as well as our jobs. For example, one aspect of noise that we tend to ignore, and perhaps even consider acceptable, is in the use of certain kitchen appliances. The electric can opener, dishwasher,

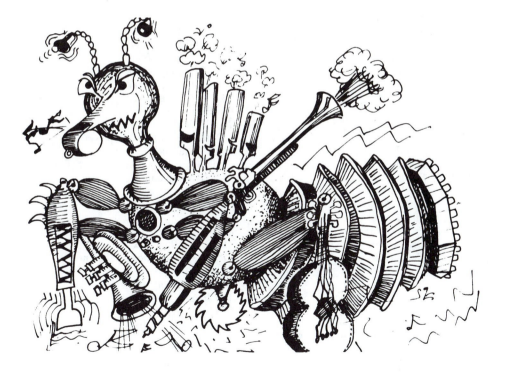

## NOISIUS RACKETUS ( The Noise Bug )

**FIGURE 11-1** **Noisius Racketus: The virus (?) that destroys hearing in the presence of noise. (Courtesy of Dr. David Lipscomb)**

blender, table saw, and electric drill often produce considerable noise when doing their assigned tasks. Table 11-1 lists the sound levels of some common appliances and tools. Because of the high intensity of some of these devices, the U.S. Environmental Protection Agency looked in to home appliances as a source of noise and, therefore, as a potential source of noise-induced hearing impairment. The result was an EPA regulation on the subject providing manufacturers with specific controls. However, most homemakers are unaware of the regulations, and consequently the EPA effort often has little effect upon what happens in the home.

Sometimes economics really overrides common sense. Farmers purchase tractors by the number of horsepower, that is, the higher the horsepower, the higher the price. Mufflers that

**TABLE 11-1    Sound output levels of appliances and tools.**

| Appliance/Tool | Output Level |
| --- | --- |
| Vacuum cleaner | 80 dBA (carpet) |
| Vacuum cleaner | 82.5 dBA (bare floor) |
| Industrial vacuum | 91.5 dBA (bare floor) |
| Typewriter (electric) | 74 dBA |
| Piano | 76 dBA (average level) |
| Organ | 79 dBA (average level) |
| Television | 64 dBA (average level) |
| Stereo | 64 dBA (average level) |
| Stereo | 79 dBA (loud) |
| Stereo | 102 dBA (lease-breaking party) |
| Live rock band | 100 dBA (average) |
| Hair dryer | 88 dBA |
| Food mixer | 84.5 dBA (in liquid) |
| Food processor | 80 dBA (grating carrot) |
| Knife (electric) | 82.5 dBA |
| Shower stall | 72.5 dBA |
| Projector (35 mm) | 61 dBA |
| Drill (electric) | 95 dBA (drilling 2" x 4") |
| Hammer (manual) | 116 dBA (impact noise of nailing) |
| Circular saw | 99 dBA (1/4" plywood) |
| Saber saw | 98 dBA (1/2" plywood) |
| Radial arm saw | 103 dBA (2" x 4") |
| Lawn mower (gas) | 92 dBA |
| Lawn mower (electric) | 81 dBA |
| Lawn trimmer (electric) | 83 dBA |
| Chain saw (gas) | 106 dBA (4" log) |
| Chain saw (electric) | 99 dBA (4" log) |
| Snow blower (gas) | 108 dBA |
| Studding gun | 122 dBA (impact noise of metal or concrete) |
| Automobile | 84 dBA (100 km/hr—windows up, heater fan on maximum) |

With permission of Gordon Whitehead, Nova Scotia Hearing and Speech Clinic, Halifax. This table also appeared in *Acquired Hearing Impairment In the Adult*, Health and Welfare, Canada.

reduce noise levels also reduce effective horse power. Many farmers, therefore, will purchase a smaller tractor than is required and remove the muffler, thus beefing up the power of the unit and defeating noise control regulations. There are similar behavior patterns by others as well. Hunters refuse to wear earplugs because they must hear their game. Given the effects of a shotgun blast on the hair cells and the number of hunters with noise-induced hearing loss, that argument seems a bit foolish. Some municipal agencies (e.g., Boulder, Colorado; Santa Clara County, California) have imposed community noise regulations. However, the few scattered reports are not encouraging, suggesting that regulations are not well enforced. Law enforcement agencies claim that they have neither the time nor the personnel to pursue violators of noise ordinances, and that there simply is not enough public outcry to merit the financial and time commitment necessary for the enforcement of the regulations.

Occupational noise has been with us since the Industrial Revolution in the nineteenth century. Historically, this has been the most quantitively important cause of noise-induced hearing loss over the past one hundred years.

## *Auditory Pathology*

Like all biological insults, the effects on any individual organism from exposure to excessive noise levels are extremely variable and relatively unpredictable, especially at moderate exposure levels. Although many theories and suggestions have been made for this variability, with variations in intrinsic protective responses coming in for recent scrutiny, a satisfactory explanation is still lacking (Henderson, Subramaniam, and Boettcher, 1993). However, there is no doubt that with increasing exposure to excessive noise levels, the occurrence of noise damage becomes inevitable. It is generally agreed that sound levels below about 80 dB are unlikely to cause any damage to the human ear no matter how long one is exposed to them. Sounds of 130 dB or greater will damage the auditory mechanism after very short periods of exposure in almost all repeatedly exposed individuals. Between these two extremes, the safe period of exposure decreases as the sound level increases, although the degree of noise damage displayed by any one individual is variable and relatively unpredictable as a result of natural biological variability (Alberti, 1987; NIH, 1990; Saunders, Dear, and Schneider, 1985).

### *Role of the Middle Ear*

Although the tympanic membrane may be damaged and the ossicles dislocated by a high impulse noise such as an explosion, in general, it is the cochlea that is the site of the pathologic manifestations of noise damage. Unless there is a signal in excess of 160 dB SPL, the middle ear will appear unaffected by the noise (Eames et al., 1975). However, the middle ear does play a significant role in determining the effects of excessive noise exposure. The frequency response characteristics of the middle ear are such that low frequency tones are damped while middle to high frequency signals are transmitted to the organ of Corti with great efficiency. The result is a high pass filter that limits those frequencies of sound that are potentially damaging to the cochlea.

The middle ear reflexes, notably the stapedius muscle reflex, provide some protection for the cochlea by stiffening the response characteristics of the conductive mechanism and, thus, preventing the transmission of sound into the cochlea. However, the attenuation is primarily in the lower frequencies, about 1000 Hz and below. Further, the extent of the reflex is limited, so that the protective function is effective over only a limited range of intensities (Dallos, 1964). Further, the reflex will decay, that is, cease to function in a continuous noise environment. Finally, the stapedius reflex itself is delayed in its onset by nearly 10 ms (Salomon and Starr, 1963), and thus its protection also is delayed in onset. In reality then, the middle ear reflexes offer protection but only of a limited and minimal nature.

In truth, the contribution of the middle ear structures, the pinna, the ear canal, and so forth, in the attenuation of excessive noise, should not be taken lightly nor overlooked; but, at the same time, those structures should not be considered adequate to protect the cochlea from excessive noise or the ear from suffering a hearing loss.

## *Damage to the Cochlea: Temporary Threshold Shift*

Exposure to excessive noise levels of insufficient duration to cause permanent threshold shift (PTS) is likely to cause temporary threshold shift (TTS). TTS is a temporary worsening of the hearing thresholds and is as familiar to most people as tinnitus (ringing in the ears) following exposure to loud noise (Alberti, 1987). TTS tends to be maximal at one half to one octave above the frequency of the stimulating sound (McFadden and Plattsmier, 1982), although that may not be the case for low frequency stimulating sounds (Burdick et al., 1977). TTS increases in response to increasing intensity and duration of exposure in an asymptotic fashion. That is, once a certain degree of TTS has been reached, further increases are so slow that effectively there are no further threshold shifts. This maximal TTS is also thought to represent the maximum permanent shift that can occur at that frequency (Alberti, 1987). It has also been suggested that individuals who have suffered prolonged noise exposure demonstrate less TTS than do nonexposed individuals with the same audiometric thresholds when both are exposed to the identical noise. This may reflect altered metabolic processes (NIH, 1990) or protective mechanisms (Henderson, Subramanian, and Boettcher, 1993). There is also evidence that a combination of sound and vibration will produce a greater TTS than exposure to the same sound alone. TTS by definition will recover and tends to do so in an exponential and predictable fashion. It is probable that repeated exposure to enough noise to cause TTS ultimately leads to a permanent threshold shift. A predictive link between PTS and TTS has long been sought and although a relationship does exist, it is not strong enough to allow predictions of an individual's PTS based on TTS patterns (Burns, 1973; Glorig, Ward, and Nixon, 1961).

Despite many histological analyses, few consistent and definitive structural features have been associated with TTS, although there is some evidence of subtle intracellular changes in the hair cells, a decrease in the stiffness of the stereocilia, and a swelling of the auditory nerve endings. As might be expected from a temporary change, all these characteristics appear to be reversible and can be considered as metabolic exhaustion of the sensory cells (Alberti, 1987; NIH, 1990; Saunders, Dear, and Schneider, 1985).

## *Damage to the Cochlea: Permanent Threshold Shift*

Permanent threshold shift reflects irreversible damage to the cochlea and is invariably associated with structural damage. It appears that the sensory hair cells are most susceptible with initial damage to the rootlet structures that anchor the stereocilia to the cell body, particularly those of the outer hair cells in row 1. With continued exposure, the stereocilia can become floppy, fused, or eventually disappear. These changes are associated with various intracellular changes such as lysosomal and nuclear swelling, mitochondrial changes, and vacuolization of the smooth endoplasmic reticulum. Ultimately, there is cellular degeneration. Once lost, these sensory cells are not replaced (Alberti, 1987; NIH, 1990; Saunders, Dear, and Schneider, 1985). As the damage progresses, these changes spread to involve the other two rows of outer hair cells and the inner hair cells, which are affected along with the supporting cells. More extreme changes include rupture of Reissner's membrane and damage to the stria vascularis (Alberti, 1987; NIH, 1990; Saunders et al., 1985). With loss of sufficient sensory cells, there is often degeneration of the central neural pathways (Alberti, 1987; NIH, 1990; Saunders et al., 1985). Regardless of the frequency of the damaging noise, it seems that in the human it is the basal turn of the cochlea that is most prone to noise damage.

This early susceptibility of the outer hair cells in row 1 is almost certainly due to their position over the middle of the basilar membrane where its excursion and the resulting shear forces are greatest and to their firm attachment to the overlying tectorial membrane. The susceptibility of the basal turn is less well understood but possibly relates to preferential frequency amplification by the external and middle ears of the usually broadband sound. There is evidence that long-term exposure to a tonal sound can lead to a hearing loss at the place on the basilar membrane serving the frequency half to one octave higher, regardless of its position in the cochlea (Alberti, 1987). Figure 11-2 illustrates the hair cell destruction in the cochlea of a patient exposed to an intense noise and the associated audiogram. It shows that there are islands of profound damage where the tissue is missing entirely.

In permanent threshold shift (PTS), as would be expected with an initial loss of the outer hair cells and consequent cochlear fine tuning, one of the earliest complaints is reduced speech discrimination, particularly in background noise (Alberti, 1987; NIH, 1990). This can be measured by a marked reduction in performance on tests involving the detection of competing signals or signals in noise. Any reduction in speech performance is usually out of proportion to the pure tone audiogram. Early noise-induced hearing loss (NIHL) displays itself as a dip in the pure tone audiogram in the region of 3000 to 6000 Hz, which is the frequency range served by the basal turn of the cochlea. However, as the damage progresses, there is progressive hearing loss in the frequencies on either side of this region, with the higher frequencies being more severely affected. Figure 11-3 illustrates a typical audiogram from a patient with a noise induced hearing loss. Note how the noise-induced notch seen in the right ear at 4000 Hz has increased to include a broader spectrum of frequencies in the left ear. Typically, the patient complains of becoming progressively hard of hearing and that progression is usually accompanied by increased difficulty in communication in occupational, social, and domestic environments. This may result in social isolation, domestic disharmony, strained relationships, and depression (Lalande, Lambert, and Riverin, 1988; Stephens, 1980).

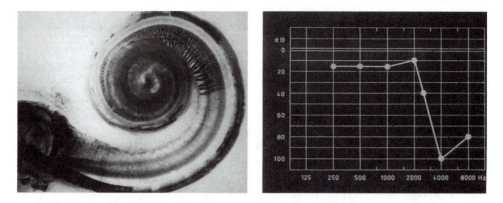

**FIGURE 11-2    Cochlea of a patient with noise-induced hearing loss. Note the rather selective and frequency-specific damage to the hair cells as reflected in the accompanying audiogram. (Permission by Dr. R. A. Tange; published in *The Inner Ear*, Duphar, 1984)**

## Associated Pathology

To this point, only damage to the middle ear and cochlea caused by excessive noise has been described. There is an additional set of pathologies, defined as physiologic or psychologic reactions to excessive noise, which are called extra-auditory effects of noise. These physical and mental health disturbances are well documented and have been clearly described by Cohen (1975), who suggested that they fall into four categories:

1. General stress reactions
2. Physical disorders
3. Mental and emotional difficulties
4. Special problems

### General Stress Reactions

A most obvious general stress reaction to noise is vasoconstriction of the small blood vessels of the extremities that becomes greater in the presence of greater intensity. The result of a constriction of the blood vessels is an alteration of arterial blood pressure. Cohen suggests this is the result of the heart compensating to overcome the constriction. Another stress reaction to noise is an increase in corticosteroids and urine released into the blood. This may signify the release of hormones from certain glands, indicating that the body is preparing a defense mechanism to respond to a threat (Cohen, 1975; Welch and Welch, 1970). In accordance with the bodily defense mode, the respiratory rate often decreases in response to loud sound. We are all familiar with the gasp and holding of breath that accompanies a startle response to a loud sound. However, long-term change in respiratory rate in response to noise is different. There is apparently reduced salivary and gastric secretion

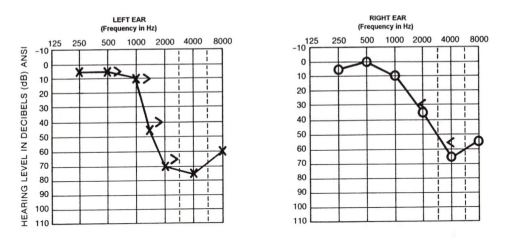

**FIGURE 11-3    Audiogram of patient with a bilateral noise-induced hearing loss. Patient worked in a warship's boiler room and also served in the weapons section.**

production, which means that digestion also is slowed. This may be accompanied by a tightening of body musculature, an increase in general body tension, and alterations in several aspects of body chemistry associated with those actions (Lipscomb, 1978; Welch and Welch, 1970).

## *Physical Disorders*

Within the category Cohen has called physical disorders, lie such serious complications as cardiovascular disease, tissue damage to kidneys and the liver (Zondek and Tamari, 1960), hoarseness and laryngitis from shouting above the noise levels, and equilibrium disturbances (U.S. Air Force, 1966; U.S. Navy, 1957). In 1929, Tullio demonstrated that presenting a high-intensity sound to pigeons could upset their vestibular system and make them fall over. His birds became dizzy and disoriented. The response of the human anatomy to intense sound is similar. Workers often report dizziness and nausea. Occasionally, noise exposure will lead to true vertigo. There is some question as to the intensity of sound required to elicit this response. Cohen (1975) refers to a series of studies (U.S. Air Force, 1966; U.S. Navy, 1957) demonstrating that humans lose their balance in the presence of noise exposure at 125 dB or greater, particularly if the noise stimulation is unequal at the two ears. It has also been suggested that individual susceptibility of the worker will determine the sound level required to trigger the response (McCabe and Lawrence, 1958).

No discussion of the physical effects of noise on the ear would be complete without reference to tinnitus. Most workers initially exposed to noise trauma report their tinnitus to be a ringing in the ears. They often comment that it comes and goes, returning as they return to work and leaving in the evening or over the weekend. Some workers and hunters have reported that an "attack of ringing" will come on suddenly, last for several hours, and then seem to disappear spontaneously. Others have reported that the ringing is constant. Some clinical staff have suggested that the pattern is related to the type of trauma and impact noise resulting in the hearing loss. In any case, there can be little doubt that a constant ringing or buzzing in the ear, day and night, everywhere and every time, is irritating and stress provoking.

## *Mental and Emotional Difficulties*

Thus far the discussion has focused on stress reactions and physical difficulties associated with excessive noise exposure. Clearly, the impact of those problems on the mental and emotional status of the individual should not be underestimated. A worker whose physical state is threatened by cardiac, liver, or biochemical changes is an individual incapable of working to full potential. A worker experiencing constant tinnitus or whose TTS or PTS cause communication problems at home and with friends is not a happy person. Thus, irritability, fatigue, difficulty sleeping, and tension can become constant companions. There is no evidence to suggest that this state of mind, or noise exposure by itself, will lead to mental illness. However, the result can be personal and social conflict. If the tinnitus and hearing loss begin to seriously interfere with communication, the worker may begin to withdraw from everyday situations. Productivity at work will be reduced and the situation at home may become tenuous, at best. Although life style, socioeconomic factors, family history, and so forth also play major roles in determining an individual's response to these phenomena, marriage or family problems, self-image, and interpersonal interactions are often affected. It is difficult to measure and quantify the mental and social turmoil a worker may experience as the result of noise exposure. Family and friends can almost always describe a change in behavior or an all too familiar pattern of response. It is obvious that the effects of noise are not limited to the physical structure known as the ear. Part of the case history of a patient reporting noise exposure should include a pertinent social history.

## *Special Problems*

Noise may also affect other parts of our anatomy, completely independent of the question of hearing. Memory function, visual acuity and tracking, tactile sensation, and cognitive and psychomotor skills have all been studied in the presence of noise and with various results. Interestingly, not all the effects are negative. For example, psychology literature abounds with studies that demonstrate that some activities, such as reading and studying, are enhanced in the presence of certain background sounds (e.g., music). Recently, recordings of the sounds of the sea have been selling to ease us into sleep, while the internal sounds of a woman's uterus supposedly calm a crying baby. On the other hand, vigilance activities suffer severely in the presence of high (but not damaging) noise levels. This can reduce productivity, negatively affect quality control, and increase the number of accidents on the job (Broadbent, 1957; Kryter, 1970). The important issue here is to be aware of noise, its intensity and its impact.

## *Prevention*

Noise-induced hearing loss can and should be prevented. To do so, a hearing conservation program including the following basic parameters must be in place:

1. Measures of existing sound levels
2. Rules and regulations limiting allowable levels of exposure to harmful noise
3. Mechanisms for reducing exposure to the levels specified in the regulations
4. Monitoring programs to ensure safety and compliance
5. Treatment and follow-up programs for those who suffer damage despite precautions

The role of the audiologist in these programs is paramount. In fact it is so great that an entire branch of the field called industrial audiology has developed.

### *Measures of Existing Sound Levels*

The ear is one of the best measuring devices for detecting excessive noise. Unfortunately, one must endanger the ear if it is to be used as a measuring system. Furthermore, as indicated earlier, "excessive noise" is really a subjective term. What may be an important sound to one person may be unpleasant and excessive to the next. Symphonies and tractors both make beautiful music to some listeners and a racket to others. Finally, the frequency components of the signal, which affect the pleasantness or unpleasantness of the signal, are not as important as the intensity characteristics. Intensity can be objectively measured on a device called a sound level meter. Containing a microphone to detect sound and to convert it to an electrical signal, an amplifier to boost the electrical energy to the point at which it can drive a meter, and a meter to reflect signal intensity, the sound level meter can provide a precise measure of the pressure of a signal. Most sound level meters have built in weighting networks labeled A, B, and C (Figure 11-4). These are used to change the responsivity of the meter to low frequency noise and thus to view the noise in a manner similar to the human ear. Although these scales provide an overview of the sound energy, when a device called an octave band filter is attached to a sound level meter, it allows the user to view slices of sound at discrete points along the frequency spectrum from low to high frequency. This enables the examiner to determine if the noise has greater energy in any one particular part of the spectrum, information that is valuable in planning a total hearing conservation strategy.

Most sound level meters are also able to provide either a slow or fast speed reading of the sound energy. This capability is important when measuring impact noise because it has a rapid buildup and sudden energy (fast speed) compared to an ongoing steady state noise with infrequent variation (slow speed). With a good sound level meter and appropriate attachments, noise levels can be measured in a workplace, and high-risk work areas can be identified easily. Industrial audiologists, engineers, architects, acousticians, health and safety officers, and many others can perform these measures accurately and rapidly.

It is important to note here that sound level readings for industry are only half of the story. If we acknowledge that noise is constantly around us, both inside and outside the walls

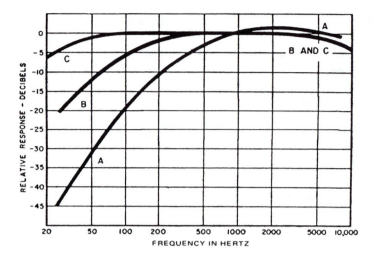

**FIGURE 11-4    The A, B, and C weighting scales for sound level readings. Note that the primary difference between these scales is limited to the very low frequency sounds.**

of the factory, it is easy to understand that rules and regulations to limit noise and noise exposure must include everyday activities and locales as well as the work environment.

There are rules and regulations that limit allowable levels of exposure to harmful noise in Canada, the United States, Sweden, and many other industrialized nations (Acton and Grime, 1978). In the United States, three federal agencies, the Environmental Protection Agency (EPA), the military, and the Occupational Safety and Health Administration (OSHA), have imposed regulations upon the makers of industrial, occupational, and community noise. In Canada, the provinces and the Government of Canada (Health and Welfare Canada), have legislation related to noise in the workplace. As expected, there is significant similarity among the rules and regulations in both countries, although they are not identical within or across borders. Table 11-2 displays current allowable levels of exposure for hazardous noise as set by the American Conference of Governmental Industrial Hygienists (1994–1995). Regulations, which are based on the physiologic response of the ear, allow for a trade-off between sound intensity and the duration of continuous exposure. That is, they permit exposure to high-intensity noises for only a brief period, as compared to a longer exposure to lower intensity sounds. The more intense the noise, the briefer the exposure permitted. Regulations in most jurisdictions in Canada, including Health and Welfare Canada and the Canada Labor Code, use the same values as those expressed in the OSHA standards, although some provinces allow a top level exposure of 90 dBA.

In the United States, the military has expressed particular concern over the noise situation, perhaps because noise reduces the efficiency of the fighting soldier, and perhaps because of the enormous economic cost associated with compensation payments to veterans whose hearing has been damaged by aircraft, artillery, engines, explosions, and the general mayhem associated with war. In a most extensive study of its kind, Gerber (1965) examined 82,000 audiograms on 59,000 different military and civilian employees of the U.S. Air Force and found that it was often impossible to distinguish between those who claimed to wear ear protection and those who did not. The hearing losses were about the same. Certainly, one might conclude from the investigation that, even though the Air Force exposes more people to more noise than anyone else and is fully aware of its own regulations, it didn't enforce its

**TABLE 11-2   Allowable sound exposure times.**

| Sound Level Intensity in dBA | Maximum Hours of Exposure Per 8-Hour Workday |
|---|---|
| 80 dBA | 24 hrs. |
| 82 dBA | 16 hrs. |
| 83 dBA | 12 hrs., 40 mins. |
| 84 dBA | 10 hrs, 04 mins. |
| 85 dBA | 8 hrs. |
| 86 dBA | 6 hrs., 21 mins. |
| 87 dBA | 5 hrs., 03 mins. |
| 88 dBA | 4 hrs. |
| 89 dBA | 3 hrs., 10 mins. |
| 90 dBA | 2 hrs., 31 mins. |
| 91 dBA | 2 hrs. |
| 92 dBA | 1 hr., 34 mins. |
| 93 dBA | 1 hr., 16 mins. |
| 94 dBA | 1 hr. |
| 95 dBA | 48 mins. |
| 96 dBA | 38 mins. |
| 97 dBA | 30 mins. |
| 98 dBA | 24 mins. |
| 99 dBA | 19 mins. |
| 100 dBA | 15 mins. |
| 101 dBA | 12 mins. |
| 102 dBA | 9 mins., 6 secs. |
| 103 dBA | 7 mins., 30 secs. |
| 106 dBA | 3 mins., 45 secs. |
| 108 dBA | 1 min., 52 secs. |
| 112 dBA | 56 secs. |
| 115 dBA | 28.07 secs. |
| 118 dBA | 14.03 secs. |
| 121 dBA | 7.01 secs. |
| 124 dBA | 3.31 secs. |
| 127 dBA | 1.45 secs. |
| 130 dBA | .52 secs. |
| 133 dBA | .26 secs. |
| 136 dBA | .13 secs. |
| 139 dBA | .06 secs. |

(From the American Conference of Governmental Industrial Hygienists, 1994–1995)

regulations about the use of ear protection. Such a conclusion is sad indeed, especially because occupational noise control is easy to effect and it is inexcusable to fail to employ it.

It is important to understand that noise regulations have not just simply appeared. They have evolved over years of study and analysis of what is harmful and what is acceptable. Court decisions based on challenges of leniency in the regulations by unions or stringency and the economic cost of the regulations by management have strongly influenced standards (Suter, 1985). These standards are living, guiding principles for human health. Federal agencies have the authority to prevent employers from subjecting their employees to too much noise. OSHA has fined and even threatened to close the plants of individual manufacturers for failure to comply. But, is that enough? Probably not. As we learn more about the effects of noise, what is an acceptable risk will probably not be an acceptable risk tomorrow. Nevertheless, knowledge of today's noise regulations and limitations is vital to prevention of hearing loss. Whether it is the "Noise Police" patrolling the streets of one of the cities of Texas, OSHA fining a factory, or the military giving a contract to a supplier for a new ship's engine based on noise abatement in the engine room, regulations must be in place so that they can be enforced and people protected.

## *Means to Reduce Hazardous Exposure*

It is unfortunate that the first thought that comes to mind when we think of reducing noise exposure is the use of some type of ear defender by the employee. That is backward thinking. In any program of noise control, the highest priority or first choice is to stop making the noise or to abate it at its source. Obviously this can be done by using quieter equipment, redesigning the process to eliminate noise, or by using less noisy materials. Sometimes simple maintenance of aging equipment accomplishes the same thing, and not only helps the workers, but prolongs the life of the machinery. While these methods are obvious, they are not always possible. Economics or the simple fact that quieter mechanisms are not readily available to carry out a specific process may mitigate improvement.

The next alternative is to reduce the noise by modification at its source. This is not as improbable a solution as it may seem. For example, some manufacturing processes can be done electrically rather than pneumatically. Lower speed machines can be used. If the equipment rests on a vibrating surface, bracing and increasing the mass of that surface may help. Placing a vibration damping surface between the equipment and the vibrating source may also work and lead to a concomitant reduction in the noise that is generated. Acoustical engineers are among the resources well equipped to offer solutions and ideas to manufacturers. The use of an appropriate consultant, and a few dollars spent early in the game, will save thousands in compensation claims later, not to mention the value saved in reducing human suffering.

If abatement cannot be achieved, the next step is to separate the workers from the noise by putting the noise source in some kind of a controlled environment (e.g., to use a special room or to enclose the equipment in a sound box) or by having the workers perform the job remotely. Manufacturing equipment that is noise producing can be enclosed in containers made of sound-absorbing material. It can be installed in such a way as to permit the worker to operate the machine while outside the enclosure. Besides, or instead of, covering the noise, it may be possible to locate the worker away from the source of the noise. This is done routinely in other hazardous occupations; for example, workers who handle radioactive material are completely removed from exposure.

A reduction in the duration of noise exposure can also be achieved, often simply by designing the work schedule to ensure that employees are in the dangerous area less frequently or for shorter periods of time and with quiet breaks between sessions. There is a number of commercial devices available to help monitor the individual's exposure to noise. Called dosimeters, these devices allow the employee to self-monitor exposure and to assume some responsibility for leaving the dangerous area when legal limits are surpassed. In that regard, these devices are quite similar to those used by x-ray technicians and employees in chemical factories. When a specific level of exposure is attained, the employee can be encouraged to work in another area of the company. Rotating employees through two different locations not only protects the worker for excessive exposure, but helps to make a job interesting and can lead to a happier and more productive workforce.

The final option, and least desirable alternative, in a hearing conservation program is personal ear protection; that is, requiring workers to protect themselves with ear muffs or earplugs. Those devices are effective, but less so than making less noise in the first place. There are ear protectors made of rubber, silicone, various fibers and wools, foam, and other materials. Some enjoy an excellent reputation as proper ear defenders, while others are sold cheaply at the local store and do little more than provide a false sense of protection to the user. The *attenuation characteristics*, that is, the reduction of sound level achieved by the defender, will vary if it is improperly fit or is, for example, the wrong type for the particular work environment. The appropriate choice of ear defender should be based on the noise level, frequency characteristics, and environmental factors faced by the user. The user should be properly fit by someone who knows how to do it, and should be given specific instructions as to the use, benefits, and advantages and disadvantages of the particular device in use. Certain occupations demand the use of individual ear protection rather than noise abatement at the source. For example, ground crews at airports are pretty well limited to the use of ear muffs to attenuate aircraft noise since the mobility of both the workers and noise source dictates that a portable, lightweight method is required.

In most industrial settings, however, one of the other alternatives to noise control is usually a better choice than ear defenders. That is true because many workers resist wearing earplugs, claiming that they are uncomfortable, not manly enough, or that it is important that they be able to communicate with their fellow workers. There is the fear that wearing ear plugs will prevent workers from hearing their fellow employees, managers, or important signals from machinery. This is a false fear. The wearing of sun glasses is a good analogy. It is well-known and accepted that it is easier to see objects in bright light while wearing sun glasses because the glasses filter out certain light rays that interfere with vision. The same is true for the ability to communicate in noise. That is, certain sounds are filtered out by the wearing of earplugs, and it is actually easier to communicate in the presence of most noises. Both sunglasses and earplugs improve the signal-to-noise ratio. Most industrial workers, if asked to stare at the sun for a period of time, would justifiably insist that they could not for fear of hurting their eyes. However, the same issues apply to hearing. That is, by having both ears continually exposed to high-level noise, they are hurting their ears.

### Monitoring Programs to Ensure Safety and Compliance

A monitoring program demands knowledge of the starting or baseline hearing level of all employees and a careful monitoring of their hearing at regular time intervals to look for shifts in their audiometric thresholds. Therefore, all new employees should have their hearing screened the day they start to work at the company. Further, baseline audiograms should be determined for existing employees. Testing should always be done only after a rest from noise exposure. The maintenance of detailed and specific audiometric records that are easily retrievable and properly interpreted by someone knowledgeable about hearing and hearing conservation is essential. This is important, not only from the point of view of an effective hearing protection program, but also from a legal perspective. Audiometric records developed as part of a hearing conservation program play a critical role in claims by noise-injured employees against employers, insurance companies, and worker's compensation. Those records can be equally important in litigation between employees and their employers.

According to standard guidelines, workers whose audiograms show the following changes should be referred to an ear specialist for investigation of a hearing problem:

1. Change of more than 15 dB at 500, 1000, or 2000 Hz
2. Change of more than 20 dB at 3000 Hz
3. Change of more than 30 dB at 4000 or 6000 Hz

When comparing previous or baseline audiograms to the current patterns, the elapsed time between testing should be no more than two years.

Other criteria that indicate the need for referral to a specialist include:

1. Average hearing level greater than 30 dB at 500, 1000, 2000, and 3000 Hz
2. A single frequency loss greater than 55 dB at 3000 Hz or greater than 30 dB at 500, 1000, or 2000 Hz
3. A difference in average hearing level between the better and poorer ear of more than 15 dB at 500, 1000, and 2000 Hz, or more than 30 dB at 3000, 4000, and 6000 Hz
4. Unusual hearing loss curves or inconsistent responses

This last group of patterns is normally seen in specific industrial settings or under unusual circumstances of employee sensitivity to noise.

All testing should be performed by a properly trained and certified industrial hearing screening technician using equipment that meets federal, state, or provincial standards. Further, all testing should be done in a proper environment and, if a problem is confirmed, the worker should be referred to an otologist and audiologist for evaluation.

In addition, the employee should be referred directly to an otologist if any of the following symptoms are present, despite the employee's status on the hearing screening test:

1. Active drainage from the ear within the previous 90 days
2. Sudden or rapidly progressive hearing loss
3. Acute or chronic dizziness or tinnitus

4. Unilateral hearing loss of sudden or recent onset
5. Significant air-bone gap
6. Visible evidence of cerumen accumulation or a foreign body in the ear canal

## *Treatment and Follow-Up Programs*

All persons whose hearing changes as a result of exposure to noise should be referred to proper medical and audiological treatment and follow-up programs. One cannot design a hearing conservation program without including a final referral source for those whose hearing changes. While there is no specific medical treatment for noise-induced hearing loss, it should not be assumed that all changes in hearing occur from noise. Medical evaluation is necessary to confirm that there are no other factors involved. Further, many of these patients may demonstrate tinnitus, recruitment, and vertigo. Medical treatment for those symptoms will usually provide relief, even if only until the worker mistakenly reenters the noisy work environment. The physician's counsel and advice are also certainly critical, especially where job change or reorganization becomes a forced choice for the worker. It is important to understand the role of the medical profession in working with a patient with a noise-induced hearing loss.

## Comment

The primary rehabilitation of this disorder falls almost entirely within the purview of the audiologist. Industrial noises tend to contain little low-frequency energy relative to the amount of the middle and high-frequency energy. Consequently, when noise-induced hearing loss does occur, generally it is restricted to high frequencies. One thing that tends to distinguish these from other sensory losses is a characteristic notch in the air conduction audiogram at 4000 Hz. This notch might be quite narrow and deep, or it may be broad, depending upon the spectrum of the noise producing the loss and the amount of time that the ear has been exposed to that noise. For example, in Figure 11-5 the notch for the left ear was the result of impact noise associated with the regular use of a shotgun by a young (22-year-old) farmer. He aims the weapon with his right eye, placing his left ear closest to the shell chamber. His right ear is protected slightly from the noise as it is attenuated by his head. The right ear pattern of this same young man reflects exposure to a steady state noise. He holds the steering wheel of his tractor in his right hand and looks over his left shoulder at the patch behind him as he is ploughing. The exhaust of his tractor is on the front of the vehicle (the muffler has been removed). Consequently, his right ear is exposed to the steady loud noise of the vehicle.

Noise-induced hearing impairments occur in the company of other things, such as disease or age, other factors that affect our hearing. For that reason, an audiogram may have the expected notch, even as great as 40 to 50 dB, reflective of a noise loss and also may show some other low- or high-frequency components related to the other pathology. Further, the severe and restricted threshold shift seen in noise-induced hearing loss can have quite a marked effect on speech discrimination, even in ears in which the speech reception threshold is nearly normal. This is because there is normal or nearly normal hearing for most

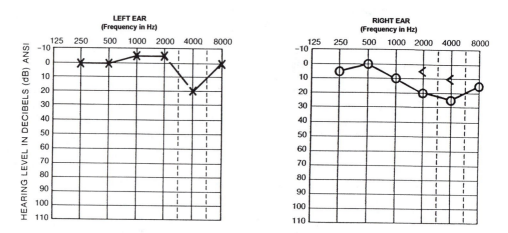

**FIGURE 11-5** **Audiogram of a 22-year-old male from a farm environment with a background in hunting and use of an unmufflered tractor.**

frequencies, and the ability to receive speech is only mildly affected compared to the impairment of the ability to understand speech. Most of the information of speech is carried by consonants, which are characterized by high-frequency information (Gerber, 1974). The information pertinent to sorting one phoneme from another may be lost in the presence of a noise-induced hearing loss. Thus, employees who work in noisy situations have more difficulty communicating than even they appreciate. This is not only because of the noise, but also because of an ever-increasing reduction in their auditory acuity. As discussed later, the problem can be compounded if the employee is showing any of the signs of an aging ear (*presbycusis*), in which case speech discrimination may be further affected because of the symptoms of that disorder. The site of the lesion for a noise-induced hearing loss is primarily in the cochlea. Therefore, the results of special audiometric tests will often indicate recruitment and, as already indicated, reduced speech discrimination. By contrast, results of central auditory system tests are usually normal as are tests of cortical function. The audiometric configuration, the case history, and the difficulty in communication usually make the audiological diagnosis of noise-induced hearing loss relatively straightforward.

Noise-induced hearing loss per se is irreversible and therefore technically untreatable. Treatment, or more accurately management, involves efforts to prevent any further hearing loss either by more aggressive use of personal hearing protection or by removing the affected individual from the noisy environment. If a worker is susceptible to the effects of noise and then is removed from further noise exposure, there is usually no additional hearing impairment. However, if the worker is not removed from further exposure, destruction of hearing will continue and even begin to accelerate. Noise-induced hearing loss is cumulative and irreparable. Each exposure leads to more destruction, and each destruction exposes the next set of hair cells, removing protection from the next frequency and the balance of the remaining structures.

Noise-induced hearing loss is unnecessary. The audiologist's responsibility in public education, particularly with workers in noisy industries, is self-evident. One important area of education is to teach that noise exposure does not produce immunity from additional loss. Another educational stress is that it is never too late to protect whatever hearing remains. Rehabilitation involves making maximum use of residual hearing (auditory training), amplification (hearing aids), and the use of environmental clues to help with understanding speech. Speech reading training is helpful as well. Counseling is often required, as is psychological support during any time of domestic and psychological disturbance resulting from the noise-induced hearing loss.

# Chapter *12*

# *Presbycusis*

Presbycusis is the reduction in auditory sensitivity that occurs with age. It is the most common cause of an acquired sensorineural hearing loss. The term "presby" means elder. The word "presbycusis" literally means the acuity of the elder. The longer we live, the more likely we will be adversely affected by presbycusis. Some are affected sooner than others, depending on individual susceptibility and a host of other factors, but, eventually, the aging that affects all parts of the body will affect the ears.

## *Demographic Background*

### *Prevalence*

There is a review in the United States called the National Health Interview Survey that, through self-report and household survey, explores the prevalence rates of various disorders. Hearing impairment is considered annually. For several years, the estimate for general hearing impairment in the U.S. population has been around 7.1 percent (National Center for Health Statistics, 1988). In 1987, results indicated that almost 21 million persons, or 8.8 percent of the population, reported hearing problems. The 1987 estimate seems high in light of previous reports and may be an artifact, or it may be a function of more recent awareness of hearing loss in the aging and the effects of noise in the environment.

Of greater interest, however, is the section on reported prevalence by age group. It has been suggested that persons 65 years and older are over seven times more likely to be hearing impaired than those under 45 (Figure 12-1). Furthermore, an estimate of the expected prevalence of hearing impairment through the year 2015 projects an increased rate per thousand in the total population from 70 in 1970 to 110 by 2015 (Figure 12-2). These estimates are predicated on the aging of our population and increased exposure to noise and chemical pollution. The fact is, we are an aging society. Currently, in Canada, 11.8 percent of the population is above age 65. By the year 2000 it is predicted to increase to 12.6 percent, and by the year 2016 it should reach 15.7 percent of the total population.

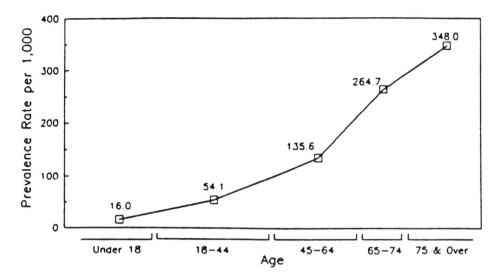

**FIGURE 12-1    Prevalence of hearing loss by age. (U.S. National Center for Health Statistics, Data from the National Health Interview Survey, 1988)**

Therefore, we must expect an increase in the number of persons seen in our clinics with presbycusis.

We know prevention is superior to treatment and cure, and it would be wonderful to prevent presbycusis, but we cannot. The normal life cycle involves a continuous process of cell death and replacement; a process that slows down with time, eventually stopping and culminating in death. Aging is that gradually increasing loss of cellular production accompanied by an accumulation of other materials such as cholesterol and lipids (Hinojosa and Naunton, 1991). Both noise-induced hearing loss and ototoxicity result in destruction of hair cell and nerve cell tissue. In some cases of ototoxicity, the tissue has disappeared entirely. Not so with presbycusis—the histopathology is recognized as one of tissue change as well as tissue loss.

## Contributing Factors

There are many factors that contribute to the progress and effects of presbycusis in each individual, but no specific element has been identified as its cause. There is probably a genetic component. When sensory hearing impairment occurs in a person in middle age in the absence of any evident cause, the paradoxical term *early* presbycusis is often invoked. Usually, this hearing pattern has occurred elsewhere in the family as well. Thus it seems evident that some individuals seem more susceptible to the hearing loss of aging than others. No doubt other factors play a major role in presbycusis. There are metabolic effects due to lifetime diet, environment, and habits. Further, arteriosclerosis due to dietary habits is a frequent

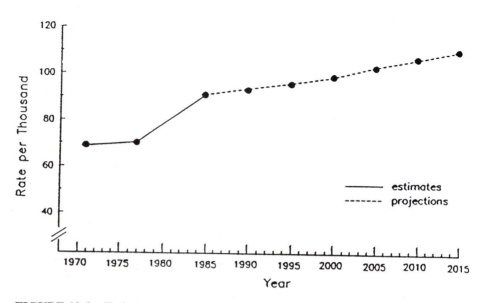

**FIGURE 12-2    Estimates and projections of the reported prevalence of hearing impairments in the population, United States, 1970–2015. (U.S. National Center for Health Statistics, Data from the National Health Interview Survey, 1988)**

adjunct of aging in Western society. A consequent interference with blood supply throughout the body, particularly the auditory nervous system, may play a significant role in presbycusis.

It is difficult to separate the effects of presbycusis from the effects of the noise of the society in which we live. There are very few places in the world where a population can be found that has not been exposed to even a small amount of noise. Such a group would be essential to studying the effects of noise and the effects of aging as independent variables. In an attempt to do such a study, Rosen and colleagues (1962) studied the Mabaans of the Sudan. The Mabaans live in a most rural part of that country and have been a society without industrial technology and its associated noise. It was the specific purpose of the investigation to determine the relationship between aging and hearing loss in a society in which noise could be ruled out as a contributory factor. Despite a number of methodological difficulties, not the least of which was trying to make an accurate determination of age of the subjects, the results certainly indicate a progressive worsening of hearing thresholds with the passage of time. As always with biological phenomena, there was great variation among individuals as to the degree of severity of the process.

Glorig, Ward, and Nixon (1961) found similar patterns for Americans in Wisconsin when they evaluated a large random population at the State Fair. Figure 12-3, based on those findings, illustrates the changes in median hearing levels one might expect through the various decades of life from age ten years to seven-nine.

Finally, it is highly likely that not all of what we have called presbycusis is due to age alone. Whether our society hastens the onset of presbycusis or increases its effects through

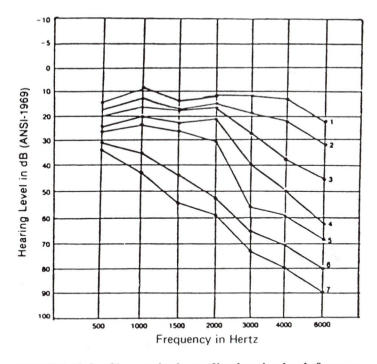

**FIGURE 12-3** **Changes in the median hearing levels from age 10 (curve 1) to age 79 (curve 7). These data are adapted from those reported by Glorig et al., 1957.**

environmental noise, or whether the two have a cumulative result, has yet to be determined. Conjecture suggests that either or both may be true, but continued research is necessary to accurately answer the question.

## Pathology

Throughout this text many of the pathologies one can acquire as an adult have been considered. While the aged are more susceptible to some of the diseases and disorders reviewed, and some are definitely associated with changes in cell structure, very few of them are specifically considered disorders of age. The purpose of this section is to discuss some of the more common ear problems seen among the aged.

### The Outer Ear

Changes in the physical structure of the pinnae because of age are often easy to see. Older people seem to have bigger ears. It is interesting to speculate if the Buddha, the great Indian philosopher who lived to be nearly ninety and whose statues all show him with elongated lobules, may have developed those lobules with age. Some Buddhists associate large ears with longevity of life and wisdom (Figure 12-4). That notion is certainly not contradictory to such a suggestion.

The physical structure of the outer ear begins to change as early as thirty years of age (Fowler, 1944). The skin becomes less resilient, perhaps because of exposure to the elements as well as aging. These changes are seen earlier and more often in men than in women. Initially, the pinnae appear to elongate, probably due to lengthening and widening of the lobule. Over time, the entire pinna is enlarged because of skin elasticity, muscle tonicity, and gravity. Hair growth may increase along the edge of the helix and at the tragus. Skin color may change to a duller appearance as the surface cells die and lose their sensitivity. There is some question how much effect these changes will have on hearing. The known high-frequency amplifying characteristics of the pinna will certainly be affected by changes in skin surface and pinna shape. Whether those changes are of a nature significant enough to cause a decrease in hearing is debatable. Furthermore, the neural damage associated with presbycusis is so great that interpretation of any changes in the role of the pinna would be very difficult.

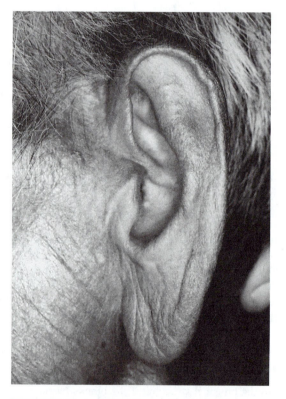

**FIGURE 12-4   "Buddha ear" of an older patient. (Courtesy of Dr. Michael Hawke)**

Among the changes that may occur within the ear canal are increased hair growth, relatively drier cerumen, and a collapsing ear canal. The combination of greater quantity and thicker hair and drier wax may interfere with the normal shedding of cerumen. This may result in a wax buildup in the canal. If not alleviated, the wax may eventually block the canal and affect hearing. A collapsing ear canal can occur when the cartilage of the external auditory meatus loses its elasticity. This may affect hearing, depending on the extent of the blockage. Although this is not a common problem associated with aging, it does happen. Chandler (1964) suggested that when it does, the result is an attenuation of high-frequency sounds. A collapsed ear canal also can result when pressure on the ear during earphone placement flattens the tragus and pinna, closing off the opening to the canal. It is a problem common to all age groups, but for reasons already discussed, it is more likely in the elderly population. Hearing is affected by a collapsed canal; sound transmission is blocked directly by the cartilaginous structures of the tragus and the pinna and an erroneous audiogram may result. Such a possibility is cause for vigilance by audiological examiners.

## *The Middle Ear*

Just as there are histopathologic changes seen in the tissue structures of the outer ear and external auditory meatus, there are associated changes in the structures of the middle ear. The tympanic membrane becomes more rigid. Schuknecht (1955) and Goodhill (1979a) refer to reduced elasticity and atrophy of muscle tissue within the middle ear, including structures associated with the tympanic membrane. The ossicles, the only bones to remain unchanged in size throughout life, do change in density and flexibility. They move from a softer spongy bone to a harder lamellar bone. The Eustachian tube may be less flexible because the tissues of the nasopharynx are less elastic and moist. These changes are seen more frequently, and to a greater degree, in smokers and those exposed to other oral toxins. The mucosal lining of the middle ear itself may show similar changes.

There has been some discussion of hearing loss associated with aging changes to the middle ear. Glorig and Davis (1961) and Nixon, Glorig, and High (1962) suggested that a conductive loss might result because of changes to the ossicles and the tympanic membrane. Called conductive presbycusis, it was based on findings of an apparent air-bone gap at 4000 Hz that increased with age and on the theory that a loss of energy across the ossicles would further reduce high frequency responses (Maurer and Rupp, 1979). Subsequent research failed to confirm the presence of the 4000-Hz air-bone gap (Etholm and Belal, 1974; Jerger, Jerger, and Mauldin, 1972; Sataloff, 1966). The question of degree of loss, no matter how mild, associated with changes in the middle ear is less clear. It is difficult to ignore that there are changes in the middle ear associated with aging that may interfere with hearing. Any hearing test of the aged must routinely include measures of middle ear function, even when visualization suggests tympanic membrane structure and the middle ear appear normal.

## *The Inner Ear*

Regardless of the other changes previously described in this section, it is the cochlea and its connections that bear the brunt of the pathology in presbycusis (Figure 12-5). Both the peripheral and central components of the system are affected, and the deterioration appears

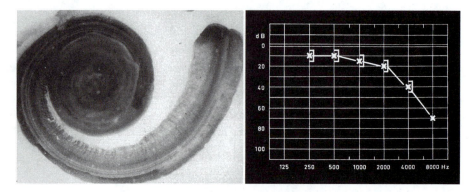

**FIGURE 12-5    Presbycusic cochlea. Note the generalized loss of hair cells in contrast to the frequency-specific patterns seen in ototoxic and noise-induced hearing losses. (Courtesy of Duphar International, Amsterdam)**

to become more rapid with increasing age. Peripheral degeneration is reported to be responsible for at least two-thirds of the clinical features of presbycusis. A variety of possible mechanisms for this destruction exists. For example, cellular degeneration reduces the number of inner and outer hair cells, particularly at the basal end of the cochlea. This can lead to secondary neural degeneration in the spiral ganglion. Further, circulatory changes such as arteriosclerosis, atrophy of the stria vascularis, and sludging of the red blood cells can lead to metabolic upset and further cell death (Salomon, 1991).

A number of investigators have tried to classify various different types of presbycusis. Schuknecht (1964) studied the histology of the disorder, considered the various clinical signs and behaviors noted, and after examining the auditory tracts of cats, concluded that presbycusis could be categorized into the four types of changes he noted within the auditory system:

1. Sensory, characterized by atrophy of the organ of Corti at its basal end
2. Neural, characterized by a reduction of the number of neurons in the auditory pathway
3. Metabolic, typified by atrophy of the stria vascularis affecting the contents of the cochlear duct
4. Mechanical, identified by a calcification and stiffening of the basilar membrane and a consequent alteration of cochlear mechanics.

Hinchcliffe (1962) also developed a model for possible mechanisms responsible for age-associated hearing loss. Although quite similar to the Schuknecht classifications, it combines two groups and adds another etiological factor—biochemical. The Schuknecht system separated sensory and neural sites. Hinchcliffe combined them and cited neural noise and cellular degeneration within the cochlea, spiral ganglion, and brain as the specific etiological factors in that grouping. What Schuknecht had called metabolic factors, Hinchcliffe calls biochemical mechanisms. Both authors use the term mechanical factors, but again, Hinchcliffe is more specific, focusing on tympano-ossicular degeneration, basilar membrane stiffening, hyperostosis of tractus spiralis foraminosus (bony changes affecting the fibers of the inner ear), spiral ligament atrophy, and cochlear duct occlusion.

Note that both models include suggested areas of destruction at several sites along the auditory tract from the cochlea to the cerebral cortex. It is evident from this why it is difficult to define a single pathology or response pattern associated with presbycusis. Regardless of the description of the pathology, the end result is similar. There is an elevation of hearing thresholds and a loss of frequency selectivity. Degeneration in the central pathways leads to a reduction in performance in terms of signal processing. Test results on elderly persons who were evaluated using a variety of audiological procedures have shown a mixture of characteristics typical of cochlear, retrocochlear, and central lesions (Arnst, 1985; Marshall, 1981; Maurer and Rupp, 1979).

## *Clinical Features*

Presbycusis differs from other hearing disorders in that its pathology is far more widespread. First, presbycusis has to be bilateral: after all, one ear is the same age as the other. The hearing loss may be truly sensorineural because the auditory nerve in a given ear is the same age as the cochlea of that ear. However, it may be sensory and not neural because the organ of Corti may be affected first. Presbycusis is uncommon before the age of fifty, but then the prevalence rises steeply. Moderate hearing impairment (>45 dB HL averaged over 0.5, 1, 2 and 4 kHz) occurs in 4 percent of the age group 51 to 60, but rises to 18 percent of those aged 71 to 80. Men and women are both affected, although men's losses tend to be slightly worse for the same age group.

Patients typically complain of being hard of hearing, but they note that the deficit is often worse in the presence of background noise and that recruitment is a problem. Although frequently present, recruitment is usually less than in noise-induced or ototoxic losses. This is true, again, because the inner hair cells are the same age as the outer hair cells, and change and/or destruction is equal for both sets of cells. Hearing impairments that accompany aging tend to develop from high frequencies to the lower ones. Consequently, presbycusis is characterized by a high frequency hearing loss. It is also characterized by a slowly progressive nature in which the high frequencies are more and more affected with time, and the lower frequencies become involved more gradually. Von Békésy (1956) calculated that auditory sensitivity is reduced 80 Hz from the higher end of the frequency spectrum every six months of life. Audiometric tests at very high frequencies are not usually done; but, if they were done on children, the results would undoubtedly confirm von Békésy's notion.

Because presbycusis seems to affect the high frequencies first and then progresses to the low frequencies, the description of a specific pure tone audiogram is difficult, as the different stages of the process will reflect differences in hearing. It has been reported that there is an apparent increase in the rate of presbycusis around age 43 years in American males and about age 48 in American women (Corso, 1963). That increased process of degeneration seems to slow down in the decade of the fifties. Clearly, the typical audiogram in our North American society is affected by noise, diet, and lifestyle, but it also reflects changes that occur within the auditory system that are purely a function of age (Figure 12-6).

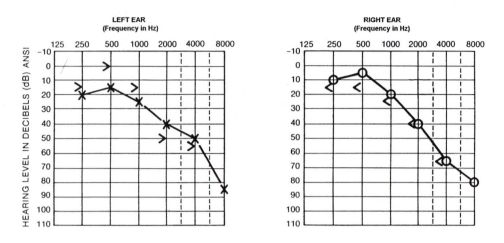

PURE TONE AUDIOGRAM

**FIGURE 12-6   Audiogram of presbycusic patient.**

The presbycusic audiogram may be quite similar to one that accompanies noise-induced hearing loss, with the notable exception that instead of a notch indicating a frequency-specific hearing loss, sensitivity continues to decrease as frequencies increase. However, because most of us are subject to both age and noise, it is not always easy to make a distinction among the types of hearing losses. The distinction between presbycusis and noise-induced hearing losses sometimes can be made based only on family and occupational history. In the absence of a history of occupational noise exposure, the typical presbycusis audiogram will show an increased hearing loss, continuous with frequency, up to an extreme of 15 dB per octave at advanced age. Tinnitus may occur, even though the origin of the disorder is not irritative.

Speech discrimination is generally worse than would be expected from the pure tone audiogram. Sometimes it is so markedly reduced it becomes a significant problem for the patient. This phenomenon has been called phonemic regression. The reduction of speech discrimination ability seems to bear no relationship to mental capabilities, appears more frequently in persons over fifty years of age, and is limited to a yet undefined subgroup of persons who have presbycusis.

Tests of higher auditory function will usually yield poorer results for the presbycusic than for the younger individual with the same audiogram. That result, coupled with the unusual speech discrimination problems seen with this pathology, suggests that the disorder involves higher auditory centers. It is difficult to determine how much of presbycusis is of cochlear origin—whether due to noise or age—and how much is the result of pathology in higher auditory centers.

## *Medical Management of the Presbycusic Patient*

One of the major clinical responsibilities associated with care of the presbycusic patient centers on confirming the diagnosis and excluding any associated aural or alternative causative pathology. If any other pathologies do exist, they should be treated vigorously by medical, surgical, or whatever appropriate means to avoid additional compromise of the patient's hearing levels. In addition, any coexistent impairments that may further disable the individual must also be identified. The classic example is that of coexistent visual impairment. In the same fashion as there may be degeneration of the cochlea with age, so there may be degeneration of ocular tissues and an associated impaired visual acuity. Finally, there is a significant role for the physician and the audiologist as educator and counselor. It is important to explain to the patient the process of presbycusis and the absence of any more serious pathology. It is important to advise the patient on appropriate care of residual hearing (e.g., avoiding excessive noise exposure) and how to maintain of a healthy lifestyle. These steps are only the beginning, however, as the principal audiological consideration for presbycusis is rehabilitation.

Older people can and do benefit from rehabilitative audiology. It is a fallacy, often perpetrated, that the aged can receive only limited benefit from amplification. Indeed, they can benefit dramatically from amplification, given that it is appropriate and correctly fitted, and that they are properly educated in the use of the hearing aid. It must be understood that a hearing aid is exactly what it says it is, an aid. Just as they should find their vision to be improved with properly fitted lenses, they should find their hearing improved with properly fitted hearing aids and education about the use of the device. Unlike eyeglasses, however, a hearing aid does not suddenly restore hearing to its former state or to normal function. Its purpose is to maximize use of residual hearing. To reach that goal will take a significant learning period as the individual readjusts to the new auditory signals. Those with presbycusis will rarely adjust to a hearing aid immediately and initially find it to be unsatisfactory. However, that must not prevent a patient from using an amplification device. They must learn how to use it. That often requires patience and a good clinical teacher.

Group rehabilitation sessions for the aged are very useful and are usually seen by that clientele as a highly valuable experience. Besides auditory training and speech reading sessions, as well as information on successful hearing aid use, the sessions usually focus on daily living and communication. The social and counseling aspects of rehabilitation groups cannot be overstressed. It is important for the hearing-impaired aged person to encounter other hearing-impaired people, to communicate with them, and to share common problems and solutions.

## *Comment*

As a result of presbycusis and some of its associated problems, many seniors become socially isolated and even depressed. They know that there is nothing that can be done medically or surgically to cure presbycusis (Goodhill, 1979b). The diagnosis is normally fairly straightforward in the presence of an appropriate audiogram and, in the absence of other aural pathology, the diagnosis is confirmed; that is, there is a sensorineural hearing loss that will continually progress and will gradually remove speech understanding and communication. No wonder these folks become depressed!

Further, the elderly are also often disabled by visual impairments, primarily a problem called presbyopia, a name and visual deficit similar to their auditory problem. As an individual ages, he doesn't hear as well as he did, he doesn't see as well as he did, he doesn't walk as well as he did, and many other bodily functions don't do as well as they did. The older the individual, the more disabling the presbycusis and the visual deficits. Whatever else may be happening with the patient, it is also well-known that a decrease in these two critical sensory modes contributes markedly to aging. The patient must receive ongoing ophthalmologic, otologic, and audiologic care (e.g., removal of cerumen) to ensure that there is no other additional handicap. Admittedly, some people are more adversely affected by aging and its disabilities than others. The clinician's role is to treat and refer those who need medical care and to guide the others to proper rehabilitative services.

Keep in mind that the elderly are not exempt from other forms of ear disease. Goodhill (1979b) has cautioned that many disorders and diseases that produce hearing losses can be mistaken for presbycusis. He suggested the term pseudopresbycusis as a useful concept for differential diagnosis of those diseases of the ear that cause hearing loss, particularly in the sixth, seventh, eighth, and ninth decades of life. He recommends careful consideration of genetic diseases, otomastoiditis, otosclerosis, ossicular fixations, temporal bone dystrophies, tumors, direct trauma, barotrauma, acoustic trauma, ototoxic drugs, syphilis, labyrinthine membrane ruptures, viremias, vascular lesions, and other causes before a specific diagnosis of presbycusis is applied. He suggested that the label "presbycusis" is tenable only when no other cause of the hearing loss can be found.

What is perhaps most important is to properly counsel the patient concerning the disorder, contributing factors (e.g., noise exposure, etc.), and what can be done about those factors. The patient must be taught that some presbycusis derives from the ailments that affect all of us as we get older, and therefore such things as routine monitoring may help to alleviate it. The patient must be taught to avoid excessive noise exposure so as to preserve residual hearing. The patient should be made aware of the fact that although there is no medical or surgical treatment for the problem, an audiologist can alleviate the communicative symptoms.

Presbycusis is the most common form of hearing loss. The longer we live, and the more of us who live longer, the more presbycusic patients there will be. It is especially important that each of us be aware that the presbycusic patient can be helped. It is also important that the elderly person be made to understand that the hearing problem can be alleviated by amplification and education and rehabilitation. For that reason, it is inexcusable for there to be a failure to provide treatment for the aged. Aged persons should not be required or allowed to be without communication with their peers for the remainder of their lives. At a time when people are living longer lives—and those lives are productive much, much, longer—the audiologist has an obligation to insure adequate auditory rehabilitative services for the presbycusic patient.

Chapter *13*

# Disorders of the Auditory Nerve and Brain Stem

There is a number of disorders affecting the auditory nerve and its connections to the central nervous system, located at the level of the brain stem. These may be separated by cause or etiology. Typical divisions include congenital, infective, inflammatory, traumatic, degenerative, et cetera. Probably the most common group to affect the nerve and its connections are the degenerative processes of presbycusis. These and most of the other disorders have been discussed in previous chapters. One pathology not discussed in any detail, however, is the neoplasm or tumor. This group of disorders is a relatively uncommon cause of auditory nerve dysfunction and is represented almost exclusively by the diagnosis of acoustic neuroma. Despite its relatively low incidence, this tumor has played an important role in the historical development of investigative audiology; many of the specialized audiometric tests were developed to help diagnose this pathology.

## *Acoustic Neuromas*

### *Pathology and Clinical Features*

The acoustic (vestibulocochlear or eighth cranial) nerve passes from the brain stem in the cerebellopontine angle to reach the internal auditory canal. It then passes through this bony canal along with the facial nerve to reach the inner ear. In the canal the nerve exists as three separate components: the cochlear nerve and the superior and inferior vestibular nerves. The lateral portion of these nerves (in the bony internal meatus), similar to other peripheral nerves in the body, is covered by a protective layer of Schwann cells. An acoustic neuroma is a benign tumor of the Schwann cells occurring most commonly on the superior vestibular nerve, followed by the inferior vestibular nerve and rarely on the cochlear nerve. Technically therefore, these tumors should be called vestibular Schwannomas. However, old habits die hard and it would seem that the term acoustic neuroma will remain for the foreseeable future. In deference to history, that title is used throughout this discussion (Roland, McCrae, and McCombe, 1995).

Acoustic neuromas represent 8 percent of all intracranial tumors and 80 percent of cerebellopontine angle tumors . Men and women are equally affected; the tumors are rare before the age of thirty, presenting most commonly between the ages of forty and sixty years. They are invariably unilateral and of unknown etiology. In about 5 percent of cases they may be bilateral, but this is usually associated with multiple neurofibromatosis type 2 (NF2) due to an aberration on the long arm of chromosome 22.

Although these tumors are histologically benign, unfortunately, they occur in a confined space, the bony internal auditory canal. As a tumor invariably expands out of the internal meatus and into the cerebellopontine angle, it enters a secondary confined space, that of the bony skull. Consequently the effects of these tumors relate to pressure on surrounding structures, as they grow and fill the available space. The symptoms can therefore be divided into two phases: an otologic phase in which a tumor compresses structures in the internal auditory meatus, and a neurologic phase in which a tumor compresses other intracranial structures.

Among the otologic symptoms, unilateral deafness is the most common presenting complaint. Often this is associated with tinnitus and is usually of less than ten years in duration. Vertigo is uncommon because the slow rate of growth of these tumors usually means that central compensation can easily keep pace with the neuronal destruction. The facial nerve seems remarkably resistant to the pressure of these tumors, and thus a facial palsy is extremely rare.

As the tumor expands intracranially, neurologic symptoms will begin to appear. For example, the trigeminal nerve may be compromised, resulting in alterations of facial sensation. Loss of the corneal reflex is an early sign of this type of damage. Irritation of the dura in the posterior cranial fossa often leads to headache and pain in the ear and mastoid region. As the brain stem and cerebellum become compressed, the patient may become unsteady, hoarse, and have difficulty swallowing. Finally, if the tumor is very large, intracranial pressure may be elevated and coma and death will ensue.

Figure 13-1 is an MRI (magnetic resonance image) of a true eighth cranial nerve acoustic tumor. These tumors are most often found on the vestibular branch of the nerve. However, in this case, an 86-year-old male with a bilateral presbycusic type hearing loss whose primary symptom was a more rapid degeneration of the hearing on the left side compared to the right, the tumor actually originated on the auditory branch. It can be clearly seen in the MRI that the internal auditory meatus has been eroded away and that the opening had become enlarged. These tumors grow quite slowly, and because of his age, this gentlemen was not considered a surgical candidate. Upon his death, due to a completely unrelated cause, the skull was opened to examine the tumor. The entry was made by removing the occipital lobe, exposing the brain stem and internal auditory meatus from a superior view. The photograph in Figure 13-2 was taken during the autopsy and clearly shows the tumor on the left auditory nerve. This is a remarkable photograph as it could not be obtained from a living subject. Figure 13-3A is a close-up of the tumor still in situ, while Figure 13-3B and C permit an accurate presentation of its size and shape.

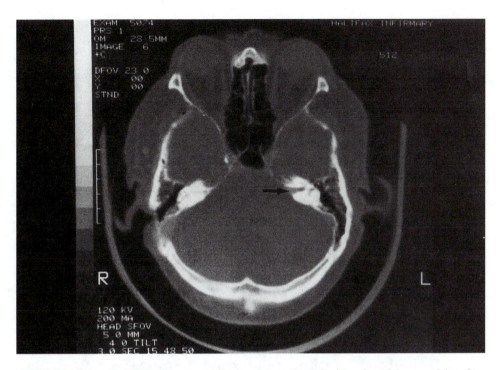

**FIGURE 13-1    An MRI of an acoustic tumor on the left side of an 86-year-old male. Note the widening of the internal auditory meatus (arrow). (Courtesy of Dr. George Novotny)**

## *Audiological Considerations*

The role of the audiologist in this condition has traditionally been twofold: diagnosis and rehabilitation. The final diagnostic role, to some extent, has been superseded by radiographic technology. However, CT and MRI scanners are expensive and are by no means universally available. Further, because of their cost and availability, those techniques are usually applied only when there is reasonable suspicion of an acoustic neuroma. That usually occurs as a result of questionable results on the initial audiological assessment. Finally, the rehabilitative process for these patients starts with a thorough assessment of their audiological status and difficulties.

An audiological diagnosis of acoustic neuroma is one of the most difficult to make. Because loss of hearing is not a common complaint of typical patients with small tumors of the auditory nerve, the audiologist may not be approached for evaluation or consultation until the tumor has grown to the point that it is causing a severe hearing impairment. Actually, nearly half of a group of patients whose acoustic neuromas were surgically confirmed had not demonstrated a hearing loss at all during pure tone air conduction audiometry (Johnson, 1968). This is an enormously significant observation for the audiologist. It underlines

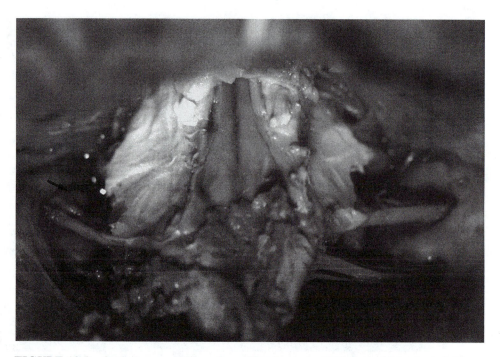

**FIGURE 13-2    Superior–posterior view of brain stem of 86-year-old male patient with left eighth cranial nerve tumor on the auditory branch (arrow). (Courtesy of Dr. George Novotny)**

one of the most important concepts to learn: *pure tone air conduction audiograms are not sufficient hearing tests.* A pure tone audiogram is only one small part of a total hearing assessment, and if it is normal in a patient who is complaining of auditory or vestibular problems, further tests are required.

It is here that the complete electrophysiologic test battery available to audiology becomes very useful. The audiologist can introduce an auditory signal at the ear, normally a click, and measure the time it takes for the electrophysiologic response associated with that stimulus to travel through the conductive and sensorineural mechanisms. Table 13-1 illustrates the most frequently used wave forms and their associated normal time delays. If a signal travels to one level at its expected rate, but is delayed in reaching the next level, the examiner can begin to pinpoint the reason for that delay, usually the lesion causing the auditory deficit. Auditory brain stem responses (ABR) are the most frequently used electrophysiologic measure because they are easiest to obtain and interpret, and they emanate from the section of the auditory nerve that passes through the cerebellopontine angle. That is where most postcochlear pathology is usually found (as were the tumors in Figures 13-2 and 13-3). Figure 13-4 is a typical ABR tracing from a normal ear. Measures of that tracing include an

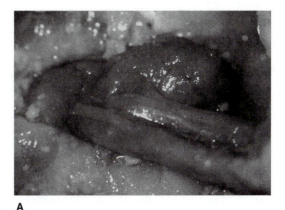

A

**FIGURE 13-3A    Close-up of acoustic tumor in situ at cerebellopontine angle.**

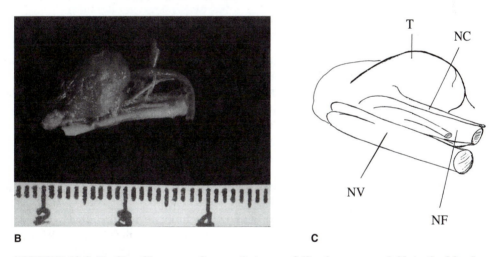

B                                               C

**FIGURE 13-3 (B, C)    Close-up of acoustic tumor following removal. Note the blood supply and its comparative size. Note also how the tumor (T) has invaded the facial (NF), cochlear (NC), and vestibular (NV) nerves. (Courtesy of Dr. George Novotny)**

analysis of the latency (delay) of the signals between the various key waves as marked with a I, III, and V.

In a typical case, the audiologist should expect to find a patient complaining of a progressive hearing loss of gradual onset, perhaps extended over as long as one or two decades. For example, Mr. W., age 39, complained of having a hearing loss and tinnitus in his right ear for almost twenty years. However, he told the audiologist that in the two or three years

**TABLE 13-1  Summary of primary auditory-evoked potentials.**

| Potential | Latency | Electrode Placement | Origin |
|---|---|---|---|
| Electrocochleography | 2.4 ms | Middle ear at the promontory; ear canal near the tympanic membrane | Cochlea; eighth cranial nerve (action potential) |
| Auditory brain stem response | 15.0 ms | Vertex to earlobe or mastoid | Eighth cranial nerve (action potential); brain stem nuclei and tracts |
| Middle latency response | 50–100 ms | Vertex to earlobe or mastoid | Thalamus, primary auditory cortex |
| Late potentials ($N_1 - P_2P_3$ ... Contingent Negative Variation) | >100 ms | Vertex to earlobe or mastoid | Primary auditory and association cortex |

before his first visit to the clinic, the hearing in his right ear worsened. In fact, masked bone conduction thresholds were beyond the limits of the audiometer for the right ear. When white noise masking was introduced contralaterally, a speech reception threshold (SRT) could not be obtained due to poor speech discrimination. Unmasked speech discrimination at 10 dB was fair at 70 percent, and remained at about that level at 20, 30, 40, and 50 dB. However, at 40 dB, with effective contralateral masking, the discrimination score was reduced to 28 percent. Threshold tone decay testing with masking showed 35 dB of decay at 2000 Hz and 30 dB of decay at 4000 Hz. Audiometric testing of the left ear revealed hearing of pure tones to be within normal limits. SRT was consistent with the pure tone audiogram. Speech discrimination was good.

Mr. W. was referred to otoneurology for further evaluation. Radiographic, electronystagomographic, and additional audiometric studies determined that Mr. W. did indeed have an acoustic neuroma. It was surgically removed, but it was necessary to destroy the cochlea. Mr. W. made a remarkable surgical recovery, had virtually no dizziness afterward, and was fitted with a hearing aid that provided the contralateral routing of signals from his deaf side to his normal ear (a CROS aid). Auditory training was very effective, and Mr. W.'s localization ability now approximates normal.

In another case a sixty-three-year-old male with a noise-induced hearing loss complained of a change in the hearing in his left ear. He was also having balance problems. Figure 13-5 illustrates the changes that had occurred over a period of three years.

As is quite evident from this last example, the hearing impairment is unilateral and characterized by marked difficulty understanding speech in the involved ear. The patient often exhibits what has been described by the peculiar term phonemic regression. It is difficult to accurately describe what is meant by that term, but the most frequent observation is that the patient has extremely poor speech discrimination, inexplicably so in view of the results of other hearing tests. Phonemic regression is probably due to distortion of the neural

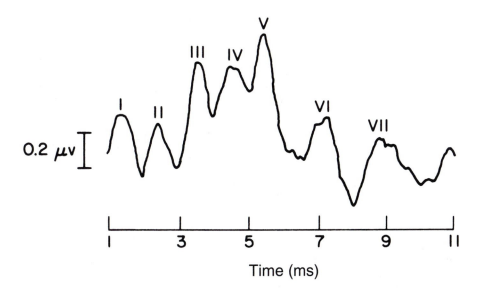

**FIGURE 13-4** **Normal auditory brain stem response (ABR) tracing. Note how waves I, III, and V are easily delineated.**

signal as it passes through the cochlear portion of the nerve. As an example, one of the patients of Weaver and Staller (1984) had a speech reception threshold of 35 dB but a speech discrimination score of only 34 percent. Phonemic regression does occur in other pathologies, notably presbycusis.

The investigator must always be careful as there are audiometric signs that suggest neuroma, but are similar to and easily confused with signs of Ménière disease. These include vertigo, tinnitus, and hearing loss. Recruitment is less likely to occur with an eighth cranial nerve pathology than in Ménière disease, but tinnitus is common even in the absence of hearing impairment. Among the five eighth cranial nerve patients described by Weaver and Northern (1976), one presented with a complaint of tinnitus and two did not complain of hearing loss at all. The acoustic neuroma patient may report tinnitus, numbness of the face, and sometimes a sense of fullness in the ear.

Medical and audiological diagnosis is based on the "Rule Out" principle. That is follow a sequence of procedures that rules out certain pathologies and leads the diagnostician to the most probable cause of the symptoms. Therefore, audiological considerations include use of all tests and procedures that eliminate from the potential diagnosis those things that may be confused with acoustic neuroma, such as brain disease, Ménière disease, and cerebral arteriosclerosis. Studies of the electrical activity of the auditory brain stem are a potentially diagnostic discriminant of eighth cranial nerve tumors. The use of ABR in diagnosis has been described at length by Abramovich (1990), who considered the ABR to be an excellent test for detection of acoustic tumors. He reported 90 to 100 percent of confirmed cases to be positive by ABR testing. Notable differences between the two ears may appear in the ABR

## Audiological Results

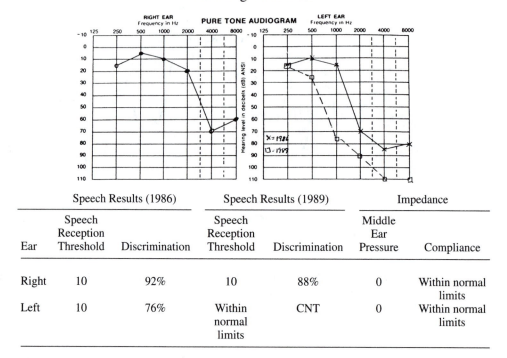

| | Speech Results (1986) | | Speech Results (1989) | | Impedance | |
|---|---|---|---|---|---|---|
| Ear | Speech Reception Threshold | Discrimination | Speech Reception Threshold | Discrimination | Middle Ear Pressure | Compliance |
| Right | 10 | 92% | 10 | 88% | 0 | Within normal limits |
| Left | 10 | 76% | Within normal limits | CNT | 0 | Within normal limits |

Acoustic reflexes present 500–2000, absent 4000–STIM Right, Elevated 4000–STIM Left

**FIGURE 13-5    Audiograms of a patient with a slow-growing acoustic neuroma on the left side. The patient also has noise-induced hearing loss, making differential diagnosis quite difficult. Note how the hearing in the affected ear decreased in three years.**

due to the presence of a tumor in one ear (Thomsen, Terkildsen, and Osterhammel, 1978). In general, these take the form of relative latency shifts that differ between the two ears (Figure 13-6).

## *Medical Considerations*

There are no ear problems, per se, that are specific to eighth cranial nerve disorders. The patient usually complains to a physician or audiologist because of hearing loss, dizziness, or tinnitus. Referral to otology, neurology, or neurosurgery for further evaluation often follows. Some otologists now limit their surgical practices to neurotology, that is, surgery for these types of neural disorders of hearing.

The first role of the specialist physician is to confirm a final diagnosis. Historically, this is done with the cooperation of audiology through the use of speech audiometry, stapedial

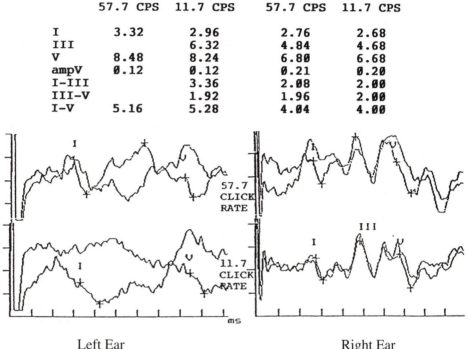

Left Acoustic Neuroma

|  | 57.7 CPS | 11.7 CPS | 57.7 CPS | 11.7 CPS |
|---|---|---|---|---|
| I | 3.32 | 2.96 | 2.76 | 2.68 |
| III |  | 6.32 | 4.84 | 4.68 |
| V | 8.48 | 8.24 | 6.80 | 6.68 |
| ampV | 0.12 | 0.12 | 0.21 | 0.20 |
| I–III |  | 3.36 | 2.08 | 2.00 |
| III–V |  | 1.92 | 1.96 | 2.00 |
| I–V | 5.16 | 5.28 | 4.04 | 4.00 |

Left Ear                                    Right Ear

**FIGURE 13-6   ABR tracings of patient with left acoustic neuroma. Testing was done at two different click rates, as is often the case when trying to verify and clarify test results. Note the difference in the latency of the wave I to wave V interval in the normal ear (4.00 ms) compared to the ear with the tumor (5.28 ms).**

reflex decay measurements, measures of recruitment, and auditory brain stem response audiometry and other special tests. Recently, the ease of diagnosis has become significantly improved through new radiologic techniques. Traditionally CT scanning was used, but with the advent of MRI, this has now become the investigation of choice. In the presence of an asymmetrical pure tone audiogram and other audiological results indicating a suspect sensorineural hearing loss, the next step would now be a gadolinium-enhanced MRI scan. The sensitivity and specificity of this test in diagnosing an acoustic neuroma is superior to other tests.

The second role of the surgeon is to decide on the most appropriate treatment. In the absence of any contraindications, this will often be surgical removal of the structure. The surgery to remove eighth cranial nerve tumors is truly neurosurgery and therefore carries a significant risk to the postoperative neurologic functioning of the patient. Further, because these types of tumors grow very slowly, there is often some question on the application of surgery for the aged patient. There is often reasonable expectation that the patient will live out his life before the tumor causes any major neurologic or life-threatening problems, except for, of course, unilateral hearing loss.

A prerequisite to the actual procedure itself, and important for deciding which surgical approach to use, is the gathering of information about the size, and effects of the tumor. Information from the audiologist about hearing, from the radiologist about the position, size, and shape of the internal auditory meatus, and from the neurologist regarding the neurological signs suggestive of involvement of other cranial nerves or areas of the brain would be critical. In addition, information concerning the likelihood of associated damage or dysfunction that might occur as a result of the surgery would be considered. All the material would be combined to permit the best informed decision to be made by the patient, the family, and the surgeon.

Finally, the role of the surgeon is to perform surgery. The aim of surgery is to remove the tumor while avoiding damage to adjacent structures. In particular, the surgeon will try to avoid damage to the facial nerve. There are three ways to approach this tumor, depending on its size and extent. The translabyrinthine approach is the most frequently used. It involves drilling through the bony labyrinth to reach and remove the tumor. Unfortunately, although the facial nerve can be preserved, all hearing (and vestibular function) in the ear will be lost. The posterior fossa approach involves removing a window of bone at the back of the patient's skull and attacking the tumor from behind. This is probably the most versatile technique, in that even large tumors can be dealt with, and both hearing and facial nerve function can be preserved. It demands the cooperation of a neurotologist and a neurosurgeon. It is also more threatening to the patient's outcome. The middle fossa approach involves removing a window of bone in the skull just above the ear. Both hearing and facial nerve can be preserved, but access is limited and only small tumors can be approached by this route.

## von Recklinghausen Disease

This unusual disease is distinguished by the development of many small tumors that seem to appear along various peripheral nerves. As they grow, they result in a variety of sensory and motor dysfunctions. When the tumors occur initially on the eighth cranial nerve or at the cerebellopontine angle, the disease first may be mistaken for an acoustic neuroma. The rate of growth of von Recklinghausen tumors is also comparatively slow, but the tumors can become malignant and lead to death. The disease is autosomal dominant and therefore inherited. When the small tumors develop on the auditory or vestibular branches of the eighth cranial nerve, the patient may exhibit a progressive hearing loss or equivalent deficit in balance. This disease has been mistaken for a typical eighth cranial nerve Schwannoma in its initial stages of development. Bilateral tumors are common in this condition. The normal treatment for this disease is genetic counseling and, as appropriate, surgery.

A clinic recently reported a twenty-three-year-old woman who developed a unilateral progressive hearing loss with some tinnitus. As the loss progressed the patient also developed vertigo. Initially, it was thought she had a Schwannoma. However, she gradually began to develop similar symptoms in the other ear, and it was discovered that she had multiple small tumors throughout her cranial cavity. She was taken to surgery to remove the tumors from her auditory nerves since they were the most life threatening because they were space-occupying and therefore pressing against the cerebellum and causing her respiratory difficulties. Unfortunately, she died immediately postoperatively. Approximately four years later, her younger sister came to the clinic with a unilateral progressive sensorineural hearing loss. She was immediately referred to neurology and, unfortunately, also diagnosed with von Recklinghausen disease. It was suggested that she undergo surgery to remove the initial tumor before it became a threat to her. In view of her family history, she refused.

## Brain Stem Lesions

Occasionally, relatively uncommon tumors that are difficult to diagnose appear in the brain stem at levels superior to the eighth cranial nerve. Unfortunately, patients with this type of lesion often go to their death with the tumor undiagnosed because they are so rare. The tumor may be situated at the level of the cochlear nucleus or anywhere above, with one of the most common sites being the inferior colliculus. Obviously, although most of these tumors are benign, there is always the danger that a large enough lesion will eventually lead to death for the same reasons an expanding acoustic neuroma can cause neurologic damage and death. A tumor of the brain stem at a region higher than the level of the auditory nerve may result in disabling effects not appreciably different from those of eighth cranial nerve lesions. If the tumor has grown to an extensive size, there may be hearing loss, facial nerve involvement, and respiratory or cardiac difficulty. Further, if the tumor is recognized and surgical intervention is attempted, there is always the possibility of a postsurgical disabling effect. Naturally, the larger the tumor, the greater the risk of a postsurgical deficit. Unfortunately, tumors deep in the brain stem or mid-brain are frequently not operable.

Alternatively, higher level tumors may lead to more central processing difficulties rather than hearing difficulties, and in brain stem lesions there may be more subtle audiological considerations. A report by Bocca and Calearo (1963) demonstrated that patients with tumors of the brain stem may suffer a disability of binaural fusion. Binaural fusion is the normal process within the auditory nervous system that makes it possible for us to function in a reverberant world. Our ears are bombarded by multiple reflections of sound in any live acoustic space. A signal, speech or otherwise, generated in or into that space reflects off walls, floors, ceilings, furniture, other people, and so forth. The result is that, at any given moment, the acoustic waveform at one ear differs from the acoustic waveform at the other ear. Yet, we are never conscious of that difference. The auditory nervous system, due in part to its bilateral representation, renders a single percept from the two acoustic events. This function occurs in the brain stem and, if pathology exists, a test for binaural fusion may reveal a deficit in that function. The next chapter focuses on these types of disorders. However, from an audiological perspective, it is important to understand the role of binaural fusion in hearing.

The test to examine for an intact auditory system is relatively simple. If a recording of speech were played to a normal listener through earphones so that all the information below a certain frequency was presented to one ear while all the information above that frequency was presented to the other ear, only one signal would be perceived by that listener. That is, the two entirely different signals would be heard as one and would render 100 percent discrimination or understanding of speech processed in that way. The listener would not notice or be aware that signals in one ear had differed from that of the other. Not so with the patient who has a lesion of the upper brain stem. If that patient were to listen to either one, but not both of the signals, the result would be a speech discrimination score consistent with the information received in only one ear. However, when the patient is required to respond to both ears with the signal filtered as described above, speech discrimination drops markedly. This is due to the failure of binaural fusion. That is, the two signals interfere with one another rather than add to each other. It is important to always keep in mind the possibility of a brain stem lesion when a patient presents with odd auditory complaints. Suspect patients should have a routine screening of their ability to use binaural fusion.

## Comment

Of all the pathologies affecting human hearing, the eighth cranial nerve tumor remains one of the most dramatic and interesting for the clinician. To find and identify one is rare, but it is one of the most satisfying aspects of a standard professional routine. The patient's complaints may not provide any clues, or they may offer a beacon to follow. Test results may be ordinary or extraordinary. In short, as Davis (1978) warned: "We must expect that the effects of brain stem lesions will not be clearly predictable and will often be quite bizarre. This very feature may distinguish lesions of such a small, compact, complicated piece of nervous tissue in which so many neuro-physiological functions are carried out."

Aside from the question of diagnosis, there is the question of rehabilitation. The patients may be left with the knowledge that they have a tumor growing inside their head. That thought is terrifying, even if the tumor is benign and growing extremely slowly. The patient may be left with ever-increasing symptoms of tinnitus, vertigo, and hearing loss. The patient may experience progressive hearing loss on the affected side, and if a senior citizen, may also have presbycusis in the remaining good ear. That combination may lead to depression and markedly reduced communication. Of course, if surgery has occurred, the patient may be left with a dead ear, not to mention a facial paralysis or other neurologic signs. If the cochlea is destroyed as a necessary concomitant of the surgery, and there is no hearing at all on that side, the patient may find the unilateral loss significant. In one of the case reports in this chapter, the patient is a police officer for whom the ability to localize sound was critical, certainly far more important than it is for most of us. The patient's auditory rehabilitation program consisted of two hours per week for over one year, during which time he relearned localization. Other rehabilitative measures, including the provision of appropriate hearing aids such as a contralateral routing of signal (CROS) aid and vestibular rehabilitation to improve balance and mobility after the loss of vestibular function, are very important.

Audiology is recognized as having four primary components: identification (screening), diagnosis, treatment, and rehabilitation. It is easy to follow each of these components and to recognize the contribution of the profession when discussion centers around the identification and management of the newborn hearing-impaired child. It is also relatively easy to recognize these roles in the industrial setting or when confronting the geriatric population. Unfortunately, there are very few programs for audiological treatment and rehabilitation of the adult adventitiously hearing impaired, most notably, those whose ears are affected by eighth cranial nerve pathology. Audiology has tended to leave management to the medical and surgical team. However, this is a population requiring audiological counseling, information on localization and making maximum use of residual hearing, amplification, protection of the ear and hearing, and in some cases, assistive devices, auditory training, speech reading and so on. Their numbers are small, but their needs are great.

Chapter *14*

# *Auditory Processing Disorders*

Historically, several more or less equally confusing terms have been employed to label those kinds of situations in which the patient seems to sense the signal adequately, but is unable to process it. Davis (1978) liked the broad term "central dysacousis," while others have employed central deafness, auditory agnosia, word deafness, receptive aphasia, and autism, to name just a few. Katz, Stecker, and Henderson (1992) defined auditory processing as what we do with the signal once heard. They observed that a variety of learning and communicative problems have become associated with central auditory processing disorders. The fact is that these may or may not be terms describing the same behavior (Chermak, 1996).

In general, experimentally induced lesions at specific locations in the brain result in specific peculiarities in behavior (Penfield and Roberts, 1959). It is also generally true that the more narrowly restricted the lesion, the more narrowly restricted the aberrant behavior. However, clinical lesions are rarely specific or so clearly defined, so it is nearly impossible to use them to impart specific diagnostic information or meaning. It is necessary to consider the pathology and etiology in each case to be able to discriminate among the several possible behavioral sequelae. It is a clinical irony that, in practice, it may not be important to be so discriminating. The effects or symptoms of many central pathologies are overtly similar, as are the treatments, regardless of the site or etiology of the disorder. Sometimes, only the fine nuances of a test for central auditory pathology can distinguish among them. Further, assessment of the patient with a central auditory deficit is not an easy task. The patient will usually pass all the conventional audiometric tests, and it is often a specific referral for additional information about central processing that encourages the astute clinician to pursue the matter further. The case history is the key, not the audiogram. The young patient in educational difficulty, the hyperactive child, the adult with a headache, the dizzy patient, and sometimes as little as a statement such as "I keep forgetting what I am told," should be enough to trigger an investigation.

## *Pathology and Etiology*

Usually, auditory processing disorders arise from cerebral lesions with the site of the pathology often being the temporal lobe. Sometimes these disorders are due to improper connections between the auditory area of the temporal lobe and other motor, sensory, or integrating areas of the brain. Auditory processing disorders may also arise from a pathology in those structures that connect the two hemispheres of the brain. Figure 14-1 illustrates the location of the principal areas of the auditory nervous system.

There are connections between the two hemispheres indicating the flow of acoustic information from one side to the other. There will be differences in behavior as a function of which of these areas is damaged and to what degree, and at what age or stage in develop-

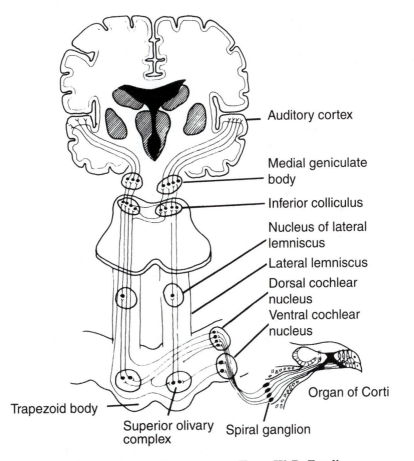

**FIGURE 14-1    Central auditory system. (From W. R. Zemlin,** *Speech and Hearing Science*, **3rd ed. Englewood Cliffs, NJ: Prentice-Hall, 1988)**

ment the lesion occurred. Further, deficits will be a function of the severity of any lesion, regardless of the age of onset. Finally, two generalizations can be made about the effects of pathology upon the central auditory system:

1. Lesions occurring after language development will usually result in a relatively specific and identifiable language deficit.
2. Lesions occurring before the onset of language development will result in more subtle and generalized deficits that are not so easily identified.

The various disorders may be considered along a continuum. One approach is in terms of their prelinguistic and postlinguistic onset. In effect, the difference is a congenital versus an acquired pathology. That artificial and arbitrary division follows the pattern established throughout this text and is designed to simplify understanding of a complex subject and not result in any misconceptions about central pathologies.

## Prelingual Disorders

Congenital malformations or disorders of the central auditory system may be so subtle that they go unnoticed for a lifetime. On the other hand, they may be so dramatic as to cause severe retardation, seizures, or what appears to be a total agnosia (cortical deafness). Aside from the intellectual and scientific knowledge gained from associating a site of lesion with a specific pathologic behavior, if one could be found, information concerning the locus of a congenital central disorder is of small clinical treatment value. Chief among the prenatal and natal factors associated with central deficits have been toxoplasmosis, hyperbilirubinemia, trauma at birth, a prolapsed cord or the umbilicus tightly wrapped around the throat causing a severe or prolonged oxygen deprivation (asphyxia). Asphyxia seems to have the greatest potential to produce damage to the brain including the auditory nervous system. Robertson (1978) singled out oxygen deprivation as a major cause of hearing impairment and motor disability in the newborn. Deprivation of oxygen associated with environmental toxins may also have widespread neurologic sequelae. It should also be noted that asphyxia is one of the high-risk items from the register for early detection of congenital sensorineural hearing losses (Joint Committee on Infant Hearing, 1994).

Almost all the factors that may result in a congenital deafness are also likely to produce processing difficulties, even in the absence of an actual hearing loss (Gerber, 1977). For example, Tooley (1973) has indicated that infants with hemolytic disease and respiratory distress in the early neonatal period often have somewhat lowered IQs when measured at age three years. They also had mild to moderate language disturbances when examined at age seven years. Leopold (1979) found that neonatal asphyxia had occurred frequently in the histories of children with language delay.

Mencher et al. (1978) reported that many children on a high-risk register for hearing loss, who had failed the high-risk screening but who had normal hearing, had physical and mental anomalies, as well as decreased performance in the school environment. Some people who have difficulty reading or spelling have an inability to make the connection between auditory input and verbal output. Certainly that type of processing disorder, while not a hearing loss in the customary sense of the word, is an auditory system processing deficit. The audiologist must be aware of the relationship between hearing and auditory processing and, of course, the possibility that some learning disorders are really disorders of auditory processing.

For auditory stimuli to be meaningful, there must be an intact auditory perceptual system that transmits, processes, stores, and retrieves information provided by the peripheral hearing mechanism. It is the perceptual system that permits focusing on specific stimuli while blocking out irrelevant auditory information. It is the perceptual system that enables identification of a voice or that permits recognition of "sit" as one of the "it" words that rhymes with "hit." Auditory perceptual disturbances involve the entire communication cycle, interfering with the complex interdependence of auditory sensitivity, auditory perception, language, and speech. The acoustic world is not perceived normally by children with deficits in these areas. The result is that the delicately balanced relationships between cognition and language and between language and subsequent academic behavior are disturbed.

The general term auditory perception, used for lack of a better one, encompasses several subareas: auditory discrimination, auditory association, auditory closure, auditory memory, auditory localization, and auditory figure-ground perception. Disruption of one or more of these perceptual skills may result in a moderate to severe learning disability. Although each of the subareas may be considered independently, in reality they are very interdependent. Deficits rarely appear in one subarea alone.

## Auditory Discrimination

Auditory discrimination is the ability to recognize acoustic similarities and differences. Phoneme combinations are meaningless or confusing in the presence of this type of deficit. A disorder may be manifested by the inability to differentiate contrasting vowels and consonants (e.g., set from sit, peg from keg, and pick from pit). This disorder should not be confused or equated with the reduction of speech discrimination ability in cochlear pathology involving the destruction of the hair cells of the organ of Corti. In contrast, this problem is quite similar, if not identical, to that seen as phonemic regression in the presbycusic patient. Abnormal auditory discrimination due to central deficit is the consequence of a distortion of speech sounds at the cortical level. The patient (usually a child) is unable to learn the correct association of visual and auditory symbols, and, as a result, has difficulty learning to read aloud.

## Auditory Association

Auditory association is the ability to relate meaning to particular environmental sounds or spoken words. A child with this problem may recognize the sound of a bird (auditory discrimination and auditory sensitivity) and be able to differentiate between a bird whistle and a human whistle. However, such a child is unable to recognize the significance of either signal. Similarly, he or she may be able to hear speech, but be unable to relate a combination of specific sounds to an appropriate referent (be it a word, phrase, or entire idea or concept). Abstraction ability is hampered, and thoughts are visually concrete. The ultimate result is a reduction in the ability to manipulate symbolic ideas. When an auditory stimulus cannot be linked to a previous experience, the individual may respond in an inappropriate manner, or fail to respond at all.

## *Auditory Closure*

The ability to complete the missing part of a verbally presented message is called auditory closure. For example, "_uper _arket" may be difficult for a child with a closure problem to recognize aurally as "supermarket." Good auditory closure is necessary for the development of the phonetic skills required in sound blending and is thus closely tied to the child's ability to read, spell, speak, and write. In addition, a child with such a difficulty might not be able to fill in a word missing in a sentence (e.g., Answer the _____ when someone knocks on it). Auditory closure enables correct analysis of the signal and filling in when a portion of the message is not heard or perceived. Without closure skills, the sequencing of events becomes extremely difficult and auditory imagery will either be distorted or will be impossible to achieve. Relationships between ideas often become irrational or non-existent. The patient's speech may become dysfluent and hesitant, and it becomes difficult to use oral language as a medium for thought.

## *Auditory Memory*

The ability to recall a sequence of information presented acoustically is called auditory memory. Short-term memory is concerned with retention over a period of seconds, or, at the very most, a few minutes; while long-term memory refers to storage of auditory information over an extended period. The capacity for storage is usually quite variable, dependent upon the uniqueness of the material, the frequency of exposure, and the individual's interest and skill. Typically, deficits are manifested by an inability to recall previous events and to associate them with current experiences. There may also be a parallel deficit in auditory sequencing. That is, the person may be unable to order events correctly. The result of these multiple problems will be a variety of order errors in sound blending (e.g., fist becomes fits) and many letter reversals when writing.

## *Auditory Localization*

Spatial orientation, or auditory localization, refers to the ability to locate the source of a sound in the environment. Skill in that area is expected as early as three or four months of age. Even children as young as one day will shift their eyes in the direction of a sound (Brazelton, 1969). Most children with auditory perceptual localization difficulty remain undetected because their audiograms and general auditory behavior are normal. Only in specific situations, often involving physical safety where the direction of a danger is critical, does the disability become evident. Rapid changes in the direction of a sound generate anxiety, creating chaos in the learning situation.

## *Auditory Figure-Ground Perception*

The ability to isolate relevant sounds from background noises and to separate them meaningfully requires figure-ground perception. The cocktail party effect (Cherry, 1966), which is the ability to tune into a conversation when there may be another, perhaps closer and louder competing conversation nearby, illustrates this skill. Because they are unable to screen out irrelevant stimuli satisfactorily, those with inadequate auditory figure-ground balance often appear distractible. Their attention is pulled from one stimulus to another, depending on which is dominant. They react to both important and unimportant auditory stimuli. Such children are often deemed to be hyperactive and poorly disciplined and are often classed as having behavior problems.

# *Postlingual Disorders*

Due to the relative plasticity of the developing infant central nervous system, if the damage occurs prelingually, there is greater opportunity for recovery or compensation through the extended use of other central areas. On the other hand, because the neural pathways and connections are relatively fixed by the time normal growth and development reach the postlingual state, damage occurring at that time seems to have less opportunity for recovery or compensatory use of other central areas.

The etiologies producing acquired central auditory pathology are as diverse as the processing disorders themselves. These may range from tumors to trauma and infections to inflammations. The results of cortical lesions will vary depending upon their location and severity. Pathologic lesions of the central nervous system may be simply destructive or they may destroy and simultaneously irritate the surrounding tissue. In the latter case, epilepsy, whether localized or generalized, is a common accompaniment to the destructive effect. Destructive lesions in the temporal lobe will have more serious effects on audition than lesions of the occipital or parietal lobes because the auditory cortex resides in the temporal lobes. Further, lesions of the left cerebral hemisphere will have more serious effects on audition than lesions of the right hemisphere; and, of course, a lesion affecting both hemispheres is far more serious than a unilateral problem.

For most people (whether right-handed or left-handed), language function predominates in the left cerebral hemisphere (Wada and Rasmussen, 1960). Consequently, the processing of speech is more severely impaired by left-side lesions than by right-side lesions. Damage to the left hemisphere leads to those disorders classically and traditionally described as aphasia, that is, the loss or diminution of the ability to process or produce meaningful spoken language. If the language system is seen as a flow of processed information from interacting auditory, sensorimotor, and visual systems, and an associated feedback mechanism for each of these channels, it is easy to conceptualize aphasia as an inability to use one or more of the information systems along with the others (Schuell, 1965). The more specific and singular the damage to a particular sensory system, the more clearly defined is the linguistic disorder; and the more restricted are abstractions, generalizations, and discriminations. It is not entirely clear what happens to auditory processing in the case of lesions to the right cerebral hemisphere. It may be that damage to the right side of the brain leads to auditory processing difficulties for acoustic events not related to speech.

A more generalized disorder related to aphasia is auditory agnosia. The patient with auditory agnosia is unable to discriminate acoustic events from one another, whether or not they include speech. That is, the ear can hear the sounds, but the brain cannot decode them. In the extreme, a pure auditory agnosia would involve a total word deafness in which the ear receives and transmits a signal, but the brain cannot relate it to auditory memory, to previous linguistic experience, or to clues from other sensory modes. The inability to monitor one's own verbal output through one's own auditory channel, an extremely critical factor in verbal interaction, is destroyed. The obvious consequence is the loss of aural and oral communication.

## *Neoplasms*

One of the most dramatic and feared lesions of the central system is a brain tumor. These tumors, usually named after their cellular structure, are called by such names as glioma, astrocytoma, blastoma, et cetera. A meningioma, as discussed earlier, is a tumor of the meninges, the layers of tissue that cover the brain and spinal cord.

A tumor located in or on the temporal lobe may cause auditory hallucinations and seizures. In addition, if the tumor is on the left side, it is highly likely there will be an interference with speech and language production or reception. One patient reported hearing a Beethoven symphony during a seizure, while another recalled radio broadcasts first heard as a child thirty years earlier. What mechanism triggers these auditory memories is not known. The treatment for these tumors usually involves radiation, chemotherapy, and surgery. The ototoxic effects of chemical treatments have already been discussed, and the reader will undoubtedly recall that they can lead to significant hearing loss. Surgical intervention, which involves opening the skull and removing the tumor, will usually relieve the symptoms. Generalizations are very difficult where brain tumors are concerned, but tumors near or on the surface of the brain are usually more successfully removed than those deep within its substance. Unfortunately, even if the patient survives the surgery, damage to the surrounding cortical tissue will often result in some permanent deficit. Surgery cannot always entirely remove some of these structures, and sometimes the residual effects are devastating. The tumor may continue to grow, the patient may die, or the effects of the surgery may leave the patient with limited function. Make no mistake, these surgeries are undertaken to preserve life, and surgical skill is improving dramatically. More of these patients are now surviving. That is a tribute to our surgical colleagues, but it does mean that audiologists and speech–language pathologists are beginning to see more and more of these patients in their facilities.

## *Diseases*

Chief among the diseases causing auditory deficits are meningitis and encephalitis. Syphilis is now a less frequent cause of central neurologic pathology, although it does occur. Briefly, these diseases cause diffuse infective inflammation of brain tissue. The infection is rarely uniform, and some areas of the brain may be more severely affected than others. These infections may therefore result in deafness in the usual sense, an auditory perceptual deficit, or some combination of the two. The perceptual deficit will depend on the degree and location of the neurologic damage.

Multiple sclerosis is an excellent example of another type of disorder involving the central auditory pathways. This disease is characterized by plaques or islands of demyelination throughout the central nervous system, usually at axonal points. Demyelination impairs neural function by interfering with the electrical transmission of signals through the central nervous system. Lesions are frequently found on the optic nerve, in the brain stem, the cerebellum, or the pyramidal motor system. Early signs of the disease may include transient weakness, minor gait disturbances, vertigo, or visual involvement (diplopia and blurring). If the temporal lobe or other auditory areas become involved, the patient may show an apathy and lack of judgment not previously seen, seizures, and alterations in speech and understanding. There may be scanning speech, dysarthria, and a very slow speaking rate. These may be accompanied by word-finding difficulties; sometimes the pattern resembles stuttering. Speech discrimination and perception become markedly reduced when there is a great deal of background noise present. That is a typical sign of central auditory pathology.

## Vascular Events (Cerebrovascular Accidents)

A cerebrovascular accident (CVA) or stroke, is, without doubt, the most common reason for cerebral damage. A CVA may be caused by one of three mechanisms:

1. A thrombosis or blood clot may occur in any cerebral blood vessel. The clot then obstructs the flow through the vessel and the area of the body it supplies becomes ischemic (suffers from lack of oxygen) and ultimately dies. This is the single most common cause of CVA and is associated with increasing age, high blood pressure, smoking, and other evidence of atherosclerosis (hardening of the arteries).

2. An embolus or blood clot that has formed somewhere else may pass into the cerebral blood vessels, become trapped, and block the blood flow through that vessel. If the clot is very small, the block may be temporary, and the clot may pass on. The ischemic effects usually recover completely and the diagnosis is a so called transient ischemic attack (TIA). The usual source of an embolic clot is the heart (often following a recent heart attack) or one of the carotid arteries.

3. A hemorrhage occurs when a blood vessel bursts and bleeds. This is the least common occurrence and causes damage for two reasons. First, the blood itself is an irritant and damages surrounding neural tissue. Second, the affected blood vessel usually goes into spasm, effectively cutting off the blood supply to distal areas.

Regardless of the mechanism, the end result is very similar and the degree of damage will depend on the size of the vessel affected and consequently the volume of brain that is damaged. In severe cases, the degree and extent of brain damage will be fatal. In other cases, a small vessel supplying one of the silent areas of the brain may be affected and the patient may be symptomless. Usually, the end result is somewhere between these two extremes. If a portion of brain that carries some of the auditory pathways is affected, there may be auditory symptoms. Typically, if the left temporal lobe is involved, a dysphasia or aphasia will result.

## Head Trauma

Any serious head trauma can result in a central auditory processing disorder. Again, this will depend on the degree, site, and severity of the brain damage. Unfortunately, unless the damage is localized, there is usually fairly global trauma and the patient is likely to have many other neurologic problems such as memory, motor, and general awareness disorders. Consequently, rehabilitation with these patients is extremely hard work and often very sad, as they are often relatively young. There is a more detailed discussion of head trauma in Chapter 9.

## Iatrogenesis

Some trauma to the brain may be iatrogenic, that is, doctor-caused. These lesions usually result from brain surgery performed to alleviate other problems or symptoms. For example, removal of a cyst or tumor that has grown within the head may require the loss of or damage to cortical tissue or may result in the development of scar tissue. As is the case with all central disorders, the exact deficit will depend on the region of the brain that is affected, and the degree it has been damaged. An excellent example for study was a child who developed a large cyst (the size of a man's fist) on the left parietal lobe. In order to remove the cyst, and in subsequent operations to remove scar tissue, most of the parietal lobe and much of the left temporal lobe were removed. Eventually the entire left hemisphere was removed. The child's language function was disturbed in a very peculiar way. After recovering from the surgery and returning to school, he greeted all the teaching and rehabilitative staff by title. He went from room to room in his wheelchair identifying each person by occupation; for example, "You are physical therapy." He was right, too. However, he knew no one's name after the surgery, even though he had known them all quite well before the operations. The point to be made here is that the behavior seen in this child whose etiology is iatrogenic actually differs very little from some stroke patients, head trauma patients, or even from those who seem to have been born with a central processing disorder.

# Identifying Central Auditory Pathology

It is the educational, speech–language pathology, and audiological centers that carry the primary clinical burden for most of these patients. The initial referral is often to audiology because the patient does not seem to respond to auditory stimuli, and the assumption is that a hearing loss is present. Hearing testing is appropriate and important but may not be fruitful. Patients in this group may not suffer from impairment of auditory sensitivity. It is only through special tests designed to probe auditory perceptual skills under various conditions that the examiner can see patients with central deficits display their special disabilities. Most procedures for differential diagnosis of these disorders involve analysis of a patient's ability to process verbal signals that have been distorted. Distortions are accomplished by altering the signals through filtering, speeding them up, slowing them down, competing with them, alternating them between the ears, or delaying their normal feedback rate to the patient's ears. The patient with a central auditory lesion will have difficulty processing any or all of these combinations, depending on the type, extent, and location of the lesion. Most of the common procedures have been described in detail in other sources (Chermak, 1996; Katz, 1977; Keith, 1977).

Various combinations of the distortion techniques are used to localize behavioral deficits in distinct areas of the brain. Accordingly, tests for central auditory pathology may be grouped into three main categories, each aimed at detecting lesions in a fairly limited area of the brain. The first category involves techniques of binaural fusion, a procedure Matzker (1959) related to lesions in the brain stem and discussed in detail in Chapter 13. In a typical test sequence, the patient will be asked to integrate high-frequency information presented to one ear with low-frequency information presented to the other ear. That is, some high-frequency components of a spondee will be received in one ear, while some low-frequency components of the same word will be presented simultaneously to the other ear. Neither portion of the word carries enough information to make the word meaningful to a normal listener, but normals can easily understand the word when both halves are presented. Patients with brain stem lesions cannot do so easily (Ivey, 1969).

The second category of tests involves techniques of alternation. A sentence is presented to the patient via earphones, with the signal alternating between the ears every 300 ms (Figure 14-2). Patients with diffuse central pathology, as may be seen in children with auditory perceptual disorders or those with brain stem lesions, do not perform well on this type of task. That is, they cannot interpret a signal presented to the two ears into a single message (Willeford, 1977).

The third category of tests involves techniques of filtering. In one such test, the patient is presented with a sequence of words in only one ear. The filter attenuates frequencies above 500 Hz at a rate of 18 dB per octave. Patients unable to identify and repeat words presented in this fashion may have lesions in the temporal lobe.

Some other tests reviewed here are presented only as examples. The important concept is not the tests per se, but how similar the tests are to the disorders considered under both the headings prelingual and postlingual disorders. For example, the section on postlingually acquired disorders contains a discussion of a problem called auditory figure-ground perception. One test procedure, dichotically competing messages, is quite useful in identifying the child with a figure-ground deficit. In this type of test, competing messages are presented, one to each ear at different sensation levels. The patient is asked to repeat both messages, a task that requires separate interpretation of the competing signals. That procedure is put to excellent application when used to evaluate an adult patient suspected of having a temporal lobe tumor. As indicated earlier, neither the age of onset of the disorder nor the medical terminology is as important as the behavior of the patient.

Another example of an excellent procedure for assessing a central disorder is the staggered spondaic word (SSW) test, first described by Katz in 1962. It is a competing message test. A spondee is presented to each ear at a 50-dB sensation level, and the patient is required to repeat both of them. A great deal has been written about the interpretation of SSW test data. We are not going to summarize all that information here, but response patterns seem to

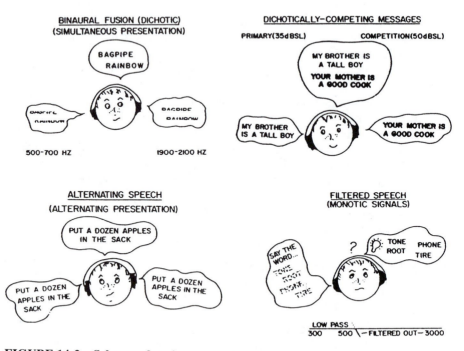

**FIGURE 14-2   Schema of various central auditory test procedures.**

reflect surprisingly specific sites of brain lesions. The SSW is now considered an effective, standardized, and versatile test of central auditory function. However, it is sufficiently complex in its interpretation that one requires special training to employ it.

## Treatment and Management of Central Processing Disorders

In dealing with auditory processing disorders, the discussion is not concerned specifically with ear disease, the principal domain of the otologist. However, that does not mean that the otologist should not be involved or attend to central problems. Psychiatrists, pediatricians, and neurologists are more usually presented with these problems. Because the otologist is the physician most concerned with hearing, that specialty is frequently one of the first to have contact with a patient who has a central processing disorder. Usually an appropriate referral to audiology follows. Central disorders, exclusive of those related to disease and surgical intervention, present a new area for most medical practitioners, but one that is worthy of attention and demanding more and more of it (Huttenlocher, 1987). Medical treatment is primarily drug oriented to control seizures, motor disorders, and aberrant behavior. Surgical management is obviously required in a number of cases, particularly in neoplastic disease.

For the young child, the burden of responsibility has fallen to the educational audiologists, psychologists, teachers of the hearing impaired, teachers of the learning disabled, speech pathologists, pediatric neurologists, and activist parents who have grown tired of having their children shuffled back and forth among the specialists. With the exception of a few centers specializing in children with these difficulties, treatment and management have been limited to those with an interest and the time. Educational approaches include use of alternate sensory modes (visual versus auditory), drug therapy, reduction of motor activities during communication, limited expectations and educational goals (sometimes in spite of above average intelligence), repetition of messages via recorded programs, and other similar methods. Rapin and Ruben (1979) have proposed that children with "auditory verbal agnosia" be educated as though deaf, that is by total communication. Some of these children are already in classrooms for the hearing impaired. Some are given amplification via auditory trainers in the classroom, and some even get hearing aids. Unfortunately, that sometimes occurs because the child's lack of auditory response is mistaken for a peripheral hearing loss. Be advised: It is the patient's behavior that is most important therapeutically and not the diagnostic label.

The adult fares no better. Deficits frequently go untreated unless displayed as something as dramatic as aphasia or agnosia. Treatment by speech–language pathology will then usually follow. If the problem is subtle, treatment is typically non-existent.

## *Comment*

This chapter has only touched on the question of auditory processing disabilities. This is a relatively uncharted area for many specialties, including audiology, but one that is worthy of attention and is demanding more and more of it (see Chermak, 1996). The child who has even a little trouble with comprehension, attention, distractibility, perception, or language needs help. It is inadequate to examine only for a peripheral auditory disorder. The possibility of a deficit in central auditory processing must also be considered. A treatment regime in which other avenues of input are employed and special teaching devices and methods are used is necessary to compensate for the impaired auditory channel. Such a child must, and can, be allowed to develop to his or her fullest potential.

It is important to keep in mind that many of the children discussed in this chapter, who were described as learning disabled or as suffering from an auditory processing disorder, have similar language difficulties, and in addition, difficulties that are sometimes closer to adult patterns than to other children. In other words, the etiology and age of onset may be different, but the overt problems are quite similar. This further illustrates that the decision to separate central auditory processing disorders into categories based on age of onset (prelingual vs. postlingual), type of trauma (intrinsic vs. extrinsic), or location of lesion (e.g., temporal lobe vs. parietal lobe) is purely arbitrary.

One last word of caution. Unfortunately, many audiology centers do not have the capability to diagnose or treat central disorders. In some cases, a referral and normal audiogram lead to case dismissal, even in the face of parent or patient complaint of difficulty processing auditory signals. This suggests that too many of these patients are being missed in the standard audiological facility. That is particularly true where adults are concerned. It is important that audiologists and otologists become increasingly involved with the diagnosis and treatment of auditory processing disorders, and that audiology centers have available a complete procedure for diagnosing these disabilities in both children and adults. Equally important, there should be programs for their treatment and management. As continued research develops new procedures for diagnosis and treatment, more and more of the audiologist's time will be spent in identification, diagnosis, and treatment of these types of patients.

# Chapter 15

# *Hearing Loss Management in Children and Adults**

The American Speech–Language–Hearing Association (1984) position on the definition of and competencies for aural rehabilitation indicates the need for professional preparation and experience in identification and evaluation of sensory capabilities; interpretation of evaluation results, counseling, and referral; and intervention for communication problems resulting from hearing loss. The process of aural rehabilitation may best be described as one of hearing loss management. Hearing loss management is guided by codes of professional ethics, principles of preferred practice, and federal laws protecting and ensuring the rights of disabled individuals. Minimal compliance with Principle of Ethics I of the ASHA Code of Ethics is demonstrated by providing services competently, without discrimination, using every available resource and only when the outcome of such service can be measured and determined to be of benefit (ASHA, 1993b). Preferred practice guidelines in aural rehabilitation assessment and treatment are offered by the American Speech–Language–Hearing Association (1993a). Clinical services are to be provided on the basis of an assessment of rehabilitative need. The clinical process should focus on treatment of communication problems and include informative and supportive counseling. The treatment program should include selection and use of sensory aids in a controlled environment. All appropriate records need to be maintained and, overall, it is expected that the program will result in improved communication ability.

Federal laws that apply to hearing-disabled individuals include the Rehabilitation Act of 1973, or the "Bill of Rights" for disabled individuals. This law ensures that individuals will not be excluded on the basis of hearing disability from participation in or benefit from programs or services receiving federal funds. Public Law 94-142, also known as the Education for All Handicapped Children Act of 1975 and renamed the Individuals with Disabilities Education Act (IDEA) in 1990, ensures hearing-impaired children from age five

---

*This chapter was written by Dean C. Garstecki and Susan F. Erler.

to twenty-one years the right to a free and appropriate public education. It provides for identification of hearing-impaired children, determination of the need for amplification, provision of communication problem assessment and treatment, implementation of individualized educational plans (IEP), institution of hearing conservation programs, and counseling. The rights of parents of hearing-disabled children also are protected by this law. In 1986, Public Law 99-457 was enacted to expand previous legislation to provide services to preschool children with disabilities. This law calls for states to develop and implement programs to provide services to infants and toddlers. These services include a comprehensive multidisciplinary assessment of the child as well as a determination of the family's strengths and needs. As a result of this evaluation, an individualized family service plan (IFSP) is developed. The IFSP includes child and family goals, evaluation criteria, designation of a case manager, and identification of services required by the child and family. Public Law 101-336, the Americans with Disabilities Act (ADA) of 1990, guarantees equal opportunity for disabled individuals, including those with a hearing disability, in employment, public accommodations, state and local government services, and transportation. Title II (Public Services) of the ADA ensures that hearing-disabled individuals will be provided with necessary auxiliary aids and services for communication access.

Finally, all hearing loss does not result in a handicapping or disabling condition. The following definitions may be helpful when considering matters relating to hearing loss management. Hearing loss or disorder refers to a pathologic condition of the auditory mechanism. Hearing impairment refers to abnormal function of the auditory system. Hearing disability refers to an individual's reduced ability to carry on life's everyday activities as a result of hearing loss. Hearing handicap implies a need for extra assistance as a result of hearing loss (Davis, 1983).

This chapter reviews the impact of hearing loss on basic communication and learning processes and information about the unique personal characteristics of hearing-impaired individuals. It includes a decision tree diagram illustrating the scope of rehabilitative services for hearing-impaired children and adults. This is followed by discussion of sensory aid, communication, and counseling considerations as they relate to evaluation and treatment of hearing-impaired children and adults.

## Impact of Hearing Loss on Communication, Learning, and Personal Development

### Effect on Speech

Hearing loss filters the distinctive properties of auditory signals. Children with mild to moderate hearing loss typically follow the same developmental pattern in speech sound acquisition as those with normal hearing, but at a slower rate. It is difficult for these children to perceive weaker speech elements such as consonantal word endings and voiced fricatives (West and Weber, 1974). Consonants typically contain more high frequency and lower intensity acoustic energy than vowels. Since most hearing loss conditions result in greater residual low-frequency hearing, problems with perception and production of consonants are likely to precede those with vowels. Consonant perception and production errors among the hearing impaired are well-documented (Davis and Hardick, 1981; Hudgins and Numbers, 1942). Davis and Hardick reported that segmental errors reflect relative differences in speech signal audibility and visibility. Highly visible and audible front, voiced consonants (e.g., /m/, /b/, and /v/) are more likely to be articulated correctly than less audible and visible consonants (e.g., /g/, /k/, /h/). Individual consonants may be missing in two- or three-element blends or a neutral vowel may be inserted between adjoining consonants within a cluster (e.g., puhlease). A neutral vowel may be added to consonantal word endings (e.g., rockuh), and voiced and voiceless cognates (e.g., /t/, /d/) may be confused.

In addition to difficulty in consonant perception and production, individuals with profound hearing loss may demonstrate problems in vowel perception and production. Vowel production may become neutralized, that is, only slight variations may be made in production across all vowels. Because vowel production generates tactile resonance cues, severely hearing-impaired individuals may prolong vowel production in an effort to monitor vocal output (Davis and Hardick, 1981). For the same reason, vowels may sound like diphthongs, and natural diphthongs may be prolonged or neutralized (Laughton and Hasenstab, 1993).

In addition to segmental errors, severely hearing-impaired individuals may produce suprasegmental errors. A tendency toward incoordination of phonation and consonant production may cause inappropriate voicing (Ling, 1989). Poor breath stream control may result in expending the entire breath supply in one or two syllables or speaking on inhalation, interrupting the flow of spoken messages and decreasing intelligibility. Resulting voice quality may be described as breathy, harsh, strident, and strained. Adding a characteristically high vocal pitch, monotone, lack of rhythm or inappropriate rhythm, and loud and hypernasal production creates what is termed deaf speech.

Most hearing-impaired individuals have the potential to develop not only functional, but refined, speech production skills (Moeller, Osberger, and Morford, 1987). Because production error patterns are similar regardless of degree of hearing loss, similar approaches to remediation may be applied across a range of hearing-impaired groups (Gold, 1980). Procedures for improving the speech intelligibility of those with impaired hearing remains a matter of concern to educators, clinical investigators, and hearing-impaired individuals.

## *Effect on Language and Learning*

Verbal communication occurs when a sender formulates ideas, requests, or comments and selects, arranges, and presents words and sentences to a receiver. When a receiver hears and understands the words and intent of the message, communication takes place. Key to this process is a common language. Bloom and Lahey (1978) defined language as a "code whereby ideas about the world are represented by a conventional system of signals of communication" (p.4). Children with normal sensory function and exposure to fluent, consistent communication acquire language in a seemingly effortless manner (Quigley and Paul, 1984). But for the child with a hearing loss, language acquisition and cognitive development may be anything but effortless.

In the process of learning how to use language, the child tests self-formed hypotheses regarding word selection and combination. An expression is tested, reinforced, or revised through mature-user feedback. Unfortunately, evidence suggests that hearing impairment alters communicative interaction (MacTurk et al., 1993). In the absence of an auditory feedback system, the hearing-impaired child reduces his vocal play, in turn providing less reinforcement of the parents' attempts to communicate with the child.

When a child is hearing impaired, the language-learning process is affected by the degree and duration of hearing loss, use of amplification, intellectual capabilities, additional handicapping conditions, commitment to habilitative efforts, style of communication, and the quality of language stimulation and instruction. The hearing-impaired child's language development is likely to be delayed, disordered, or otherwise different from that of normally-hearing age peers. Even mild and moderate hearing losses may place a child at risk for "delayed development of verbal skills and reduced academic achievement" (Davis et al., 1986).

Up to the age of six to nine months, hearing-impaired babies demonstrate vocalization patterns similar to their hearing counterparts. Phonemes first produced by hearing-impaired children are similar to hearing infants. Other prelinguistic behavior is exhibited by the use of informal gestures and pointing, demonstrating the child's need to interact with the people in the environment (McAnally, Rose, and Quigley, 1987). Infants exposed to American Sign Language reportedly produce their first signs before the first spoken words of hearing babies, some as early as five months (Bonvillian, Orlansky, and Novack, 1983; Litowitz, 1987). This precocious language milestone appears to reflect a maturation of motor skills for gesture occurring earlier than those for speech. By eighteen months of age, hearing-impaired children may have an expressive vocabulary of fewer than ten words compared to twenty to fifty words for normal hearing peers (Schafer and Lynch, 1980). Semantic studies indicate reduced knowledge and greater inappropriate use of vocabulary among the hearing impaired. More often than those with normal hearing, they demonstrate difficulty understanding the multiple meanings of words. While their storehouse of vocabulary items increases at a fast pace, their sophistication in use of these items remains slow to develop. Hearing-impaired children often find it easier to use known vocabulary to refer to the immediate event rather than to use vocabulary in an abstract sense. The gap in word usage skill between normal-hearing and hearing-impaired children tends to increase rather than close over time. The average vocabulary level of eighteen-year-old hearing-impaired individuals may not exceed the fourth to sixth grade level (Cooper and Rosenstein, 1966; DiFrancesca, 1972).

At the morphological level, the most significant problems for hearing-impaired children are attributed to the relative low audibility and visual obscurity of bound morphemes (i.e., plurals, possessives, comparatives, superlatives, and agent endings). In general, hearing-impaired children apply morphological rules poorly, with their knowledge of inflectional endings (such as past tense and plural markers) being superior to derivational rule usage (changing words from one class to another, e.g., sad to sadly) (Cooper, 1967). For those children who communicate principally through use of American Sign Language, nonfamiliarity with use of morphological markers is a major deterrent to their acquisition (Easterbrooks, 1987). Alternatively, Gilman and Raffin (1975) reported a positive correlation between morpheme rule usage and a hearing-impaired child's exposure to manually coded English that includes morphological markers. Children using spoken English appear to acquire morphological markers in the same order as their hearing peers, but at a much slower rate (Presnell, 1973). In general, hearing-impaired children demonstrate a tendency to confuse noun–verb agreement, tense markers, and use of possessive forms (Taylor, 1969) and to omit, overgeneralize, or incorrectly use word endings (Easterbrooks, 1987). In most instances, receptive knowledge of morphological rules is considered to be superior to that demonstrated expressively (Cooper, 1967).

Syntactic skills among hearing-impaired children have been found to be delayed in comparison to normal hearing peers. Engen and Engen (1983) reported delays approaching three years in seven-year-old hearing-impaired children. Hearing impairment affects acquisition of grammatical rule usage in both spoken and written form and the rate of development appears to be related to degree of hearing loss (Davis and Hardick, 1981). Sentences produced by these children tend to be loaded with content words, especially nouns, and arranged in subject–verb–object order regardless of the intent of the message. According to Russell, Quigley, and Power (1976), the tendency to process sentence information using a linear rather than hierarchical structure accounts for many of the hearing-impaired child's difficulties with English.

Pragmatic skill development in hearing-impaired children has not been extensively investigated. Kretschmer and Kretschmer (1978) found that hearing-impaired children were capable of understanding the same pragmatic language functions as normally hearing children. Curtis, Prutting, and Lowell (1979) determined that hearing-impaired babies were capable of expressing pragmatic intentions. Studies of adult–child interaction reveal hearing mothers of deaf children use more tutorial strategies than spontaneous verbalization and verbal praise (Gross, 1970; Meadow et al., 1981). Hearing-impaired children exposed to oral language develop communication intents similar to normal-hearing children (Curtis, Prutting, and Lowell, 1979). In addition, hearing-impaired children often demonstrate difficulty in entering a conversation by using attention-getting strategies (McKirdy and Blank, 1982).

Cognition is the complex ability to acquire and organize knowledge and use knowledge through thinking, recalling, and reasoning. Unfortunately, research examining the cognitive development of hearing-impaired children is flawed by limited control of variables such as mode of communication, method of assessment, and interpretation of results. However, certain general conclusions can be drawn. It appears that much of the difference in cognitive development between hearing and hearing-impaired children reflects verbal influences including the language of instruction used during assessment and the child's mode of communication. Hearing-impaired children develop cognitive skills in the same sequence as normal hearing children but at a delayed rate. Examination of short-term memory suggests that performance varies with degree of hearing loss, intelligence, the communication system the individual uses, and whether the person uses a speech-based code.

While considerable information has been published, the effect of hearing loss on language and cognitive development requires further study. There is a need for more appropriate tests of language and cognitive development. Inconsistencies in educational and habilitative methods must also be resolved.

## *Effect on Personal Development*

Attempts to define a psychology of deafness have failed to identify personality traits or mental conditions that are unique to hearing-impaired individuals. Overall, hearing-impaired individuals experience the same range of emotions, behaviors, and abilities as everyone. Hearing-impaired children are sometimes described as more impulsive, passive, dependent, immature, inflexible, and egocentric than hearing children (Paul and Quigley, 1990). While these behaviors can be regarded as normal given particular circumstances, they also may be more frequently observed in both hearing-impaired adults and children than in those with normal hearing and no other disabilities. Behavioral differences are not a direct result of a hearing impairment. Rather, the impact of a hearing loss on communication, reactions to hearing loss, peer relations, and the home and learning environment will have a significant secondary influence on psychosocial development.

Despite successful use of amplification and other technical advances, hearing-impaired individuals continue to experience difficulty functioning on a par with normal-hearing individuals. Unlike others with sensory and physical disabilities, the problems experienced by hearing-impaired individuals may not be fully compensated through prosthetic intervention (Spear, 1984). Hearing loss is invisible. Although a hearing aid serves as a sign of hearing loss, it gives no indication of hearing ability. Hearing loss-related speech disorders may provide another clue but are more often attributed to some physical or mental conditions. The impact of a hearing loss may be confused with mental disorders, personality aberrations, inattention, and, among the elderly, with senility. Unlike those with visible handicaps, hearing-impaired individuals are expected to announce their communication difficulty and take responsibility for explaining to others how to accommodate their loss in order to conduct a successful conversation (Spear, 1984).

Socialization is also affected by the presence of a hearing loss. Age, gender, degree of loss, communication skill, and educational or occupational setting all influence a hearing-impaired person's social skill development. For example, the mainstreamed hearing impaired may feel that they are less popular and have more difficulty making friends. Some teachers indicate these children are likely to have greater difficulty getting along with other children (Loeb and Sarigiani, 1986). Maxon, Brackett, and van den Berg (1991) found hearing-impaired children had difficulty expressing feeling and presenting arguments. Because they are less able to verbally express anger, hearing-impaired children may be more likely to do so physically.

Hearing-impaired individuals are at a disadvantage in job competition primarily due to the academic achievement gap, particularly in reading skill between severely hearing-impaired and normal-hearing individuals (Schildroth, Rawlings, and Allen, 1991). This impacts significantly on the hearing-impaired child's ability to earn a high school degree. The National Center for Education Statistics (1989) reported that essentially 25 percent of all eighteen- and nineteen-year-olds do not earn a high school degree. This rate is as high, if not higher, for ethnic minority and disabled populations (Butler-Nalin, Marder, and Padilla, 1989). However, opportunities for employment of severely hearing-impaired high school graduates are positively impacted by the Americans with Disabilities Act through heightened awareness of their ability to capitalize on technical advances to compensate for hearing loss. On the negative side, many of the new jobs are in lower-paying service-oriented occupations. There also has been some reluctance on the part of employers to place disabled individuals in service occupations because of their high visibility and concerns about consumer interaction (Bluestone, 1989). New jobs will require higher skills than current jobs, further increasing the need for academic and vocational training.

## The Clinical Process

Hearing loss management is based on several principles. The first is that everything should be done to minimize personal disability or handicap, with medical and/or prosthetic intervention given priority over approaches to intervention. Next, intervention must be guided by evaluation data. Clinical evaluations are needed in the selection and fitting of sensory aids, in developing the communication component of a treatment program, and to guide the counseling process. Initial intervention plans then are to be regularly reevaluated and revised. Hearing loss management is a dynamic process with changes reflecting adjustment to hearing loss and advances in hearing technology. Finally, ethical practice dictates that formal intervention occur only as long as benefit to the client can be demonstrated and that dismissal or referral is considered when appropriate. Organization of clinical procedures for hearing-impaired children and adults may be demonstrated using a decision tree diagram (Figure 15-1).

### Candidacy

Any hearing-impaired individual, regardless of degree or type of hearing loss, age at onset, benefit from sensory aids, or degree of self-perceived handicap is a candidate for participation in a hearing loss management program. Ideal candidates are new hearing aid users and newly identified hearing-impaired children. These individuals have already taken their first positive steps toward management of hearing loss. They have become acquainted with hearing aid technology and may be motivated toward considering other assistive listening devices (ALDs). Hearing-impaired individuals and their families may benefit from advice and assistance in management of hearing loss.

### Introduction and Orientation

A professional relationship is initiated during which the client grows to recognize the value of the clinician's resources, and the clinician tries to understand the unique impact of hearing loss on the client's everyday activity. The client is oriented to the clinical process and components. Options for participation are presented, the format explained, and a treatment and fee schedule is set.

### History

Reports of medical treatment for hearing loss, use of sensory aids, and training or counseling in management of hearing loss and its associated problems are reviewed. Communication skill is observed, as is the possible need for sensory aid evaluation or counseling. The

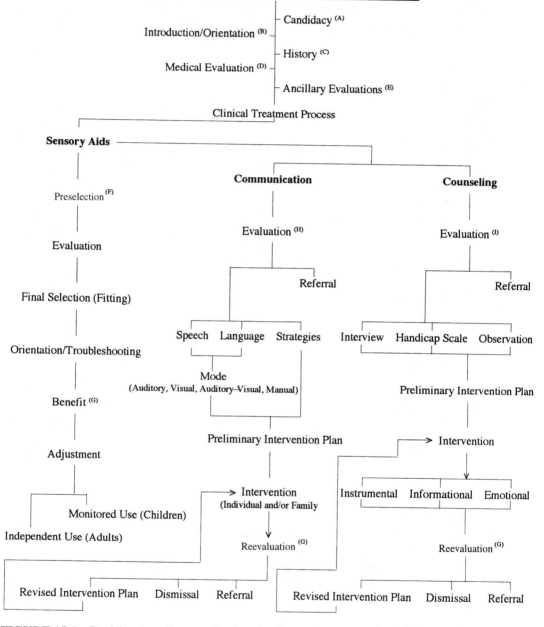

**FIGURE 15-1    Decision tree diagram for hearing loss management in children and adults.**

clinician determines what has been done to address the hearing loss and its associated problems and predicts a client's potential for success. Evidence of noncompliance with professional advice may be reason to anticipate similar reaction to the proposed program.

## *Medical Evaluation*

Examination by an otologist or other specialist is needed to identify treatable conditions. The ear specialist also rules out vestibular disorders, treats problems related to tinnitus, or prepares the ear canal for an earmold impression as part of a hearing aid fitting procedure.

## *Ancillary Evaluations*

Evaluations by other professionals may be required for some clients. These may include an academic assessment, psychological evaluation, and a speech–language evaluation.

## *Preselection of Sensory Aids*

Initial choice of a sensory aid is determined by degree of hearing loss and client preference. Hearing aids typically are the device of choice, but assistive listening devices used alone or in addition to a hearing aid may be preferred. When amplification has limited benefit, tactile aids or cochlear implants may be recommended. By considering audiological information with client lifestyle and personal preference data, the appropriate category of sensory aid can be selected.

## *Benefit and Reevaluation*

Sensory aid benefit is determined through a combination of objective and subjective means, such as real-ear measures, word recognition scores, and questionnaire data. It is equally important to establish treatment efficacy. This usually is accomplished through pre- and postintervention measures.

## *Communication Evaluation*

In children, evaluation of communication skills focuses on measures of speech sound articulation, language skills, voice, communication strategies, and ability to perceive speech aurally, visually, and through combined auditory–visual modalities. For some, evaluation of manual or total communication skills should be included. The intent is to establish the influence of hearing loss on communication for learning and interaction with the family, school, and in social settings. In adults, typically those with some degree of usable hearing or a history of auditory–oral communication ability, evaluation of communication skills focuses on ability to perceive spoken English aurally, visually, and through combined auditory–visual modalities. It also includes measures of speech intelligibility and use of communication strategies. The intent is to determine how hearing loss impacts on communication for purposes of employment and social and family interaction.

## Handicap Scales

Standardized questionnaires are available and useful for determining self-perceived hearing handicaps. These questionnaires yield prescriptive data that may be applied in counseling hearing-impaired individuals and their families as well as in planning communication remediation activities.

# Considerations in Evaluations

## Sensory Aid Benefit

To ensure that capabilities are optimized, one of the clinician's first responsibilities will be to determine whether the device is benefiting the user. There are international standards that apply to hearing aid performance measurement—e.g., ANSI S3.3-1971, ANSI S3.22-1987, IEC 118 (1959) and Hearing Aid Industry Conference (HAIC) (1961) standards. International standards for specifying the performance characteristics of ALDs are currently being developed. Specifications for each type of cochlear implant device are determined by their manufacturers.

Preferred practice guidelines for hearing aid assessment specify inclusion of behavioral measures (e.g., functional gain and word recognition measures), real-ear measures, electroacoustic evaluation, determination of earmold and frequency response characteristics, and administration of communication inventories. User benefit can be surmised from differences in performance between aided and unaided conditions (ASHA, 1993a). For ALDs, in addition to determining user benefit by noting performance with and without the device, consideration is given to hearing aid compatibility when the ALD is used to enhance hearing aid use. At this time, there are no specifications for measurement of electroacoustic characteristics of ALDs or for setting output controls (ASHA, 1993a). Preferred practice guidelines for assessment of cochlear implants suggest that benefit in their use can be determined by measures of pre- and postdevice performance on speech and nonspeech processing tasks. Use of communication inventories also is recommended (ASHA, 1993a).

Sensory aid benefit can be measured in two ways: pre and post measures of speech recognition and user survey. The ideal speech recognition test should represent conversational speech, allow for multimodality processing, be objectively scored, be reliable, and be available in multiple forms. Failing to find test materials that meet these requirements, Cox, Alexander, and Gilmore (1987) created the Connected Speech Test (CST).

Questionnaires useful for quantifying self-assessed hearing aid benefit include the Hearing Aid Performance Inventory (HAPI) developed by Walden, Demorest, and Hepler (1984), the Profile of Hearing Aid Performance (PHAP) by Cox and Gilmore (1990), and the Profile of Hearing Aid Benefit (PHAB) by Cox and Rivera (1992). The HAPI was developed to measure successful use of amplification in noisy situations; quiet situations with the primary talker nearby; situations with reduced message information; and, situations involving processing of nonspeech stimuli. The PHAB was developed to determine hearing aid benefit under selected environmental conditions (viz., Environment A scale consisting of familiar talker and ease of communication subscales; Environment B scale consisting of reverberation and reduced cues subscales; Environment C scale on background noise; and Environmental sounds scale consisting of aversiveness to sounds and distortion of sounds subscales).

The advantage of using self-report questionnaires to measure sensory aid benefit is that they enable the user to be surveyed directly. The primary disadvantage relates to the current lack of information on the clinical utility of self-report measures. There are no data to indicate how much of a difference in self-report assessment scores is required before noted changes can be considered to be clinically significant (Walden and Grant, 1993). Another disadvantage relates to the accuracy of collected information. This problem may be reduced through multiple, time-delayed re-administrations or administration to others who are familiar with the hearing-impaired individual. In all, self-report methodology is helpful for measuring benefit from use of sensory aids. While clinical research and practice have focused on measuring benefit in using hearing aids, the same word recognition comparisons and survey approaches could be adapted to determine benefit from ALDs and cochlear implants.

## *Evaluation of Communication Skills*

In addition to mandating a free and appropriate education, PL 94-142 and PL 99-457 are clear in their requirements regarding evaluation of handicapped children. Comprehensive, nondiscriminatory, multidisciplinary evaluation must be completed prior to placement in special education and must include testing of auditory abilities, intelligence, communication skills, academic performance, social-emotional status, motor skills, vision, and general health. Such evaluations are problematic because (1) most evaluative tools were designed for and normed on hearing children; (2) they often are conducted by professionals whose training and experience relate primarily to hearing children (Gibbins, 1989); and (3) they may fail to allow for needs related to use of interpreters, examiner's style of communication, and extra time needed for administration of tests. Multidisciplinary evaluation serves to identify strengths and weaknesses, assists in determining appropriate academic placement and development of an individual educational program, monitor progress, and to provide information to parents and professionals. It should include both formal and informal measurement.

The clinician's primary concern is assessment of communication skills, including the child's ability to receive, recognize, comprehend, and produce messages. Audiologic assessment helps to identify the sounds available to the child with and without a sensory aid. Benefit provided by hearing aids, ALDs, cochlear implants, or other devices must also be determined. Testing conducted under various listening conditions should approximate the child's communicative environments.

Comprehensive communication evaluations include measurement of both receptive and expressive skills as well as knowledge of the rules of communication (metalinguistics), speech, sign (if used), and written skills (Laughton and Hasenstab, 1993; Ling, 1989; Moeller and Carney, 1993; Ying, 1990). Preschool evaluations rely heavily upon information provided by parents as well as from observation of child–caregiver interactions. Kretschmer and Kretschmer (1990) argue persuasively for the need to assess hearing-impaired children naturalistically. Language sample analysis, in addition to more formal measures, should include evaluation of syntactic, semantic, morphologic, and pragmatic aspects.

Educational and therapeutic programs must be developed with an awareness and under-standing of each child's functional levels and style of learning. Even though the hearing pro-fessional may not be responsible for administering psychoeducational evaluations, it is essential to understand the purpose, administration, and interpretation of results of these instruments. Most frequently used for evaluating cognitive abilities are the Hiskey-Nebraska (Hiskey, 1966), Kaufman Assessment Battery for Children (Kaufman and Kaufman, 1983), Leiter (1979), WISC-R (Wechsler, 1974), and WAIS-R (Wechsler, 1981). Three tests normed for hearing-impaired children to assess academic achievement are the Stanford Achievement Test Battery—Hearing Impaired Edition, Metropolitan Achievement Battery, and Brill Educational Achievement Test for Secondary Age Deaf Students (Paul and Quigley, 1990).

To determine the impact of hearing loss on communication in adults, two essential steps need be followed. First, communication need should be established. Second, communica-tion ability should be measured. A needs assessment is helpful to understand an individual's usual communication situations and to identify specific tasks associated with each. In home, work, and social situations, most hearing-impaired individuals are likely to converse with family, friends, or coworkers face-to-face as well as in small group settings under quiet and noisy listening conditions, with and without the advantage of visual cues. Home communi-cation may require use of the telephone, listening to radios, listening to and watching televi-sion, and responding to alerting and warning systems such as wake-up alarms, doorbells, smoke detectors, and the like (Compton, 1993). Similar experiences may be encountered in the work setting with a need to follow office discussions, understand seminar leaders, deci-pher recorded telephone messages, understand customer complaints, and detect warning sig-nals and computer prompts. Successful communication in these circumstances is dependent on one or more of the following skills: understanding spoken messages with visual input alone; understanding spoken messages by auditory input alone; understanding with com-bined auditory–visual input; and understanding environmental sounds.

Visual-only communication skills can be evaluated through controlled presentation (e.g., video recording) of sentences materials. The Utley Lipreading Task (Utley, 1946), the Central Institute for the Deaf Sentences (Davis and Silverman, 1978), the Revised Speech Perception in Noise Test (Bilger, 1984), and the Visual Enhancement subtest of the Minimal Auditory Capabilities battery (Owens et al., 1981) may be useful for this purpose. Mont-gomery and Demorest (1988) note that because of problems with material selection and interpretation of results, most existing measures of speechreading fail to meet psychometric standards for test design. This factor should be kept in mind when attempting to measure speechreading ability. Instead, speechreading measures may be used as indicators of general ability and to help determine the need for special instruction relating to controlling speaker-viewer angle, environmental lighting, speaker mannerisms, and message visibility factors that may impact on the communication process.

Auditory-only communication skills can be evaluated through traditional audiometric measures (i.e., speech reception thresholds and word recognition scores). It is helpful to establish a profile of auditory-only performance using test stimuli that vary in amount of auditory and linguistic information. The test battery should include a nonsense syllable recognition task to assess ability to distinguish differences in acoustic properties of speech signals, e.g., the CUNY Nonsense Syllable Test (Resnick et al., 1975) and Consonant Confusion Test (Binnie, Jackson, and Montgomery, 1976). To measure the ability to use both acoustic and semantic cues, monosyllabic word lists can be presented. Northwestern University Word Test Number 6 (Tillman and Carhart, 1966), the California Consonant Test (Owens and Schubert, 1977), and selected subtests from the Minimal Auditory Capabilities battery (Owens et al., 1981) would be appropriate. Sentences provide acoustic, semantic, and syntactic cues to message perception. Central Institute for the Deaf Sentences (Davis and Silverman, 1978), the Revised Speech Perception in Noise Test (Bilger, 1984), and selected subtests from the Minimal Auditory Capabilities battery (Owens et al., 1981) may be used for this purpose. By using syllable, word, and sentence materials, the clinician not only learns about a hearing-impaired individual's ability to distinguish acoustically similar speech signals but also about their ability to use linguistic constructs to compensate for problems in speech understanding.

Auditory–visual communication can be evaluated through auditory–visual presentation of the other evaluation materials. The same caveats that apply to speechreading tests apply to measures of auditory–visual communication skill. Nevertheless, such information can be useful in determining the relative contribution of combined modality presentation to message perception and for developing a remediation plan.

Understanding of environmental sounds can be measured using the Everyday Sounds subtest of the Minimal Auditory Capabilities Test battery (Owens et al., 1981). Results from this measure will be useful in developing strategies for monitoring and managing everyday alerting needs.

Finally, it is also helpful to use hearing handicap scales to evaluate communication problems. For example, the Hearing Performance Inventory (Lamb, Owens, and Schubert, 1983) contains subscales regarding self-perceived handicap with and without visual cues in everyday communication situations. There also is a subscale dealing with understanding messages of low intensity and others that request information relating to self-perceived communication handicap in social and occupational settings. Together, needs assessment information, single and combined modality speech recognition data, environmental sound recognition data, and hearing handicap scale information can provide a comprehensive picture of the hearing-impaired adult's communication ability.

## *Evaluation of Counseling Needs*

ASHA's 1993 statement of preferred practices, identifies four aspects of counseling to be addressed by audiologists: assessment of needs; provision of information; use of strategies to modify the client's behavior and/or environment; and development of coping mechanisms and systems for emotional support. Nowhere is the need for counseling more apparent than in the case of hearing-impaired children and their families. Traditionally, parent reaction to a child's hearing loss has been described in terms of a mourning process (Atkins, 1994; Kricos, 1993; Luterman, 1979; Mencher, 1996; Mindel and Feldman, 1987). Most parents experience an initial state of shock. Periods of denial, guilt, anger, bargaining, and depression may follow. Fortunately, for most families, the hearing loss is accepted and constructive action is undertaken. How an individual family reacts will reflect their personal resources, experiences, support from extended family and friends, availability of professional services, and socioeconomic status. The diagnosis of hearing impairment of any degree is an emotional, intimidating, and, in some ways, threatening experience. The clinician must be prepared to provide ongoing assistance to the child's family.

A number of surveys have identified audiologists as the primary source of information counseling on the diagnosis of hearing loss, its impact, and treatment (Haas and Crowley, 1982). However, audiologists continue to report lack of confidence in providing emotional counseling (Flahive and White, 1981) and lack of academic training in counseling techniques (Oyler and Matkin, 1987). When surveyed, parents of hearing-impaired children appear to support these findings. While expressing satisfaction with overall audiological care, parents report the need for more emotional counseling (Bernstein and Barta, 1988; Sweetow and Barrager, 1980). With the emphasis of PL 99-457 on family-based intervention, it seems clear that the need for effective family counseling will increase in the areas of establishing a trustful rapport between the audiologist and the family, providing informational and emotional support, facilitating acceptance of the child's hearing loss, creating a supportive setting for expressing concerns, and determining needs for referral to other professionals.

Assessing the counseling needs of families with a hearing-impaired child should be an ongoing process. The effective counselor will assess needs by collection of actual and observational data as well as through active listening and responding. Data collection begins with the child's medical and social history before the confirmation of the child's hearing loss. This provides information about the family's structure, intellectual and economic resources, presence of other chronic stressors, the child's overall development, and what actions on the child's hearing have already been taken. During all contact with the family, the clinician must be aware of parent–child and parent–parent interactions. Before testing, the clinician should determine what has brought the family to this point—what are their suspicions and what behaviors have they observed? If possible, parents should either participate in or observe clinical evaluations. As a team, the parents and clinician discuss the testing process and share their observations. Expressions of confirmation, or sometimes denial, help the clinician determine the family's level of understanding and acceptance. During all contacts with the family, but especially during this initial diagnostic session, Luterman (1991) encourages the parents to express "what they need to know now" and "how they feel." In this way the clinician can respond to the individual needs of a particular family with follow-up appointments, contacts with other parents, information about organizations and support groups, and specific techniques on communication and hearing loss management (Clark and Martin, 1994).

Perhaps some of the insecurity clinicians experience when providing emotional counseling stems from the lack of specific assessment tools. A number of questionnaires are used with hearing-impaired adults to determine self-perceived hearing handicap. Comparable scales have not been developed for the families of young hearing-impaired children. Instead, clinicians must develop a personal counseling style, reflecting a shift from the medical model of dispensing information to an empowering model in which the professional and family work as a team.

When families experience extreme levels of distress because of their child's hearing loss, the clinician must be prepared to make a referral to mental health experts in the community. Unfortunately, few psychologists and social workers are experienced in working with hearing-impaired individuals and their families. Surveys indicate that both school and community-based professionals seldom have training related specifically to hearing impairment, and few are able to communicate manually (McEntee, 1993; Weaver and Bradley-Johnson, 1993). Although the need for counseling services among hearing-impaired individuals and their families is similar to that for hearing individuals, it is apparent that such services are at a premium.

Early formal approaches to hearing handicap measurement in adults were driven by the interests of the medical profession in developing a means of determining percentage of hearing loss for compensation purposes in medicolegal matters. In an effort to determine when hearing impairment becomes a hearing handicap, in 1979, the American Academy of Otolaryngology—Head and Neck Surgery (Melnick and Morgan, 1991) proposed a procedure for converting pure tone threshold data into percentage of hearing loss. This procedure is as follows:

1. The average pure tone threshold levels at 500, 1000, 2000, and 3000 Hz are calculated for each ear.
2. The amount by which the pure tone average exceeds 25 dB (low fence) is multiplied by 1.5 percent to determine the percentage impairment for each ear.
3. Binaural impairment is calculated by multiplying the better ear threshold by 5, adding this to the percentage for the poorer ear, and dividing by 6. For example, a 40 percent loss would indicate that on a scale where 0 percent indicates no loss/no compensation and 100 percent indicates profound loss/total compensation, an individual would be eligible to receive 40 percent of the maximum available compensation. While consideration has been given to the relevance of low- and high-frequency data, there is no universal standard for measuring hearing handicap using pure tone threshold data.

Another audiometrically based approach to hearing handicap evaluation, the Social Adequacy Index, was developed by Davis (1948b). This method involves a comparison of pure tone average and speech discrimination scores. The greater the combination of hearing loss and speech discrimination difficulty, the lower the adequacy rating for social communication. This approach was short-lived. However, the concern for hearing handicap continues to be an area addressed by hearing professionals today, although through self-assessment rather than audiometric procedures.

Bronfenbrenner, a psychologist, developed the Hearing Attitude Scale for counseling hearing-impaired World War II veterans. This 100-item survey addressed concerns in the areas of self-appraisal, depression, optimism, tension, job worry, sensitivity, cover-up, withdrawal, eccentricity, and reaction to rehabilitation (Levine, 1960). Beginning in the early 1960s, other scales were developed for self-assessment of communication problems relating to hearing loss. These scales include the High, Fairbanks, and Glorig (1964) Self-Assessment of Hearing Handicap scale, which is used for assessing difficulty in speech perception, localization, telephone usage, and communication in noisy settings; the Hearing Measurement Scale (Noble and Atherley, 1970), which is designed for victims of noise-induced hearing loss; the Social Hearing Handicap Index (Ewertsen and Birk-Nielsen, 1973), which evaluates success in individual and group conversation in quiet and noisy conditions; and, other communicative performance scales developed by Alpiner and colleagues (1974), McCarthy and Alpiner (1983), Sanders (1982), and Schow and Nerbonne (1982).

Self-assessment scales are intended to standardize the collection of interview data. By using standardized evaluation measures, information relating to hearing handicap can be collected in a uniform way and comparison of reports across individuals and by the same individuals over time can be assumed to have some level of reliability and validity. This information is important to hearing professionals in their efforts to better understand hearing loss and its personal ramifications. In order to be clinically useful, self-assessment scales must be valid instruments and provide useful, meaningful, and appropriate data from which to draw specific inferences (Demorest and DeHaven, 1993). A self-assessment scale is said to demonstrate content validity when it includes items that address the author's concern (Cronbach, 1984). For example, a survey of difficulty in telephone use must include questions dealing specifically with telephone communication. Construct validity is demonstrated by including items that potentially discriminate levels of self-perceived difficulty. Finally, a self-assessment scale must be reliable in order to be valid (Ventry and Schiavetti, 1980).

There are several hearing handicap scales that meet contemporary psychometric standards. The Revised Hearing Performance Inventory (HPI) (Lamb, Owens, and Schubert, 1983) is a 90-item inventory surveying communication conditions experienced by hearing-impaired adults. Its subscales can be administered to determine self-perceived communication difficulty when the speaker is easily seen, not seen, or when messages are of low intensity. There are questions dealing with encountering failure in a communication situation that provide insight to hearing loss management in a way that is unique from other scales. The revised HPI also includes subsets of questions dealing with personal, social, and occupational aspects of hearing loss. By surveying reaction to multiple situations that vary in complexity, the clinician is provided with a wealth of information for use in designing a remediation program that is tailored to the needs of the individual.

The Communication Profile for the Hearing-Impaired (CPHI) (Demorest and Erdman, 1986) is useful when there is concern with an individual's behavior and attitude in dealing with communication and personal adjustment problems related to hearing loss. This 145-item scale includes twenty-five subscales arranged in four categories: communication performance assessed in social, work, and home situations under average and adverse conditions; communication environment, including reaction to the behaviors and attitudes of others; verbal and nonverbal communication strategies, and personal adjustment, including anger, stress, and withdrawal; acceptance or denial of hearing loss. Communication importance is assessed in social, work, and home situations.

Other scales are noteworthy for their emphasis on special populations. For example, the Hearing Handicap Inventory for the Elderly (HHIE) (Ventry and Weinstein, 1982) is designed for self-assessment of social and emotional problems associated with hearing loss in older adults. A ten-item screening version of the HHIE, the HHIE-S, (Ventry and Weinstein, 1982) and an HHIE for younger adults (HHIE-A) (Newman et al., 1991) also have been developed. The Performance Inventory for Profound and Severe Hearing Loss (Owens and Raggio, 1984) was developed for use by those with extreme hearing loss, particularly cochlear implant candidates. Its seventy-four items are arranged into six subscales: understanding speech with or without visual cues, detection of intensity information, response to auditory failure, environmental sounds, and personal items. Raw scores from the Likert-scale are converted to percentage data and assigned descriptors for use in reporting degree of handicap.

In summary, contemporary evaluation of hearing handicap in adults incorporates use of self-assessment techniques. In doing so, the clinician is able to learn the impact of hearing loss on an individual's everyday function and to design a remediation program that is directed toward minimizing self-perceived handicap.

## Considerations in Remediation

### Sensory Aids

Sensory aids are critical tools in the rehabilitation process. For many hearing-impaired individuals, use of sensory aids obviates the need for more extensive rehabilitative intervention. For purposes of this chapter, the term sensory aid will be restricted to any electro-mechanical device that is designed to compensate for hearing loss. Most common sensory aids are hearing aids, ALDs, and cochlear implants. The most common hearing aids are miniature, personal, battery-powered amplification systems worn within the ear canal or behind the ear. Conventional hearing aids have a microphone to pick up sound from the environment and convert acoustic energy into electric energy. In the amplifier, which is powered by a battery, electric energy is increased and filtered to compensate for the user's hearing loss pattern. Then the amplified electric energy is reconverted to acoustic energy in the receiver and directed down the user's ear canal for processing by the user's auditory system (Figure 15-2). The level of amplification or gain provided by a hearing aid is adjustable, within limits, using a volume control. To most hearing aid users, an ideal aid will not only improve listening and communication, it will not call attention to itself.

Some ALDs may be used as a substitute for hearing aids or to enhance hearing aid benefit. While they have the same primary components as personal hearing aids, they take advantage of hardwire, magnetic induction, infrared light, or frequency-modulated (FM) radio waves to minimize the effects of distance and background noise on auditory signal reception (Figure 15-3). The microphone either is placed next to or hardwired into the sound source. This maximizes the signal-to-noise ratio, providing amplified sound directly to the user's ear with minimal interference. For example, using an FM system, a speaker standing 300 feet away from a hearing-impaired listener in a noisy crowd will sound as

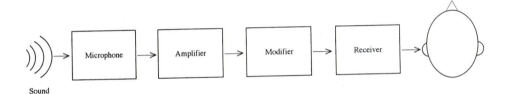

**FIGURE 15-2   Typical signal path for a conventional hearing aid.**

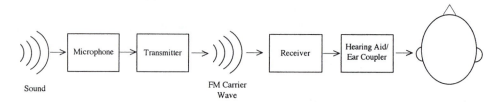

**FIGURE 15-3    Typical signal path for an FM interpersonal communication device.**

though he is speaking directly into the receiver's ear. Most users of assistive devices have overcome initial concerns with vanity and are concerned with maximizing their communication potential.

A cochlear implant differs from a hearing aid or ALD in that it includes both external and surgically implanted internal components in a system that is designed to improve speech recognition augmented by speechreading. In the typical system, sound is captured by a microphone, converted to an electrical signal, and directed to a speech processor (Figure 15-4). In the speech processor, sound is converted into a distinct electrical code that is programmed by the audiologist. The electrically coded speech signal is sent to the implanted receiver through the user's skin. The receiver decodes the signal and sends it to the electrode array placed in the bony shell of the cochlea. The electrode array distributes the signal and stimulates auditory nerve endings. The resulting impulses are delivered to the brain where they are interpreted as sound. Cochlear implants are designed to restore ability to detect sound. Vanity is a lesser concern for the motivated implant user.

All sensory aids improve potential for understanding spoken messages and increase the ease of everyday interpersonal communication. In doing so, their users may experience improved social communication, emotional adjustment, auditory learning potential, and personal affect. However, sensory aids will not restore lost sound quality. Their use may draw attention to a hearing deficit that may, in turn, be interpreted as a sign of weakness or aging. Another potential drawback is cost.

There are benefits and limitations that are specific to each type of aid. For example, hearing aids increase the audibility of speech, yet their limited frequency range impacts on sound fidelity. They are custom-fitted to the user's ear(s), which maximizes the benefit one might receive from sound being injected into a closed ear canal. The amplified signal is not lost to the listening environment. On the other hand, any distortion of the amplified signal created by hearing loss or background noise is not eliminated by the hearing aid. Finally, hearing aids have small controls making them difficult to manipulate by those with arthritic fingers or poor vision.

ALDs have the amplifying benefits of hearing aids, with the additional advantage of improving listening capability over distance and in noise. However, ALDs tend to be bulky units that vary widely in quality (Fikret-Pasa and Garstecki, 1993). Unlike hearing aids, there are no standards specifying the electroacoustic characteristics of ALDs or how they can be measured.

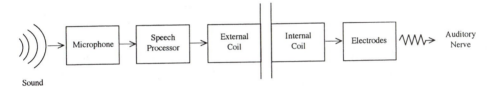

**FIGURE 15-4    Typical signal path for conventional cochlear implant.**

Cochlear implants restore sound perception capabilities and improve the audibility of high-frequency speech information over what can be accomplished by conventional hearing aids and ALDs. However, use of a cochlear implant involves the normal risks of surgery, potential infection, potential injury to the facial nerve, numbness of the scalp and ear, as well as the unknown effects of long-term electrical stimulation. Finally, successful adjustment to a cochlear implant requires extensive user experience and training.

An ear specialist should be consulted prior to hearing aid use when any of these conditions are noted (FDA, 1977):

1. Visible congenital or traumatic deformity
2. History of active drainage from the ear within the previous 90 days
3. History of sudden or rapidly progressive hearing loss within the previous 90 days
4. Acute or chronic dizziness
5. Unilateral hearing loss of sudden or recent onset within the previous 90 days
6. Audiometric air-bone gap equal to or greater than 15 dB at 500, 1000, and 2000 Hz
7. Visible evidence of significant cerumen accumulation or foreign body in ear canal
8. Pain or discomfort in the ear

Once these criteria are met, hearing aid candidacy is dependent on a combination of personal factors and audiometric information. The potential users must be motivated, personally or by the demands of their communication experiences, and psychologically ready to wear a hearing aid. The candidate must also demonstrate the potential for improved communication. For children, early binaural amplification is recommended for those with mild loss and greater, particularly to guard against any loss of auditory stimulation during critical language development years. Fitting a school-age child with mild loss may help that child overcome problems listening in classroom conditions. For all others, potential benefit increases as hearing loss increases, with maximum benefit for those with pure tone thresholds in the moderate to moderately severe hearing loss range. Beyond this level, users may reach a point of diminishing returns, a point at which there may be no benefit from amplification. This judgment is best left to the hearing-impaired individual as even those with profound hearing loss, left-corner audiograms, and only islands of hearing may benefit from selected use of an amplification system.

There are no specific candidacy requirements for use of ALDs, although the above requirements for hearing aids would apply. Candidacy for cochlear implants includes evidence of profound, bilateral sensorineural hearing loss; little or no measurable benefit from use of a hearing aid; and no radiologic, medical, or psychological contraindications. For children, there are additional recommendations relating to normal intelligence, strong family support, no significant learning disabilities or handicaps that might affect potential for success, and evidence that progress toward auditory development is not being made despite training and appropriate hearing aids (Brimacombe and Beiter, 1996).

To effectively use any sensory aid, clients must know and understand:

1. Component parts and their specific function
2. Benefits and limitations of available sensory aids
3. How to clean and maintain the aid for daily use
4. How to troubleshoot the operation and performance of selected aids (see Garstecki, 1994)
5. How to adjust the aid for everyday use
6. How to manage minor repairs
7. Who to contact in the event of a problem with the aid
8. Cost of replacement aids and batteries and how to acquire them
9. How to use aids in combination to enhance the performance over a single aid
10. Insurance and manufacturer warranty conditions
11. How to proceed if a battery is swallowed (call the National Battery Hotline: 1-202-625-3333).

In addition to sensory aids that are intended to compensate directly for hearing loss, there are other devices that may be beneficial. These include telephone amplifiers, text telephones, personal computers equipped with telephone modems, facsimile machines, and telephone relay systems. They also include television amplifying and captioning devices. Warning devices using sound, light, or vibration may alert hearing-impaired individuals to problems in their environment. These include wake-up alarm clocks, door signalers, baby monitors, building security systems, smoke alarms, and telephone alerting devices. Some individuals who must communicate in group meeting situations may benefit from real-time captioning systems that require use of a transcriber, captioning equipment, and a screen to display printed transcription of spoken messages.

## *Communication Remediation*

No single method of intervention or setting for providing services will meet the needs of all hearing-impaired children. Meeting the needs of a specific child should be an interactive, dynamic process incorporating all dimensions of the child and the child's environment. Intervention will vary according to the type, degree, and duration of hearing loss, use of sensory aids, intellectual ability, communicative style and motivation, learning style, and personality. Influencing factors within the child's environment include family support resources (both emotional and financial), availability of professional services, educational options, and family and community attitudes toward sensory impairments. The goal of hearing loss management for children is to maximize each child's potential to develop auditory, speech, language, and cognitive skills. Effective habilitative intervention demands that parents, children, and professionals work together to create trusting, supportive relationships.

Although specific skills may be taught in the course of habilitation, the emphasis should be placed on integrating audiological management, language and cognitive skill development, speech development, auditory training, academic concept development, socioemotional growth, and family counseling in treatment to address the comprehensive needs of the child. The needs of the child will best be served by identifying a case manager capable of acting as advocate, instructor, model, interpreter, counselor, and resource person (Grant, 1987). The case manager may coordinate the evaluation and intervention activities of an audiologist, speech–language pathologist, educator, psychologist, social worker, and others.

The controversy of selecting and establishing a communication system or language is well-reported. In the United States, hearing-impaired children learn to communicate using oral or manual English-based methods or American Sign Language. Oral approaches include aural–oral, auditory–verbal, and cued speech. Manually coded methods include signing exact English, seeing exact English, the Rochester method, pidgin sign English. For descriptions of these and other approaches the reader should refer to Bornstein, 1990; Goldberg, 1993; Gustason, 1983; Ling, 1984a, 1984b; Scouten, 1967; and Wilbur, 1987. Books, videotapes, discussions with other families, and visits to schools and therapy centers will help familiarize parents with communicative options. Results of audiological, speech, and language evaluations should be interpreted for the parents by the case manager and other professionals to assist in making early remediation decisions. Tools such as the Deafness Management Quotient (Northern and Downs, 1984) or the Spoken Language Predictor Index (Geers and Moog, 1987), which assess a number of child and environment factors, may also be helpful in guiding parents through their options. Regardless of educational placement, 60 percent of hearing-impaired children use simultaneous sign and speech, 39 percent use auditory–aural methods, and only 1 percent use other approaches such as American Sign Language or cued speech (Moores, 1991). Any approach requires consistent use by all the members of the child's communication environment. If, after such consistent effort, the child makes little progress in language acquisition, parents and professionals must consider other options. This should not be viewed as a failure but as a readjustment in the child's overall intervention plan.

The need for early intervention is well-recognized by audiologists, speech pathologists, and educators of the hearing impaired. PL 99-457 has reinforced this concept by requiring states to develop family-based programs for disabled children from birth to two years of age. Parent-infant programs emphasize providing guidance and counseling to the family to help them understand the child's hearing loss and its impact on all aspects of development. Parents learn to observe and evaluate their child's behavior, facilitate language and cognitive development through natural, playful interactions, and develop confidence in their ability to meet their child's needs.

The past twenty years have evidenced a dramatic shift in educational settings most frequently used by school-age hearing-impaired children. These range from residential schools for the deaf to self-contained classrooms for hearing-impaired children to various mainstream or integrated placements. As a result of the movement toward less restrictive environments, between 1979 and 1985 there was a 22.5 percent drop in residential school enrollment in the United States. Today 67 percent of all hearing-impaired children attend local schools (Allen, 1992). However, choice of educational setting will vary according to the age of the child, the degree of hearing loss, options available within the community, financial resources of the family, experience and philosophy of those providing services, method of communication, and family preference.

Clinicians will be most effective by employing a holistic approach to habilitation with hearing-impaired children. Skills should not be taught in isolation, but in meaningful play and academic contexts. Interventions can be attempted only after thorough evaluation of the child's hearing loss and fitting with appropriate sensory aids. Any residual hearing should be exploited to facilitate development of expressive and receptive communicative skills. Auditory rehabilitation involves treatment focused on developing or restoring skills that facilitate communication. Traditionally, hearing loss management in children has focused on auditory training and speechreading. The primary purpose of auditory training is to develop the ability to listen and understand environmental and speech sounds. Erber (1982) summarizes four aspects of auditory skill development: detection, discrimination, recognition, and comprehension. Laughton and Hasenstab (1993) call these stages auditory learning and expand them to include reception, processing, representation, recognition, and comprehension. Therapy materials should be developed to address the specific needs of each child. A number of auditory skills curricula has been published, including the Auditory Skills Curriculum (1976) and Developmental Approach to Successful Listening II (Stout and Windle, 1986), that can be used as a basis for auditory training activities.

With the increased use of cochlear implants, children who in the past were unable to receive benefit from traditional amplification now may have significant auditory information available. Extensive training is required to assist these children in their ability to listen to and understand sound. Robbins (1990) outlines an approach emphasizing carry-over of specific auditory skills into natural communication settings. Tye-Murray and Kelsay (1993) have developed a cochlear implant training program focused on home training and parent–child communication.

Another component of habilitation is speechreading, which combines visual information with audition to compensate for hearing loss (Mussen, 1988). For very young children, speechreading focuses on attending skills, such as localization and figure-ground attention. Older children learn to interpret facial expression, lip movement, context cues, and gestures to augment auditory information (DeFilippo and Sims, 1988).

Approaches to language intervention with hearing-impaired children have varied from analytic–structural to naturalistic–pragmatic and combinations of the two. Analytic–structural refers to a metacognitive approach, progressing from the part to the whole. Techniques such as the Fitzgerald Key and Rhode Island School for the Deaf Sentence Charts have been used to teach "the language of language." Children are taught the components of language and practice combining them into phrases and sentences of increasing complexity. Naturalistic approaches focus on normal language development sequences. Many programs for hearing-impaired children now use whole language techniques, emphasizing language learning in real-world contexts. The child learns language experientially, based on interests and communication needs (Kretschmer and Kretschmer, 1990). For additional discussion of language development and intervention techniques see Bloom and Lahey, 1978; Kretschmer and Kretschmer, 1978; Paul and Quigley, 1990; and Quigley and Paul, 1984.

Hearing loss management in children must give consideration to the child's school placement, particularly when the child is mainstreamed. The clinician may need to provide in-service training and classroom monitoring in addition to direct intervention. Room acoustics and lighting, preferential seating, provision of interpreters and notetakers, classroom or personal FM amplification systems, and adaptation of teaching methods and materials must be considered for each child (Berg, 1987; Flexer, 1993; Luetke-Stahlman and Luckner, 1991; Ross, 1990).

Hearing-impaired adults, left to their own devices, often develop personal strategies for ensuring successful communication. However, sometimes these strategies fail and there may be no obvious alternative solution. Most times, success or failure is unpredictable. When hearing-impaired adults become motivated to increase the odds of successful communication, they may seek a communication remediation program. Unfortunately, there are no universal approaches or standard treatment protocols for remediation of communication problems in adults. Usual methods carry strong face validity, but there are relatively few standardized procedures. Usual methods include speechreading and listening exercises and instruction in stage-managing difficult communication situations for personal success. As a result, performance scores suggesting levels of ability and change over time may be unreliable and of limited prescriptive value. Even so, clinical intervention focusing on remediation of communication problems is valued by program participants.

Clinicians interested in providing a communication remediation program for hearing-impaired adults might consider the following approach.

**1.** Address immediate concerns. The clinician's first priority is to learn why the program candidate believes instruction in communication remediation is indicated. What are the primary complaints? Plan to address complaints in program activities.

**2.** Determine usual experiences. Hearing handicap scales, such as the Hearing Performance Inventory (Owens and Schubert, 1977), provide an organized list of questions relating to self-perceived success in a variety of everyday communication situations. They yield information that defines the communication circumstance that is most difficult for the respondent. While at first this provides important diagnostic information, ultimately this information can be used for determining communication conditions in role playing exercises.

**3.** Identify communication abilities. Videotaped recordings of nonsense syllable, word, and sentence materials used in speech audiometry may be used for identifying communication ability. In considering results across input modalities, it is possible to determine one's ability to decipher visual speech information. If they can lipread 40 percent of a spoken passage with success, they may have no need for more formal instruction in lipreading or speechreading. This is an acceptable level of ability (Binnie, Jackson, and Montgomery, 1976). This information would be useful in predicting success in communication when severe hearing loss or background noise prevents perception of acoustic cues to message perception. It also is possible to supplement information provided by the clinical audiologist with measure of performance across presentation modes and in alternate contexts (e.g., syllables or sentences). This information would be useful in predicting potential difficulty in understanding others in face-to-face communication situations and in televised broadcasts by providing a measure of combined auditory–visual message understanding. The difference in performance between auditory-only and auditory–visual tasks will suggest the relative value of the visual component to understanding.

In considering the influence of context on spoken message understanding, it is possible to develop a profile of scores that compare success in detecting the smallest distinguishable speech units (phonemes and visemes) with possible change in ability when words are substituted for syllables, adding a semantic component to perceived acoustic cues. Then, placing test words in the context of meaningful phrases and sentences provides additional information about the contribution of syntactic information to message understanding. This progression of steps could be extended to include paragraph and story stimuli and the inclusion of external cues (e.g., pictures) that may be related to the topic of the spoken message. Garstecki (1981) describes an auditory and auditory–visual communication evaluation and remediation paradigm that incorporates speech stimuli varying in amount of linguistic content, background noise conditions, and use of situational cues.

For example, if it is determined that visual communication or speechreading skills need to be developed, the program participant's visual processing skills must be assessed. At minimum, this should involve a screening of binocular visual acuity and a survey of any known vision problems or reasons why visual skills may be ineffective. Binocular visual acuity should approximate the 20/30 level or better in order not to influence the speechreading process (Hardick, Oyer, and Irion, 1970).

**4.** Develop a routine. It is helpful to introduce the program participants to how speech sounds are articulated in order to prepare them for what they might expect in a speechreading task. If one knows /b/ is highly visible because it is a bilabial plosive and /h/ is invisible because it is a glottal, then it is easier to understand one of the limitations of speechreading. Next, speechreading principles should be reviewed. Sender, receiver, message, and environmental factors that impact on the speechreading process should be understood and suggestions made to improve success in visual message understanding (Erber, 1993). Speechreading exercises might include interaction with others in a competing noise situation, review of videotaped materials varying in message content, review of videotape recordings of "slice of life" or soap opera dialogue, and use of interactive computer software (Pichora-Fuller and Benguerel, 1991; Tye-Murray et al., 1988). Computer tasks tend to be highly analytical in nature in that they require exact identification of word elements, whereas linguistic or environmental cues facilitate word identification in an everyday communication experience.

If auditory communication skills need to be developed, exercises might involve message understanding under various listening conditions (e.g., in quiet and in noise, with different types and levels of noise, with hearing aids and ALDs, and in face-to-face as well as speech transmission system conditions). Auditory signal presentation levels may be varied to simulate near and distant listening tasks. Training stimuli may include speech as well as environmental sounds and warning signals. Live, audiotaped, and audio–videotaped presentation of materials would be appropriate.

Another approach would be to follow a plan like that proposed by Eisenwort, Brauneis, and Burian (1985) for cochlear implant recipients. The first stage involves drawing attention to temporal, loudness, and frequency differences in pure tone stimuli. The next stage involves auditory discrimination of everyday sounds and voices. The third stage requires discrimination of suprasegmental features. Identification of the number of words, the duration of words, the lengths of sentences, and sentence forms comprises this part of the program. Then, attention is focused on recognition of segmental information: syllable number, word length, length of vowels, identification of familiar words among unfamiliar words, and sentence recognition. Finally, auditory comprehension of materials varying in amount of linguistic content is exercised.

If combined auditory–visual communication needs to be developed, videotaped or laser videodisc materials would be appropriate to use in the ways indicated for auditory communication training above. By using recorded materials, stimulus presentation is constant from one administration to the next, contributing to the reliability of any treatment outcome measure. While control is important, it is also useful to incorporate interpersonal communication exercises in the remediation program to simulate the everyday communication experience. A speech tracking procedure provides a mechanism for guiding the development of skills necessary to keep pace with everyday conversation (DeFilippo and Sims, 1988). Speech tracking essentially is a timed clinical procedure during which the words and phrases of a thematic passage are presented for verbatim repetition using repair strategies (Tye-Murray, 1991). Unfortunately, again, while the intent is to develop improved conversational skills, the approach requires analysis of message elements on a word-by-word basis.

Multimodality communication exercises provide an opportunity to develop and refine rudimentary speech processing skills. It is also important to help the hearing-impaired individual understand and use appropriate anticipatory, listening, and general communication strategies. Ultimately, it will be the use of these strategies that will guarantee success outside the clinic environment. Examples of each type of strategy are provided below.

*Anticipatory strategies*

1. Plan questions to be asked and expected responses.
2. Plan to close the gap if someone is speaking at a distance.
3. Anticipate possible dialogue and its sequence.
4. Anticipate environmental conditions and how to avoid problems.
5. Consider how you can be assertive.

*Repair strategies*

1. Ask for message clarification.
2. Ask for a summary.
3. Ask for key words to be rephrased.
4. Ask the speaker to write key information.
5. Ask the speaker to use a natural pace.

*Listening strategies*

1. Read facial expression and body gesture.
2. Look for ideas rather than isolated words.
3. Combine message and environmental cues.
4. Tell others when you are having difficulty understanding them.
5. Encourage two-way conversation.

Finally, communication partners have a responsibility for optimizing the opportunity for successful communication. Erber (1993) provides suggestions on how to prepare to communicate with hearing-impaired individuals. These suggestions include maintaining a normal voice level, talking slowly, identifying any change in topic, using appropriate facial expressions and body gestures, cooperating with requests for clarification and others.

By following this format, a comprehensive program will be provided that allows for development and refinement of speech processing skills in contexts that have direct relevance to everyday communication. Furthermore, strategies will be learned and applied to ensure success in communication beyond the remediation program.

## *Counseling*

The third component of the remediation process is counseling. Counseling parents of hearing-impaired children is an ongoing process, providing support during the diagnostic process, assessing the parents' emotional state, providing an accepting atmosphere in which feelings and questions are expressed, establishing trust, and facilitating progress (Mencher, 1996). Counseling needs vary from family to family as well as throughout the course of the therapeutic process. Hearing professionals feel most comfortable and confident in their role as an informational counselor, providing interpretations of assessment results, recommending appropriate sensory aids, discussing communicative and educational options, and referring families to agencies and professionals who can provide additional services. These are essential counseling functions; however, they must be combined with appropriate emotional support (Kricos, 1993; Luterman, 1991). If families can be assisted in developing an acceptance and understanding of their child's hearing impairment, they will be better able to provide a trusting, supportive environment.

Research findings suggest that several dimensions of the family environment play a significant role in the hearing-impaired child's eventual academic achievement. Bodner-Johnson (1985) found that academic achievement is enhanced by families who accept their child's hearing loss, who set appropriate limitations, who are actively involved with their children, and who encourage achievement. Likewise, Geers and Moog (1987) identify parental understanding of the impact of a hearing loss and active support as key factors in enhancing language and academic progress. Finally, hearing-impaired children come from a variety of cultural and ethnic backgrounds. Family roles and responsibilities, attitudes about disabilities and their causes, and willingness to accept help must be considered (Yacobacci-Tam, 1987).

A critical feature of an adult's rehabilitation program is the opportunity to obtain professional advice, exchange ideas and opinions, and discuss matters relating to personal management of hearing loss. Hearing-impaired adults want to talk with someone about the way they feel about problems at home, on the job, and in interpersonal communication situations (Frankel, 1981). Hearing professionals are routinely asked information on the nature of hearing loss, its consequences, and its treatment. They may also clarify attitudes and provide assistance in emotional adjustment to hearing loss. Emotional adjustment or affective counseling may involve dealing with negative feelings of self-worth. It might emphasize development of a family or peer support system for a hearing-impaired individual. It might involve clarification or validation of personal needs or feelings resulting from hearing loss.

It also could focus on defining the roles of family members and peers in communication situations.

To understand the counseling process, it is helpful to review Wylde's (1987) proposed stages in a counseling relationship. The entry stage is the intake interview where the client explains the primary complaint, rapport is established, the clinician develops appropriate empathy, and the groundwork is laid for a trusting, open relationship. In the clarification stage, problems are defined and the impact of hearing loss is determined. The structure stage deals with the mechanics of setting up a formal counseling program. At the relationship stage, consensus is reached that counseling is needed and will be provided. In the exploration stage, intervention strategies are determined and they are implemented in the consolidation stage. Plans for program termination or referral are completed after a period of direct intervention. In the termination stage, accomplishments are summarized and the formal intervention program is concluded.

Topics addressed during counseling sessions can be categorized as addressing the need for information on general resources available for hearing loss management, tangible assistance available for hearing loss management, and personal support in emotional adjustment to hearing loss. Information counseling is cognitively based assistance. It is instruction, guidance, and expert advice. For example, helping someone develop the appropriate strategies for managing difficult communication situations is an informational counseling experience. Providing someone with information on hearing loss; medical treatment of hearing loss; sensory aids, and assistive devices; how to communicate with hearing-impaired individuals; how to conserve residual hearing, the range of community services available for hearing-impaired individuals; and the legal rights of hearing-disabled individuals also would be considered informational counseling.

Instrumental counseling relates to tangible assistance or physical support. It may include activities relating to sensory aid procurement such as petitioning third party payers or philanthropic organizations. It may involve arranging for public transportation to attend clinic sessions. It also may involve working with a nurse or personal assistant in managing daily living tasks such as helping another wear a hearing aid.

The clinician is vulnerable to possible risks associated with the provision of counseling service. One is the risk of professional malpractice. The other is the risk of burnout. Malpractice may occur when the clinician fails to properly evaluate counseling needs, provides a substandard counseling service, fails to reveal alternative solutions to concerns raised in counseling sessions, or fails to refer when alternate types of professional services are indicated. Burnout occurs when the boundaries of a counseling relationship are not clearly specified. Counseling boundaries typically are not verbalized. They often are negotiated nonverbally during the course of a professional relationship. Through clinician feedback, the hearing-impaired individual should come to realize that while it may be appropriate to discuss communication problems occurring on the job, it may not be appropriate to discuss personal finances or concerns about an unrelated illness. It is within boundaries to discuss what it is like to have a hearing impairment and outside boundaries to discuss chronic feelings of unhappiness or marital instability. By guarding against potential risks, the counseling experience can be professionally rewarding for the clinician and vital to the future happiness and welfare of hearing-impaired individuals.

## Comment

The effects of hearing loss on speech perception and production, language acquisition and growth, and personality development have been summarized in an effort to describe potential areas of concern in rehabilitative management of hearing-impaired children and adults. This chapter also describes what to do to manage problems related to hearing loss. The process has been organized by a decision tree diagram demonstrating clinical treatment components arranged in hierarchical order. Emphasis in the rehabilitation process has been directed toward maximizing sensory capability through use of conventional and advanced technology. Attention has been given to evaluation and remediation of related communication problems, as well as to the counseling needs of hearing-impaired individuals. Selected clinical materials were identified and classic and contemporary published works cited. In all, this chapter provides a comprehensive overview of the hearing loss management process, a wealth of information on selected clinical procedures and materials, and a complete list of key references for those interested in knowing what to expect and what to do once hearing loss impacts on communication and learning.

# *Epilogue*

It is fitting that the last chapter of *Audiology and Auditory Dysfunction* should bring to a close a discussion that began with identifying how we hear and what we hear, progressed to a review of the various diseases and disorders that can affect the auditory system, and finally, considered the care of the hearing-impaired individual from an educational, clinical, and psychosocial perspective. Auditory dysfunction is one of the major reasons why audiology exists.

There is no doubt that improved diagnostic techniques, amplification devices, surgery, and cochlear implants are rapidly changing the field. Consider the differences between Figure 16-1*A* and Figure 16-1*B* and *C*. No doubt, a pediatrician, family practitioner, otologist, audiologist, speech–language pathologist, prosthodontist, plastic surgeon, and social worker, have all been involved in the process to restructure the jaw line, implant a bone conduction hearing aid, and expand this lady's facial area. The result is an ear where one didn't exist and hearing where it wasn't. The result is the courage to wear outrageous earrings and to be heard as a full functioning member of society. If you, dear reader, think this

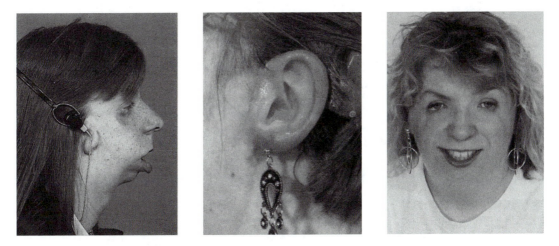

**FIGURE 16-1*A*–*C*** **Treacher-Collins syndrome pre- and post reconstructive surgery and care. (Photo courtesy of Nobelpharma, Canada, manufacturers of the prosthetic pinna).**

achievement is great, it is. But it's just the beginning. It is not beyond the realm of possibility that within our lifetime, the skilled audiologist will identify a child as hearing impaired at birth—or perhaps even before—and the skilled surgeon will be able to implant an artificial ear shortly thereafter. As our imaginary friend of the future, Captain Picard on Star Trek would say, "Make it so!"

# References

Aballi, AJ and Korones, SB (1963). The newborn infant. In JG Hughes (ed.), *Synopsis of Pediatrics* (St. Louis: The C.V. Mosby Co.).

Abd Al-Hady, MR, Shehata, O, El-Mously, M, and Sallam, FS (1990). Audiological findings following head trauma. *J Laryng Otol* 101:927–936.

Abramovich, S (1990). *Electric Response Audiometry in Clinical Practice* (Edinburgh: Churchill Livingstone).

Abrams, IF (1977). Nongenetic hearing loss, In BF Jaffe (ed), *Hearing Loss in Children* (Baltimore: University Park Press).

Acton, WI and Grime, RP (1978). *Industrial Noise: The Conduct of the Reasonable and Prudent Employer* (University of Southhampton: Wolfson Institute for Noise and Vibration).

Adams, PF and Benson, V (1991). Current estimates from the National Health Interview Survey, 1990. *Vital Health Statistics* 10: 82–128.

Ad Hoc Committee on Workers Compensation (1992). A survey of states' workers' compensation practices for occupational hearing loss. *Asha* 34 (Suppl No. 8).

Affias, S and Embil, JA (1978). Congenital infections and the TORCH syndrome. *Nova Scotia Med Bull* 57:43–47.

Alberti, PW (1987). Noise and the ear. In D. Stephens (ed), *Scott-Brown's Otolaryngology*, 5th ed., vol 2: *Adult Audiology* (London: Butterworths).

Allen, TA (1992). Subgroup differences in educational placement for deaf and hard of hearing students. *Am Annals Deaf* 137:381–388.

Alpiner, JC, Chevrette, W, Glascoe, G, Metz, M, and Olsen, B (1974). Denver scale of communication function. *J Acad Rehab Aud* 13:66–77.

Alport, AC (1927). Hereditary familial congenital haemorrhagic nephritis. *Brit Med J* 1:504–506.

American Academy of Pediatrics (1987). Statement on childhood lead poisoning. *Peds.* 79:457–465.

American Conference of Governmental Industrial Hygienists (1994–1995). *Threshold Limit Values for Chemical Substances and Physical Agents and Biological Exposure Indices* (Cincinnati, Ohio: Kemper Woods Center).

American National Standards Institute. (1969). Specifications for Audiometers. *ANSI S36–1969* (New York: ANSI).

American National Standards Institute. (1971). Specifications for hearing aid characteristics. *ANSI S3.33–1971* (New York: ANSI).

American National Standards Institute. (1987). Specifications for hearing aid measurement. *ANSI S3.22–1987* (New York: ANSI).

American Speech-Language-Hearing Association (1984). Position statement: Definition of and competencies for aural rehabilitation. *Asha* 26:37–41.

American Speech-Language-Hearing Association (1993a). Preferred practice patterns for the professions of speech-language pathology and audiology. *Asha* (suppl. No. 11) 35:21–24.

American Speech-Language-Hearing Association (1993b). Code of ethics. *Asha* (suppl.) 35:99–100.

Amstey, MS (1977). Maternal viral infection with adverse results: Cytomegalovirus and herpes virus. *Sem Perinatol* 1:1–10.

Anderson, H, Barr, B, and Wedenberg, E (1970). Genetic disposition prerequisite for maternal rubella deafness. *Arch Otolaryn* 91:141–174.

Anvar, B, Mencher, GT, and Keet, SJ (1984). Hearing loss and congenital rubella in Atlantic Canada. *Ear and Hearing* 5:340–345.

Arnst, DJ (1985). Presbycusis. In J. Katz (ed), *Handbook of Clinical Audiology,* 3rd ed. (Baltimore: Williams & Wilkins).

Atkins, D (1994). Counseling children with hearing loss and their families. In JG Clark and FN Martin (eds), *Effective Counseling in Audiology: Perspectives and Practice* (Englewood Cliffs, NJ: Prentice-Hall).

Baldursson, G, Bjarnason, O, Halldorsson, S, Juliusdottir, E, and Kjeld, M (1972). Maternal rubella in Iceland 1963–1964. *Scand Aud* 1:3–10.

Ballachanda, BB, Roeser, RJ, and Kemp, RJ (1996). Control and prevention of disease transmission in audiology. *Amer J Audiol* 5:74–82.

Barr, B (1965). Early primary screening. In H Davis (ed), *The Young Deaf Child, Acta Otolaryn Suppl* 206:45–47.

Battin, RR (1979). The effects of early middle ear problems on later learning development revisited. *Corti's Org* 4:4.

Becker, W, Naumann, HH, and Pfaltz, CR and edited by R.A. Buckingham (1994) *Ear, Nose and Throat Diseases* (New York: Thieme Medical Publishers).

Berg, FS (1987). *Facilitating Classroom Listening: A Handbook for Teachers of Normal and Hard of Hearing Children* (Boston: College-Hill Press/Little, Brown).

Berger, J (1987). Complicaciones neurologicas del sindroma de inmunodeficiencia adquirida. *Tribuna Medica* Nov (2ndo), 1–4.

Bergstrom, L (1977). Viruses that deafen. In FH Bess (ed), *Childhood Deafness* (New York: Grune & Stratton).

Bergstrom, L (1984). Congenital hearing loss. In JL Northern (ed), *Hearing Disorders,* 2nd ed. (Boston: Little, Brown).

Bergstrom, L and Thompson, PL (1984). Ototoxicity. In JL Northern (ed), *Hearing Disorders*, 2nd ed. (Boston: Little, Brown).

Bernstein, ME and Barta, L (1988). What do parents want in parent education? *Am Annals Deaf* 133:235–246.

Bess, FH (1984). The minimally hearing-impaired child. *Ear and Hearing* 6:43–47.

Bess, FH and Tharpe, AM (1984). Unilateral hearing impairment in children. *Peds* 74:206–216.

Beynon, G (1993). When is a decibel not a decibel?: The application of decibel scales and calibration in clinical audiology. *J Laryn Otol* 107:985–989.

Bilger, RC (1984). Speech recognition test development. In E. Elkins (ed), *Speech Recognition By the Hearing Impaired.* (Rockville, MD: ASHA).

Binnie, C, Jackson, P, and Montgomery, A (1976) Visual intelligibility of consonants: A lipreading screening test with implications for aural rehabilitation. *J Speech Hear Dis* 41:530–539.

Blakley, BW and Myers, SF (1993). Patterns of hearing loss resulting from cis-platinum therapy. *Otol—Head and Neck Surg* 109:385–391.

Bloom, L and Lahey, M (1978). *Language Development and Language Disorders* (New York: John Wiley and Sons).

Bluestone, B (1989). Employment prospects for persons with disabilities. In Kiernan, WE and Schalock, RL (eds), *Economics, Industry, and Disability* (Baltimore: Paul H Brookes).

Bluestone, C (1991). Physiology of the middle ear and eustachian tube. In MM Papparella et al. (eds), *Otolaryngology,* 3rd ed. (Philadelphia: W.B. Saunders Co.).

Bocca, E and Calearo, C (1963). Central hearing processes. In JF Jerger (ed), *Modern Developments in Audiology* (New York: Academic Press).

Bodner-Johnson, B (1985). Families that work for the hearing impaired child. *Volta Rev* 87:131–137.

Boedts, D (1967). La surdité dans la dysostose craniofaciale ou maladie de Crouzon. *Acta Otol Belgica* 21:143–155.

Bonvillian, J, Orlansky, M, and Novack, L (1983). Early sign language acquisition and its relation to cognitive and motor development. In J Kyle and B Woll (eds), *Language in Sign: An International Perspective on Sign Language* (London: Croom Helm).

Bordley, JE, Brookhouser, PE, Hardy, J and Hardy, WG (1967). Observations on the effect of prenatal rubella in hearing. In F McConnell and PH Ward (eds), *Deafness in Childhood* (Nashville: Vanderbilt University Press).

Bordley, JE, Brookhouser, PE, and Tucker Jr, GF (1986). *Ear, Nose and Throat Disorders in Children* (New York: Raven Press).

Bordley, JE, Brookhouser, PE, and Worthington, DL (1971). Viral infections and hearing: a critical review of the literature. *Laryng* 81:557–579.

Bornstein, H (1990). *Manual Communication: Implications for Education* (Washington, DC: Gallaudet Press).

Brackbill, Y (1987). Behavioral teratology comes to the classroom. *Topics in Early Child Spec Ed* 6:33–48.

Bradford, L and Hardy, W (1985). *Hearing and Hearing Impairment* (New York: Grune & Stratton).

Brazelton, TB (1969). *Infants and Mothers: Differences in Development* (New York: Delacorte).

Brimacombe, J and Beiter, A (1996). Cochlear implants. In SE Gerber (ed). *The Handbook of Pediatric Audiology* (Washington, DC: Gallaudet University Press).

Broadbent, DE (1957). Effects of noise on behavior. In CM Harris (ed), *Handbook of Noise Control* (New York: McGraw-Hill).

Brookhouser, PE and Bordley, JE (1973). Congenital rubella deafness. *Arch Otolaryn* 98:252–256.

Burdick, CK, Patterson JH, Mozo BT, Hargett CE, and Camp RT (1977). Threshold shifts in chinchillas exposed to low frequency noise for nine days (Abstract). *J Acoust Soc Amer*, (Suppl 1), 62:595.

Burns, W (1973). Temporary effects of noise on hearing. In W. Burns (ed.), *Noise and Man*, 2nd ed. (London: John Murray).

Butler-Nalin, P, Marder, C, and Padilla, C (1989). *Dropouts: The relationship of student characteristics, behaviors, and performance for special education students* (Menlo Park, Calif.: Stanford Research Institute).

Carhart, R (1950). The clinical application of bone conduction audiometry. *Otolaryn* 51:789–807.

Carhart, R and Jerger, J (1959). Preferred method for clinical determination of pure tone thresholds. *J Speech Hear Dis* 24:330–345.

Carrel, RJ (1977). Epidemiology of hearing loss. In SE Gerber (ed), *Audiometry in Infancy* (New York: Grune & Stratton).

Catlin, FI (1981). Otologic diagnosis and treatment of disorders affecting hearing. In FN Martin (ed), *Medical Audiology* (Englewood Cliffs, NJ: Prentice Hall).

Centers for Disease Control. (1981a). Pneumocystis pneumonia—Los Angeles. *Morbidity and Mortality Weekly Report* 30:250–252.

Centers for Disease Control. (1981b). Kaposi's sarcoma and *Pneumocystis* pneumonia among homosexual men—New York City and California. *Morbidity and Mortality Weekly Report* 25:305–308.

Chandler, JR (1964). Partial occlusion of the external auditory meatus: Its effect upon air and bone conduction acuity. *Laryng* 74: 22–54.

Chermak, GD (1996). Central tests. In SE Gerber (ed), *The Handbook of Pediatric Audiology* (Washington, DC: Gallaudet University Press).

Cherry, EC (1966). *On Human Communication* (Cambridge, Mass.: The M.I.T. Press).

Christian, MS (1983). Statement of problem. In MS Christian et al. (eds), *Advances in Modern Toxicology*, Vol. III: *Assessment of Reproductive and Teratogenic Hazards* (Princeton, NJ: Princeton Scientific Publishers).

Church, MW and Gerkin, KP (1987). Hearing disorders in children with fetal alcohol syndrome: Findings from case reports. *Peds* 82: 147–154.

Churcher, BG and King, AJ (1937). The performance of noise meters in terms of the primary standard. *J Inst Elec Eng* 81:57–90.

Clark, JG and Martin, FN (eds), (1994). *Effective Counseling in Audiology: Perspectives and Practice* (Englewood Cliffs, NJ: Prentice-Hall).

Cody, DTR (1978). Otologic assessment and treatment. In DE Rose (ed), *Audiological Assessment,* 2nd ed. (Englewood Cliffs, NJ: Prentice-Hall).

Cohen, A (1975). Extra-auditory effects of noise. In J Olishefski and E Harford (eds), *Industrial Noise and Hearing Conservation* (Chicago: National Safety Council).

Cohen, MR and McCollough, TD (1996). Infection control protocols for audiologists. *Amer J Audiol* 5: 20–22.

Compton, CL (1993). Assistive technology for deaf and hard-of-hearing people. In JG Alpiner and PA McCarthy (eds), *Rehabilitative Audiology: Children and Adults*, 2nd ed. (Baltimore: Williams & Wilkins).

Cooper, R (1967). The ability of deaf and hearing children to apply morphological rules. *J Speech Hear Res* 10:77–86.

Cooper, R and Rosenstein, J (1966). Language acquisition of deaf children. *Volta Rev* 68:58–67.

Corso, JF (1963). Age and sex differences in pure-tone thresholds. *Arch Otolaryn* 77:398–399.

Cotton, R (1977). Progressive hearing loss. In BF Jaffe (ed), *Hearing Loss in Children* (Baltimore: University Park Press).

Coulman, CU, Greene, I, and Archibald, RW (1987). Cutaneous pneumocystosis. *Ann Intern Med* 106(3):396–398.

Cox, RM, Alexander, GC, and Gilmore, C. (1987). Development of the connected speech test (CST). *Ear and Hearing* 8 (suppl.):119–126.

Cox, RM and Gilmore, C (1990). Development of the profile of hearing aid performance (PHAP). *J Speech Hear Res* 33:343–357.

Cox, RM and Rivera, IM (1992). Predictability and reliability of hearing aid benefit measured using the PHAP. *J Am Acad Aud* 3:242–254.

Cronbach, LJ (1984). *Essentials of Psychological Testing*, 4th ed. (New York: Harper and Row).

Curtis, S, Prutting, C, and Lowell, E (1979). Pragmatic and semantic development in young children with impaired hearing. *J Speech Hear Res* 22:534–552.

Dahle, AJ, McCollister, FP, Hamner, BA, Reynolds, DW, and Stagno, S (1974). Subclinical congenital cytomegalovirus infection and hearing impairment. *J Speech Hear Dis* 39:320–329.

Dahle, AJ, McCollister, FP, Stagno, S, Reynolds, DW, and Hoffman, HE (1979). Progressive hearing impairment in children with congenital cytomegalovirus infection. *J Speech Hear Dis* 44:220–229.

Dallos, P (1964). Dynamics of the acoustic reflex. *J Acoust Soc Amer* 36:2175–2183.

Davidson, T and Stabile, B (1991). Acquired immunodeficiency syndrome precautions for otolaryngology-head and neck surgery. *Arch Otolaryn* 117:1343–1344.

Davis, AC (1983). Hearing disorders in the population: First phase findings of the MRC national study of hearing. In ME Lutman and MP Haggard (eds), *Hearing Science and Hearing Disorders* (London: Academic Press).

Davis, AC and Sancho, J (1988). Screening for hearing impairment in children. In SE Gerber and GT Mencher (eds), *International Perspectives On Communication Disorders* (Washington: Gallaudet University Press).

Davis, H (1948a). *Hearing and Deafness* (NY: Rinehart).

Davis, H. (1948b). The articulation area and the social adequacy index for hearing. *Layrng* 58:761–778.

Davis, H (1978). Audiometry: Other auditory tests. In H Davis and SR Silverman (eds), *Hearing and Deafness*, 4th ed. (New York: Holt, Rinehart and Winston).

Davis, H, Gernhardt, BE, Riesco-MacClure, JS, and Covell, WP (1949). Aural microphonics in the cochlea of the Guinea pig. *J Acoust Soc Amer* 21:502–510.

Davis, H and Silverman, RS (1978). *Hearing and Deafness*, 4th ed. (New York: Holt, Rinehart and Winston).

Davis, JM, Elfenbein, J, Schum, R, and Bentler, R (1986). Effects of mild and moderate hearing impairments on language, educational and psychosocial behavior of children. *J Speech Hear Dis* 46:130–137, 1981.

Davis, JM and Hardick, EJ (1981). *Rehabilitative Audiology for Children and Adults* (New York: John Wiley and Sons).

DeBoer, E (1967). Correlation studies applied to the frequency resolution of the cochlea. *J Aud Res* 7:209–217.

DeBoer, E and Bouwmeester, J (1975). Clinical psychophysics illustrated by the problem of auditory overload. *Audiology* 14:274–299.

DeFilippo, CL and Sims, DG (eds), (1988). New reflections on speechreading [Monograph]. *Volta Rev*, 90.

Demorest, ME and DeHaven, GP (1993). Psychometric adequacy of self-assessment scales. *Sem Hearing* 14:314–325.

Demorest, ME and Erdman, SA (1986). Scale composition and item analysis of the communication profile for the hearing impaired. *J Speech Hear Res* 29:515–535.

Derlacki, E (1976). Otosclerosis. In JL Northern (ed), *Hearing Disorders* (Boston: Little, Brown).

DiBartolomeo, JR (1979). Exoxtoses of the external auditory canal. *Ann Otol Rhin Laryng* (Suppl.) 61, 88:1–20.

DiBartolomeo, JR and Gerber, SE (1977). Pathology of hearing loss. In SE Gerber (ed.), *Audiometry in Infancy* (New York: Grune and Statton).

DiBartolomeo, JR, Papparella, MM, and Meyerhoff, WL (1991). Cysts and tumors of the external ear. In MM Papparella et al. (eds), *Otolaryngology* (vol 2), 3rd ed. (Philadelphia: W.B. Saunders Co.).

Diefendorf, AO, Leverett, RG, and Miller, SM (1994). Hearing impairment. In S Adler and DA King (eds), *Oral Communication Problems in Children and Adolescents* (Boston: Allyn & Bacon).

DiFrancesca, S (1972). Academic achievement test results of a national testing program for hearing-impaired students—United States, Spring 1971. Office of Demographic Studies, Series D, No. 9 (Washington, DC: Gallaudet College).

Downs, MP (1978). The interaction of critical periods with conductive losses. Presented to the sixth annual meeting of the Society for Ear, Nose and Throat Advances in Children. Santa Barbara, California.

Downs, MP (1984). Personal Communication. XVIIth International Congress of Audiology, Santa Barbara, California.

Downs, MP and Silver, HK (1972). The A.B.C.D.s to H.E.A.R.: Early identification in nursery, office and clinic of the infant who is deaf. *Clin Ped* 11: 563–566.

Duane, DD (1977). A neurologic perspective of central auditory dysfunction. In RW Keith (ed), *Central Auditory Dysfunction* (New York: Grune & Stratton).

Dublin, WB (1976). *Fundamentals of Sensorineural Auditory Pathology* (Springfield, Ill.: Charles C. Thomas).

Eames, BL, Hamernik, R, Henderson, D, and Feldman, A (1975). The role of the middle ear in acoustic trauma from impulses. *Laryng* 85:1582–1592.

Easterbrooks, SR (1987). Speech/language assessment and intervention with school-age hearing-impaired children. In JG Alpiner and PA McCarthy (eds), *Rehabilitative Audiology: Children and Adults* (Baltimore: Williams & Wilkins).

Eichenwald, E (1979). Rationale and efficacy of antibiotics use in ear, nose and throat practice. Presented to the seventh annual meeting of the Society for Ear, Nose and Throat Advances in Children, Cincinnati, Ohio.

Eisenwort, B, Brauneis, K, and Burian, K (1985). Rehabilitation of the cochlear implant patient. In RF Gray (ed), *Cochlear Implants* (San Diego: College-Hill Press).

Engen, E and Engen, T (1983). *Rhode Island Test of Language Structure—Manual* (Baltimore: University Park Press).

Epstein, LG (1986). Manifestations of human immunodeficiency virus infection in children. *Peds* 78: 678–687.

Erber, NP (1982). *Auditory Training* (Washington, DC: A.G. Bell Association).

Erber, NP (1993). *Communication and Adult Hearing Loss* (Victoria, Australia: Claves Publishing).

Etholm, B and Belal, A (1974). Senile changes in the middle ear joints. *Ann Otol Rhin and Laryn* 83: 49–54.

Evans, EF and Wilson, JP (1977). *Psychophysics and Physiology of Hearing* (London: Academic Press).

Ewertsen, H and Birk-Nielsen, H (1973). Social hearing handicap index: Social handicap in relation to hearing impairment. *Audiology* 12:180–187.

Fauci, AS (1988). The human immunodeficiency virus: Infectivity and mechanisms of pathogenesis. *Science* 239:617–622.

Fazen, LE, Lovejoy, Jr, FH, and Crone, RK (1986). Acute poisoning in a children's hospital: A 2–year experience. *Peds* 77:144–151.

FDA (1977). Food and Drug Administration rules and regulations regarding hearing aid devices. *Federal Register* 9286–9296.

Feinmesser, M and Tell, L (1976). Evaluation of methods for detecting hearing impairment in infancy and early childhood. In GT Mencher (ed), *Early Identification of Hearing Loss* (Basel, Switzerland: Karger).

Feldman, AS (1978). Acoustic impedance-admittance battery. In J Katz (ed), *Handbook of Clinical Audiology*, 2nd ed. (Baltimore: Williams & Wilkins).

Feldman, AS and Wilber, LA (1976). *Acoustic Impedance and Admittance: The Measurement of Middle Ear Function* (Baltimore: Williams & Wilkins).

Fikret-Pasa, S and Garstecki, DC (1993). Real-ear measures in evaluation of frequency response and volume control characteristics of telephone amplifiers. *J Amer Acad Audiol* 4:5–12.

Fischer, WH and Schafer, JW (1991). Direction dependent amplification of the human outer ear. *Brit J Aud* 25:123–130.

Flahive, MJ, and White, SC (1981). Audiologists and counseling. *J Acad Rehab Aud* 14:274–283.

Fletcher, H and Munson, WA (1933). Loudness, its definition, measurement, and calculation. *J Acoust Soc Amer* 5:82–108.

Flexer, C (1993). Management of hearing in an educational setting. In JG Alpiner and PA McCarthy (eds), *Rehabilitative Audiology: Children and Adults*, 2nd ed. (Baltimore: Williams & Wilkins).

Flower, WM and Sooy, CD (1987). AIDS: An introduction for speech-language pathologists and audiologists. *Asha* 29:25–30.

Forret-Kaminsky, MC, Scherer, C, Bemer, M, Robert, V, Steinbach, G, and Poussel, JF (1991). Nocardia asteroides otitis media in AIDS. *Presse Med* 20:1512–1513.

Fowler, EP (1944). The aging ear. *Arch Otolaryn* 40: 475–480.

Frankel, BJ (1981). Adult onset hearing-impairment: Social and psychological correlates of adjustment. Unpublished doctoral dissertation, University of Western Ontario, London, Ontario.

Fraser, GR (1971). The genetics of congenital deafness. *Otol Clin N Am* 4:227–247.

Fraser, GR (1976). *The Causes of Profound Deafness in Childhood*. (Baltimore: The Johns Hopkins University Press).

Friedman, H and Prier, JE (eds), (1973). Rubella. *First annual symposium, Eastern Pennsylvania Branch, Am Soc for Microbiology* (Springfield, Ill.: Charles C. Thomas).

Fritsch, MH and Sommer, A (1991). *Handbook of Congenital and Early Onset Hearing Loss* (New York: Igaku-Shoin).

Garstecki, DC (1981). Audio-visual training paradigm for hearing impaired adults. *J Acad Rehabil Audiol* 14:223–228.

Garstecki, DC (1994). Hearing aid acceptance in adults. In JG Clark and FN Martin (eds), *Effective Counseling in Audiology: Perspectives and Practice*. (Englewood Cliffs, NJ: Prentice-Hall).

Geers, A and Moog, J (1987). Predicting spoken language acquisition of profoundly hearing-impaired children. *J Speech Hear Dis* 52:84–94.

Gelfand, SA (1990). *Hearing* (New York: Marcel Dekker).

Gerber, SE (1965). *Evaluation of Air Force Hearing Test Data* (Fullerton, Calif.: Hughes Aircraft Co.).

Gerber, SE (1974). The intelligibility of speech. In SE Gerber (ed), *Introductory Hearing Science* (Philadelphia: W.B. Saunders Co.).

Gerber, SE (1977a). Prevention of handicap by early detection. Keynote address presented at Interprofessional Forum on Learning. University of Santa Clara, California.

Gerber, SE (1977b). High risk conditions. In SE Gerber (ed), *Audiometry in Infancy* (New York: Grune & Stratton).

Gerber, SE (1990a). AIDS and otorhinolaryngology. In JJ Madriz-Alfaro (ed), (1990). *Prevention and Early Identification of Deafness*. (San José, Costa Rica: Publicaciones Ministerio de Salud).

Gerber, SE (1990b). *Prevention: The Etiology of Communicative Disorders in Children* (Englewood Cliffs, NJ: Prentice-Hall).

Gerber, SE and Mencher, GT (eds), (1978). *Early Diagnosis of Hearing Loss* (New York: Grune & Stratton).

Gerber, SE, Mendel, MI, and Goller, M (1979). Progressive hearing loss subsequent to congenital cytomegalovirus infection. *Human Comm Can* 4:231–234.

Gherman, CR, Ward, RR, and Bassis, ML (1988). *Pneumocystis carinii* otitis media and mastoiditis as the initial manifestation of the acquired immunodeficiency syndrome. *Am J Med* 85:250–252.

Ghorayeb, BY and Yeakley, JW (1992). Temporal bone fractures: Longitudinal or oblique? The case for oblique temporal bone fractures *Laryng* 102:129–134.

Gibbins, S (1989). The provision of school psychological assessment services for the hearing impaired: A national survey. *Volta Rev* 91:95–103.

Gilman, L and Raffin, M (1975). Acquisition of common morphemes by hearing impaired children exposed to the Seeing Exact English sign system. Paper presented at the meeting of the American Speech and Hearing Association, Washington, D.C.

Glorig, A and Davis, H (1961). Age, noise, and hearing loss. *Trans Am Otol Soc* 490:262–280.

Glorig, A, Ward, WD, and Nixon, J (1961). Damage risk criteria and noise induced hearing loss. *Arch Otolaryn* 74:71–81.

Goethe, KE, Mitchell, JE, and Marshall, DW (1989). Neuropsychologic-neurological function of human immunodeficiency virus seropositive individuals. *Neuro* 41:209–216.

Goin, DW (1976). Otospongiosis. In G English (ed), *Otolaryngology: A Textbook* (New York: Harper and Row).

Gold, T (1980). Speech production in hearing-impaired children. *J Comm Dis* 13:397–418.

Goldberg, DM (1993). Auditory-verbal philosophy. *Volta Rev* 95:181–186.

Goodhill, V (1979a). Otologic relationships with audiology. In LJ Bradford and WG Hardy (eds), *Hearing and Hearing Impairment* (New York: Grune & Stratton).

Goodhill, V (1979b). *Ear Diseases, Deafness, and Dizziness* (New York: Harper and Row).

Goodhill, V. and Brockman, SJ (1979). Secretory otitis media. In V Goodhill (ed), *Ear Diseases, Deafness and Dizziness*. (New York: Harper and Row).

Goodhill, V and Harris, I (1979a). Sudden hearing loss syndrome. In V Goodhill (ed), *Ear Diseases, Deafness and Dizziness* (New York: Harper and Row).

Goodhill, V and Harris, I (1979b). Peripheral vertigo, labyrinthitis, and Ménière's disease In V Goodhill (ed), *Ear Diseases, Deafness and Dizziness* (New York: Harper and Row).

Goodwin, J (1987). Acoustics and electroacoustics. In D. Stephens (ed), *Scott Brown's Otolaryngology*,

5th ed., Volume 2: *Adult Audiology* (London: Butterworths).

Gorlin, RJ, Cohen, MM, and Levin, LS (eds), (1990). *Syndromes of the Head and Neck* (New York: Oxford University Press).

Gottlieb, MS, Schroff, R, and Schanker (1981). *Pneumocystis carinii* pneumonia and mucosal candidiasis in previously healthy homosexual men: Evidence of a new acquired cellular immunodeficiency. *N Engl J Med* 305:1425–1431.

Grant, J (1987). *The Hearing Impaired: Birth To Six* (Boston: Little, Brown).

Gregg, NM (1941). Congenital cataract following German measles in the mother. *Trans Ophth Soc Aus* 3:35–46.

Groopman, J (1987). Neoplasms in the acquired immune deficiency syndrome: The multidisciplinary approach to treatment. *Sem Oncol* (Suppl. 2), 14: 34–39.

Gross, R (1970). Language used by mothers of deaf children and mothers of hearing children. *Am Ann Deaf* 115:93–96.

Gross, DJ, Parris, A, and Safai, B (1991). SIDA—una actualizacion. *Tribuna Medica* 48:35–44.

Gulick, WL, Gescheider, GA, and Frisina, RD (1989). *Hearing: Physiological Acoustics, Neural Coding, and Psychoacoustics* (New York: Oxford University Press).

Gustason, G (1983). *Teaching and Learning Signing Exact English* (Los Alamitos, Calif.: Modern Signs Press).

Haas, WH and Crowley, DJ (1982). Professional information dissemination to parents of pre-school hearing-impaired children. *Volta Rev* 84:17–23.

Haddad, J, Brager, R, and Bluestone, CD (1992). Infections of the ears, nose and throat in children with primary immunodeficiencies. *Arch Otolaryn* 118: 138–141.

Hanshaw, JB (1979). Cytomegaloviral infection. In VC Vaughn, RJ McKay, and RE Behrman (eds), *Textbook of Pediatrics* (Philadelphia: W.B. Saunders Co.).

Hanshaw, JB and Dudgeon, JA (1978). Viral diseases of the fetus and newborn. *Maj Prob Clin Ped* 17:1–9.

Hanshaw, JB, Scheiner, AP, Moxley, AW, Gaev, L, Abel, V, and Scheiner, BA (1976). School failure and deafness after "silent" cytomegalovirus infection. *New Eng J Med* 295:468–470.

Hardick, E, Oyer, H, and Irion, P (1970). Lipreading performance as related to measurement of vision. *J Speech Hear Res* 13:92–100.

Hardy, JB (1973). Fetal consequences of maternal virus infections in pregnancy. *Arch Otol* 98:218–227.

Hardy, JB, Sever, JL, and Gilkeson, MR (1969). Declining antibody titers in children with congenital rubella. *J Ped* 75:213–220.

Hardy, WG and Bordley, JE (1973). Problems in diagnosis and management of the multiply handicapped deaf child. *Arch Otol* 98:269–274.

Hart, CW, Cokely, CG, Schupbach, J, Dal Canto, M, and Coppleson, W (1989). Neurotologic findings of a patient with acquired immune deficiency syndrome. *Ear and Hearing* 10:68–76.

Hawkins, JE (1975). Drug ototoxicity. In M Strome (ed), *Differential Diagnosis in Pediatric Otolaryngology* (Boston: Little, Brown).

Hawke, M (1987). *Clinical Pocket Guide to Ear Disease* (New York: Gower Medical Publishing).

Hawke, M, and McCombe, A (1995). *Diseases of the Ear: A Pocket Atlas* (Hamilton, Ontario: Manticore Communications).

Hazell, J (1990). Tinnitus III: The practical management of sensorineural tinnitus. *J Otolaryn* 19:11–18.

Health and Welfare Canada (1988). *Acquired Hearing Impairment in the Adult* (Ottawa).

Hearing Aid Industry Conference (1961). *HAIC Standard Method of Expressing Hearing Aid Performance* (New York).

Hemenway, WG, Sando, S and McChesney, D. (1969). Temporal bone pathology following maternal rubella. *Arch Klin Exp Ohren Nosen Kehlkopf, Heilk.* 193:287–300.

Henderson, D, Subramanian, M, and Boettcher, FA (1993). Individual susceptibility to noise-induced hearing loss: An old topic revisited. *Ear and Hearing*, 14, 152–168.

Hicks, GS (1986). Hearing loss secondary to bacterial meningitis. Unpublished manuscript, University of California at Santa Barbara.

High, WS, Fairbanks, G, and Glorig, A (1964). Scale for self-assessment of hearing handicap. *J Speech Hear Dis* 29:215–230.

Hinchcliffe, R (1962). Aging and sensory thresholds. *J Geron* 73:10–12.

Hinojosa, R and Naunton, RF (1991). Presbycusis. In MM Papparella et al. (eds), *Otolaryngology,* 3rd ed. (Philadelphia: W.B. Saunders Co.).

Hiskey, M (1966). *Hiskey-Nebraska Test of Learning Aptitude: Manual* (Lincoln, Neb.: Union College Press).

Ho, DD (1992). *VIII International AIDS Conference* (Amsterdam).

Howie, VM (1975). Natural history of otitis media. *Ann Otol, Rhin, Laryn*, Suppl. 19, 85:67–72.

Howie, VM (1978). The effect of early onset of otitis media on educational achievement. Presented to the sixth annual meeting of the Society for Ear, Nose and Throat Advances in Children. Santa Barbara, California.

Hudgins, CV and Numbers, F (1942). An investigation of the intelligibility of the speech of the deaf. *Genet Psych Mono* 25:289–392.

Hull, FM, Mielke, PW, Willeford, J, and Timmons, RJ (1976). *National Speech and Hearing Survey: Final Report.* Project No. 50978. Education Office, DHEW. Cited in GT Mencher (1990). Epidemiology of Communication Disorders. In JJ Madriz-Alfaro (ed), (1990). *Prevention and Early Identification of Deafness* (San José, Costa Rica: Publicaciones Ministerio de Salud).

Huttenlocher, PR (1987). The nervous system. In RE Behrman and VC Vaughan (eds), N*elson Textbook of Pediatrics*, 13th ed. (Philadelphia: W.B. Saunders Co.).

International Electrotechnical Commission (1959). *IEC Recommended Methods for Measurement of the Electroacoustical Characteristics of Hearing Aids,* Publication No. 118 (Geneva).

Ivey, RG (1969). Tests of CNS auditory function. Unpublished master's thesis, Colorado State University, Fort Collins.

Jaffe, BF (ed), (1977). *Hearing Loss in Children* (Baltimore: University Park Press).

Jaffe, BF (1978). Topographical signs associated with congenital hearing loss. In SE Gerber and GT Mencher (eds), *Early Diagnosis of Hearing Loss* (New York: Grune & Stratton).

Jaffe, BF (1979). The life cycle of middle ear disease in cleft palate children. Presented to the seventh annual meeting of the Society for Ear, Nose and Throat Advances in Children, Cincinnati. Ohio.

Jerger, J (1970). Clinical experience with impedance audiometry. *Arch Otolaryn* 93:311–324.

Jerger, J, Jerger, S, and Mauldin, L (1972). Studies in impedance audiometry I. Normal and sensorineural ears. *Arch Otolaryn* 96:513–523.

Jerger, J and Northern, JL (eds), (1980). *Clinical Impedance Audiometry* (Acton, Mass.: American Electromedics Corporation).

Jerger, JF, Speaks, C, and Trammell, JL (1968). A new approach to speech audiometry. *J Speech Hear Dis* 33:318–328.

Jerger, S and Jerger, J (1981). *Auditory Disorders* (Boston: Little, Brown).

Johnson, EW (1968). Confirmed retrocochlear lesions. *Arch Otolaryn* 88:598–603.

Johnson, SJ (1986). Prevalence of sensorineural hearing loss in premature and sick term infants with perinatally acquired cytomegalovirus infection. *Ear and Hearing* 7:325–327.

Johnstone, BM, Patuzzi, R, and Yates, GK (1986). Basilar membrane measurements and the travelling wave. *Hear Res* 22:147–153.

Joint Committee on Infant Hearing (1994). Position Statement. *Asha* 36:38–41.

Jung, TKT and Nissen, RL (1991). Otologic manifestations of retrocochlear disease. In MM Papparella et al. (eds). *Otolaryngology*, 3rd ed. (Philadelphia: W.B. Saunders Co.).

Karmody, CS (1969). Asymptomatic maternal rubella and congenital deafness. *Arch Otolaryn* 89:720.

Kassirer, E (ed), (1988). *Acquired Hearing Impairment in the Adult* (Ottawa: Health and Welfare Canada).

Kassirer, E (ed), (1984). *Childhood Hearing Impairment* (Ottawa: Health and Welfare Canada).

Kastner, T and Friedman, D (1988). Pediatric acquired immune deficiency syndrome and the prevention of mental retardation. *Devel and Behav Peds.* 9:47–48.

Katz, J (1962). The use of staggered spondaic words for assessing the integrity of the central nervous system. *J Aud Res* 2:327–337.

Katz, J (1977). The staggered spondaic word test. In RW Keith (ed), *Central Auditory Dysfunction* (New York: Grune & Stratton).

Katz, J (1978). The effects of conductive hearing loss on auditory function. *Asha* 20:879–886.

Katz, J (ed), (1993). *Handbook of Clinical Audiology*, 4th ed., (Baltimore: Williams & Wilkins).

Katz, J, Stecker, N, and Henderson, D (1992). *Central Auditory Processing* (St. Louis: Mosby Year Book).

Kaufman, AS and Kaufman, NL (1983). *Kaufman Assessment Battery for Children* (Circle Pines, Minn.: American Guidance Services).

Keith, RW (ed), (1977). *Central Auditory Dysfunction* (New York: Grune & Stratton).

Kelemen, G (1977). Morquio's disease and the hearing organ. *ORL* 39:233–240.

Kemp, DT (1980). Towards a model for the origin of cochlear echoes. *Hear Res* 2: 533–548.

Khanna, SM, (1984). Inner ear function based on the mechanical tuning of the hair cells. In C Berlin (ed), *Hearing Science* (San Diego: College-Hill Press).

Kileny, P and Robertson, C (1985). Neurological aspects of infant hearing screening. *J Otol* (Suppl) 14:34–39.

Kim, DO (1984). Functional roles of the inner- and outer-hair cell sub-systems in the cochlea and brainstem. In C Berlin (ed), *Hearing Science* (San Diego: College-Hill Press).

Kohan, D, Hammerschlag, PE, and Holliday, RA (1990). Otologic disease in AIDS patients: CT correlation. *Laryng* 100:1326–1330.

Kohji, IJ, Yukiaki, N, and Kenji, O (1979). Congenital rubella syndrome: Correlation of gestational age at time of maternal rubella with type of onset. *J Ped* 94:763–765.

Konigsmark, BW (1971). Hereditary and congenital factors affecting newborn sensorineural hearing. In GC Cunningham (ed), *Conference on Newborn Hearing Screening* (Berkeley: California Department of Health).

Konigsmark, BW (1972). Genetic hearing loss with no associated abnormalities: A review. Part II. *J Speech Hear Dis* 37:89–99.

Konigsmark, BW and Gorlin, RJ (1976). *Genetic and Metabolic Deafness* (Philadelphia: W.B. Saunders Co.).

Koralnik, IJ, Beaumanoir, A, and Hausler, R (1990). A controlled study of early neurologic abnormalities in men with asymptomatic human immunodeficiency virus infection. *N Engl J Med* 323:864–870.

Kozlowski, PB (1992). Neuropathology of HIV infection in children. In AC Crocker, HJ Cohen, and TA Kastner (eds), (1992). *HIV Infection and Developmental Disabilities: A Resource for Service Providers* (Baltimore: Paul H. Brookes Publishing).

Krajicek, MJ and Tierney, AL (1977). *Detection of Developmental Problems in Children* (Austin: Pro-Ed, Inc.).

Kramer, RL (1978). Miniseminar on chronic otitis media. Presented to the annual convention of the American Speech and Hearing Association, San Francisco, California.

Kretschmer, RR and Kretschmer, LW (1978). *Language Development and Intervention with the Hearing Impaired*. (Baltimore: University Park Press).

Kretschmer, RR and Kretschmer, LW (1990). Language. *Volta Rev* 92:56–71.

Kricos, PB (1993). The counseling process: Children and parents. In JG Alpiner and PA McCarthy (eds), *Rehabilitative Audiology: Children and Adults*, 2nd ed. (Baltimore: Williams & Wilkins).

Kryter, KD (1970). *The Effects of Noise on Man* (New York: Academic Press).

Kwartler, JA, Linthicum, FH, Jahn, AF, and Hawke, M (1991). Sudden hearing loss due to AIDS related cryptococcal meningitis: A temporal bone study. *Otolaryn* 103:817–821.

Lalande, NM, Lambert, J, and Riverin, L (1988). Quantification of the psychosocial disadvantages experienced by workers in a noisy industry and their nearest relatives: Perspectives for rehabilitation. *Audiology* 27:196–206.

Lamb, SH, Owens, E, and Schubert, ED (1983). The revised form of the hearing performance inventory. *Ear and Hearing* 4:152–159.

Laughton, J and Hasenstab, MS (1986). *The Language Learning Process: Implications for Management of Disorders* (Rockville, Md.: Aspen Publishers).

Laughton, J and Hasenstab, MS (1993). Assessment and intervention with school-age hearing-impaired children. In JG Alpiner and PA McCarthy (eds), *Rehabilitative Audiology: Children and Adults*, 2nd ed. (Baltimore: Williams & Wilkins).

Lee, KC, Tami, TA, Echavez, M, and Wildes, TO (1990). Deep neck infections in patients at risk for acquired immunodeficiency syndrome. *Laryng* 100:915–919.

Leiter, R (1979). *Leiter International Performance Scale: Instruction Manual.* (Chicago: Stoelting).

Lempert, J (1938). Improvement of hearing in cases of otosclerosis: A new oto-surgical technique. *Arch Otolaryn* 28:42–97.

Leopold, RE (1979). A retrospective study of the relationship between perinatal anoxia and communicative disorders. Unpublished master's thesis, University of California, Santa Barbara.

Leroy, JG and Crocker, AC (1966). Clinical definition of Hunter-Hurler phenotypes. A review of 50 patients. *Am J Dis Child* 112:518–530.

Levine, E (1960). *The Psychology of Deafness* (New York: Columbia University Press).

Lim, DJ, (1986). Functional structure of the organ of Corti. *Hear Res* 22:117–146.

Lindsay, JR (1973). Otosclerosis. In MM Papparella and DA Shumrick (eds), *Otolaryngology*, vol. 2. (Philadelphia: W.B. Saunders Co.).

Lindsay, JR and Matz, G (1966). The differentiation of acquired congenital from genetically determined inner ear deafness. *Ann Otol, Rhin, and Laryng* 75:830–843.

Ling, D (1984a). *Early Intervention for Hearing-Impaired Children: Oral Options* (San Diego: College-Hill Press).

Ling, D (1984b). *Early Intervention for Hearing-Impaired Children: Total Communication Options* (San Diego: College-Hill Press).

Ling, D (1989). *Foundations of Spoken Language for Hearing-Impaired Children.* (Washington DC: AG Bell Association).

Lipscomb, D (ed), (1978). *Noise and Audiology* (Baltimore: University Park Press).

Litowitz, B (1987). Language and the young deaf child. In E Mindel and M Vernon (eds), *They Grow in Silence: Understanding Deaf Children and Adults* (Boston: Little, Brown).

Littler, TS (1965). *The Physics of the Ear* (New York: Macmillan).

Liu-Shindo, M and Hawkins, DB (1989). Basilar skull fractures in children. *Intl J Ped Otorhinolaryn* 17:109–117.

Loeb, R and Sarigiani, P (1986). The impact of hearing impairment on self-perceptions of children. *Volta Rev* 88:89–100.

Los Angeles County, Office of Education (1976). Auditory Skills Curriculum (North Hollywood: Foreworks).

Ludman, HE (1988). *Mawson's Diseases of the Ear*, 5th ed. (London: Edward Arnold).

Luetke-Stahlman, B and Luckner, J (1991). *Effectively Educating Students with Hearing Impairments* (New York: Longman).

Luterman, DM (1979). *Counseling Parents of Hearing-Impaired children* (Boston: Little, Brown).

Luterman, DM (1991). *Counseling the Communicatively Disordered and their Families* (Austin, Tex.: ProEd).

MacTurk, RH, Meadow-Orlans, KP, Koester, LS, and Spencer, PE (1993). Social support, motivation, language, and interaction: A longitudinal study of mothers and deaf infants. *Am Ann Deaf* 138: 19–25.

Madriz, JJ and Herrera, G (1992). AIDS and Deafness, Presented at XXI International Congress of Audiology, Morioka, Japan.

Manson, MM, Logan, WPD, and Loy, RM (1960). *Rubella and other Virus Infections During Pregnancy* (London: HM Stationery Office).

Marelli, RA, Biddinger, PW, and Gluckman, JL (1992). Cytomegalovirus infection of the larynx in the acquired immunodeficiency syndrome. *Otolaryn* 106:296–303.

Marshall, L (1981). Auditory processing in aging listeners. *J Speech Hear Dis* 46:226–240.

Martin, JAM (1982). Aetiological factors relating to childhood deafness in the European Community. *Audiology* 21:149–158.

Martin, JAM, Hennebert, D, Bentzen, O, Morgon, A, Holm, C, McCullen, O, Iurato, S, Meyer, L, de Jonge, GA, Colley, JRT, and Moore, WJ (1979). *Childhood Deafness in The European Community* (Brussels: Commission of the European Communities).

Marx, JL (1975). Cytomegalovirus: A major cause of birth defects. *Science* 190:1184–1186.

Maslan, MJ, Graham, MD, and Flood, LM (1985). Cryptococcal meningitis presentation as sudden deafness. *Arch Otolaryn* 6:435–437.

Mattox, DE, Nager, GT, and Levin, LS (1991). Congenital aural atresia: Embryology, pathology, classification, surgical management. In MM Papparella et al. (eds), *Otolaryngology*, 3rd ed. (Philadelphia: W.B. Saunders).

Matzker, J (1959). Two new methods for assessment of central auditory functions in cases of brain disease. *Ann Otol, Rhino, and Laryng* 68:1185–1197.

Maurer, JF and Rupp, RR (1979). *Hearing and Aging* (New York: Grune & Stratton).

Mawson, SR (1967). *Diseases of the Ear* (London: Edward Arnold).

Maxon, AB, Brackett, D, and van den Berg, SA (1991). Self perception of socialization: The effects of hearing status, age, and gender. *Volta Rev* 93:7–17.

McAnally, PL, Rose, S, and Quigley, SP (1987). *Language Learning Practices with Deaf Children* (San Diego: College-Hill Press).

McCabe, B (1963). The etiology of deafness. *Volta Rev* 65:471–477.

McCabe, B and Lawrence, M (1958). Effects of intense sound on non-auditory labyrinth. *Acta Otolaryn* 49:147–157.

McCarthy, PA and Alpiner, JG (1983). McCarthy-Alpiner scale of hearing handicap. *J Acad Rehab Audio* 16:256–270.

McElroy, EA, and Marks, GL (1991). Fatal necrotizing otitis externa in a patient with AIDS (Letter). *Rev Infec Dis* 132:1246–1247.

McEntee, MK (1993). Accessibility of mental health services and crisis intervention to the deaf. *Am Ann Deaf* 138:26–30.

McFadden, D and Plattsmier, HS (1982). Exposure-induced loudness shifts and threshold shifts. In RP Hamernik, D Henderson, and R Salvi (eds), *New Perspectives on Noise Induced Hearing Loss* (New York: Raven Press).

McKirdy, L and Blank, M (1982). Dialogue in deaf and hearing preschoolers. *J Speech Hear Res* 25:487–499.

Meadow, K, Greenberg, M, Erting, C, and Carmichael, H (1981). Interactions of deaf mothers and deaf preschool children: Comparisons with three other groups of deaf and hearing dyads. *Am Ann Deaf* 126:454–468.

Melnick, W and Morgan, W (1991). Hearing compensation evaluation. *Otolaryn Clin N Am* 24:391–402.

Mencher, GT (ed) (1976). *Early Identification of Hearing Loss* (Basel, Switzerland: Karger).

Mencher, GT (1995) Ototoxicity and irradiation: Additional etiologies of hearing loss in adults. *J Amer Acad Audiol* 6:351–357.

Mencher, GT (1996). Counseling families of hearing-impaired children: Suggestions for the audiologist. In SE Gerber (ed), *The Handbook of Pediatric Audiology* (Washington: DC: Gallaudet University Press).

Mencher, GT, Baldursson, G, Tell, L, and Levi, C (1978). Mass behavioral screening and follow-up. Presented to the meeting of the National Research Council—National Academy of Sciences, Assembly of Behavioral and Social Sciences Meeting of the Committee on Hearing, Bioacoustics and Biomechanics, Omaha, Nebraska.

Mencher, GT and Gerber, SE (eds), (1978). *Early Diagnosis of Hearing Loss* (New York: Grune and Stratton).

Mencher, GT and Gerber, SE (eds), (1981). *Early Management of Hearing Loss* (New York: Grune & Stratton).

Mencher, GT and Mencher, LS (1995). Report of a 10 year study of the Nova Scotia early identification of hearing loss program. *Report to the NSHSC and Grace Hospitals, Halifax, Nova Scotia, Canada.*

Mencher, GT and Stick, SL (1976). On beyond the cochlea: Auditory perceptual disorders. In GT Mencher (ed), *Early Identification of Hearing Loss* (Basel, Switzerland: Karger).

Meyerhoff, WL and Liston, SL (1991). Metabolic hearing loss. In MM Papparella et al. (eds), *Otolaryngology*, 3rd ed. (Philadelphia: W.B. Saunders Co.).

Meyerhoff, WL and Papparella, MM (1991). Management of otosclerosis. In MM Papparella et al. (eds), *Otolaryngology*, 3rd ed. (Philadelphia: W.B. Saunders Co.).

Mindel, E and Feldman, V (1987). The impact of deaf children on their families. In E Mindel and M Vernon (eds), *They Grow in Silence: Understanding Deaf Children and Adults* (Boston: Little, Brown).

Mishell, JH and Applebaum, EL (1990). Ramsay Hunt Syndrome in a patient with HIV infection. *Otolaryng* 102:177–179.

Moeller, MP and Carney, AE (1993). Assessment and intervention with preschool hearing-impaired children, In JG Alpiner and PA McCarthy (eds), *Rehabilitative Audiology: Children and Adults*, 2nd ed. (Baltimore: Williams & Wilkins).

Moeller, MP, Osberger, MJ and Morford, J (1987). Speech-language assessment with preschool hearing-impaired children. In JG Alpiner and PA McCarthy (eds), *Rehabilitative Audiology: Children and Adults* (Baltimore: Williams & Wilkins).

Monif, G and Jordon, PA (1977). Rubella virus and rubella vaccine, *Sem Perinat* 1:41–49.

Montgomery, A and Demorest, M (1988). Issues and developments in the evaluation of speechreading. *Volta Rev* 90:193–214.

Moore, BCJ (1989). *An Introduction to the Psychology of Hearing*, 3rd ed. (London: Academic Press).

Moores, D (1991). The school placement revolution. *Am Ann Deaf* 136:307–308.

*Morbidity and Mortality Weekly Report* (1992). 41(30), July 30.

Mussen, EF (1988). Techniques and concepts in auditory training and speechreading. In RJ Roeser and MP Downs (eds), *Auditory Disorders in School Children: Identification and Remediation* (New York: Thieme Medical Publishers).

Myers, EN and Stool, S (1968). Cytomegalic inclusion disease of the inner ear. *Laryng* 78: 1904–1915.

Nager, GT (1973). Congenital aural atresia: Anatomy and surgical management. In MM Papparella and DA Shumrick (eds), *Otolaryngology*, vol. 2 (Philadelphia: W.B. Saunders Co.).

Nahmias, AJ and Norrild, B (1979). Herpes Simplex Virus 1 and 2: Basic and Clinical Aspects. *DM* 25: 10.

National Center for Education Statistics (1989). *Profile of Handicapped Students in Post Secondary Education*, 1987, DE Publication No. CS89–337 (Washington, DC: US Government Printing Office).

National Center for Health Statistics (1988). Data from the National Health Interview Survey, Series 10, No. 166.

National Institutes of Health (1990). *Noise and Hearing Loss*. National Institutes of Health consensus development conference statement (Washington, D.C.: National Institutes of Health).

National Institutes of Health (1994). *Early Identification of Hearing Impairment in Infants and Young Children*. (Washington, D.C.: National Institutes of Health). National Institutes of Health Consensus development conference statement.

Newman, CW, Weinstein, BE, Jacobson, GP, and Hug, GA (1991). Test-retest reliability of the hearing handicap inventory for adults. *Ear and Hearing* 12:355–357.

Newman, MH (1975). Hearing loss. In M Strome (ed), *Differential Diagnosis in Pediatric Otolaryngology* (Boston: Little, Brown).

Nixon, J, Glorig, A, and High, W (1962). Changes in air and bone conduction thresholds as a function of age. *J Laryngol* 76:288–298.

Noble, WG and Atherly, GRC (1970). The hearing measurement scale: A questionnaire for the assessment of auditory disability. *J Aud Res* 10:229–250.

Northern, JL (1981). Impedance measurements in infants. In GT Mencher and SE Gerber (eds), *Early Management of Hearing Loss* (New York: Grune & Stratton).

Northern, JL (1988). Recent developments in acoustic immitance measurements in children, In F Bess (ed), *Hearing Impairment in Children* (Parkton, Md.: York Press).

Northern, JL and Downs, MP (1984). *Hearing in Children*, 3rd ed. (Baltimore: Williams & Wilkins).

Northern, JL and Downs, MP (1991). *Hearing in Children*, 4th ed. (Baltimore: Williams & Wilkins).

Oleske, J (1987). Natural history of HIV infection II, In BK Silverman and A Waddell (eds), *Surgeon General's Workshop Report on Children with HIV Infection*. (Washington: U.S. Department of Health and Human Services).

Ollo, C, Johnson, R, and Grafman, J (1991). Signs of cognitive change in HIV disease: An event-related brain potential study. *Neuro* 41:209–215.

OPS/OMS. Programa de Analisis de la Situacion de Salud y sus Tendencias. Vigilancia Epidemiologica del SIDA en las Americas. Informacion al 10 de Marzo,1992.

Owens, E, Kessler, D, Telleen, C, and Schubert, E (1981). The minimal auditory capabilities (MAC) battery. *Hear J* 34:32–34.

Owens, E and Raggio, MW (1984). *Hearing Performance Inventory for Severe to Profound Hearing Loss* (San Francisco: University of California).

Owens, E and Schubert, E (1977). Development of the California consonant test *J Speech Hear Res* 20:463–474.

Oyler, RF and Matkin, ND (1987). National survey of educational preparation in pediatric audiology. *Asha* 29:27–32.

Padmanabhan, R (1987). Abnormalities of the ear associated with exencephaly in mouse fetuses. *Teratol* 35:9–18.

Pagano, MA, Cahn, PE, and Garau, ML (1992). Brainstem auditory evoked potentials in human immunodeficiency virus seropositive patients with and without acquired immunodeficiency syndrome. *Arch Neuro* 49:166–169.

Papparella, MM (1991). Methods of diagnosis and treatment of Ménière's disease. *Acta Otolaryn* (Suppl.) 485:108–119.

Papparella, MM and Schachern, PA (1991). Sensorineural hearing loss in children—nongenetic. In MM Papparella et al. (eds) *Otolaryngology*, 3rd ed. (Philadelphia: W.B. Saunders Co.).

Parisier, SC (1993). Injuries of the ear and temporal bone. In CD Bluestone and SE Stool (eds), *Pediatric Otolaryngology*, 3rd ed. (Philadelphia: W.B. Saunders Co.).

Park, S, Wunderlich, H, Goldenberg, RA, and Marshall, M (1992). *Pneumocystis carinii* infection in the middle ear. *Arch Otolaryn* 118:269–270.

Partington, MW (1959). An English family with Waardenburg's syndrome. *Arch Dis Child* 34:154–157.

Paul, PV and Quigley, SP (1990). *Education and Deafness* (New York: Longman).

Penfield, W and Roberts, L (1959). *Speech and Brain Mechanisms* (Princeton: Princeton Universit Press).

Perkins, R (1975). Formaldehyde formed autogenous fascia graft tympanoplasty. *Trans Am Acad Ophth and Otolaryn 80:565.*

Pichora-Fuller, MK and Benguerel, AP (1991). The design of CAST (computer-aided speechreading training). *J Speech Hear Res* 34:202–212.

Pickles, JO (1988). *An Introduction to the Physiology of Hearing*, 2nd ed. (London: Academic Press).

Poole, MD, Postma, D, and Cohen, MS (1984). Pyogenic otorhinologic infections in acquired immune deficiency syndrome. *Arch Otolaryn* 110: 130–131.

Potsic, W (1978). Miniseminar on chronic otitis media. Presented at the annual convention of the American Speech and Hearing Association, San Francisco, California.

Prescod, SV (1978). *Audiological Handbook of Hearing Disorders* (New York: Van Nostrand Reinhold Co.).

Presnell, L (1973). Hearing-impaired children's comprehension and production of syntax in oral language. *J Speech Hear Res* 16:12–21.

Pressman, H (1992). Communication disorders and dysphagia in pediatric AIDS. *Asha*, 34:45–47.

Principi, N, Marchisio, P, and Tornaghi, R. (1991). Acute otitis media in human immunodeficiency virus infected children. *Peds* 88:566–571.

Proctor, C (1977). Congenital rubella and sensorineural hearing loss. *Laryng* (Suppl) 7, 87:1–60.

Pulec, JL (1984). Ménière's disease. In JL Northern (ed), *Hearing Disorders* (Boston: Little, Brown).

Quick, CA (1973). Chemical and drug effects on the inner ear. In MM Papparella and DA Shumrick (eds), *Otolaryngology* (Philadelphia: W.B. Saunders Co.).

Quigley, SP and Paul, PV (1984). *Language and Deafness* (San Diego: College-Hill Press).

Rapin, I and Ruben, R (1979). Clinical appraisal of auditory function. Presented to the symposium on developmental disabilities in the preschool child. Chicago, Illinois.

Real, R, Thomas, M and Gerwin, JM (1987). Sudden hearing loss and acquired immunodeficiency syndrome. *Otolaryn* 97:409–412.

Rene, R, Mas, A, and Villabona, CM (1990). Otitis externa maligna and cranial neuropathy. *Neurologia* 5:222–227.

Resnick, S, Dubno, J, Hoffnung, S, and Levitt, H (1975). Phoneme errors on a nonsense syllable test. *J Acoust Soc Amer* 58:114.

Rivas-Lacarte, MP and Pumarola-Segura, F (1990). Malignant otitis externa and HIV antibodies. *Ann Otorrinol Ibero-Am* 17:505–512.

Robbins, AM (1990). Developing meaningful auditory integration in children with cochlear implants. *Volta Rev* 92:361–370.

Robertson, C (1978). Pediatric assessment of the infant at risk for deafness. In SE Gerber and GT Mencher (eds), *Early Diagnosis of Hearing Loss* (New York: Grune & Stratton).

Robertson, C and Whyte L (1983). Prospective identification of infants with hearing loss and multiple handicaps: The role of the neonatal follow-up clinic. In GT Mencher and SE Gerber (eds), *The Multiply Handicapped Hearing Impaired Child* (New York: Grune & Stratton).

Roland, NJ, McCrae, D, and McCombe, AW (1995). *Key Topics in Otolaryngology, Head and Neck Surgery* (Oxford, U.K: Bios Scientific Publications).

Rose, DE (1994). Cochlear implants in children with prelingual deafness: Another side of the coin. *Am J Aud* 3:6.

Rosen, S (1953). Mobilization of the stapes to restore hearing in otosclerosis. *NY State J Med* 53: 2650–2653.

Rosen, S, Bergman, M, and Plester, D (1962). Presbycusis study of a relatively noise free population in the Sudan. *Ann Otol Rhin Laryng* 71:727–43.

Ross, M (1990). *Hearing-Impaired Children in the Mainstream* (Parkton: York Press).

Rothstein, SG, Persky, MS, Edelman, BA, Gittlemand, PE, and Stroschein, M (1989). Epiglottitis in AIDS patients. *Laryng* 99:389–392.

Ruben, RJ (1972). The external ear. In C Ferguson and E Kendig (eds), *Pediatric Otolaryngology*, vol. 2 (Philadelphia: W.B. Saunders Co.)

Ruben, RJ (1996). The pediatric otolaryngic assessment of the child with suspected hearing loss. In SE Gerber (ed), *The Handbook of Pediatric Audiology* (Washington, DC: Gallaudet University Press).

Rubin, W (1968). Sudden hearing loss. *Laryng* 78: 829–833.

Russell, WK, Quigley, SP, and Power, DJ (1976). *Linguistics and Deaf Children: Transformational Syntax and Its Applications* (Washington, DC: AG Bell Association).

Salamy, A, Eldridge, L, Anderson, J, and Bull, D (1990). Brainstem transmission time in infants exposed to cocaine in utero. *J Ped* 117:627–629.

Salomon, G, (1991). Hearing in the aged. The European concerted action project. *Acta Otolaryn*, Suppl. No. 476.

Salomon, G and Starr, A (1963). Electromyography of middle ear muscles in man during motor activities. *Acta Neuro Scand* 39:161.

Sanders, DA (1982). *Aural Rehabilitation: A Management Model*, 2nd ed. (Englewood Cliffs, NJ: Prentice-Hall).

Sataloff, J (1966). *Hearing Loss* (Philadelphia: J.B. Lippincott).

Saunders, JC, Dear, SP, and Schneider, ME (1985). The anatomical consequences of acoustic injury: A review and tutorial. *J Acoust Soc Amer* 78:833–860.

Schafer, D and Lynch, J (1980). Emergent language of six prelingually deaf children. *Teach Deaf* 5:94–111.

Schildroth, A, Rawlings, B, and Allen, T (1991). Deaf students in transition: Education and employment issues for deaf adolescents. *Volta Rev* 93:41–53.

Schow, RL and Nerbonne, MA (1982). Communication screening profile: Use with elderly clients. *Ear and Hearing* 3:135–147.

Schuell, H (1965). *Differential Diagnosis of Aphasia with the Minnesota Test* (Minneapolis: University of Minnesota Press).

Schuknecht, HF (1955). Presbycusis. *Laryng* 65:402–419.

Schuknecht, HF (1964). Further observations on the pathology of presbycusis. *Arch Otolaryn* 80:369–382.

Schuknecht, HF (1975). Pathophysiology of Ménière's disease. In JJ Shea (ed), "Symposium on Fluctuating Hearing Loss," *Otolaryn Clin N Amer* 8:507–514.

Schuknecht, HF and Karmody, CS (1965). Radionecrosis of the temporal bone. *Laryng* 76:870–880.

Schwan S, Gupta A, Myers SF, Blakley BW (1992). Physiological risk-factors for cis-platinum induced hearing loss. *J Amer Acad Aud (Poster Session)* 4:48.

Scouten, E (1967). The Rochester method: An oral multisensory approach for instructing prelingual deaf children. *Am Ann Deaf* 112:50–55.

Sever, JL (1983). Maternal infections. In CC Brown (ed), *Childhood Learning Disabilities and Prenatal Risk* (Skillman, NJ: Johnson and Johnson Baby Products).

Sever, JL and Bethesda, M (1973). Present status of vaccines for rubella. *Arch Otolaryn* 98:265–268.

Shambaugh, GE (1967). *Surgery of the Ear*, 2nd ed. (Philadelphia: W.B.Saunders Co.).

Shambaugh, GE and Causse, J (1974). Ten years with fluoride in otosclerotic (otospongiotic) patients. *Ann Otol Rhino Laryng* 83:635–642.

Shambaugh, GE and Girgis, TF (1991). Acute otitis media and mastoiditis. In MM Papparella et al. (eds), *Otolaryngology*, 3rd ed. (Philadelphia: W.B. Saunders Co.).

Shapiro, AL, Shechtman, FG, Guida, RA, and Kimmelman, CP (1992). Head and neck lymphoma in patients with the acquired immune deficiency syndrome. *Otolaryn* 106:258–260.

Shih, L, Cone-Wesson, B, and Reddix, B (1988). Effects of maternal cocaine abuse on the neonatal auditory system. *Intl J Ped Otolaryn* 15:245–251.

Shulman, JB (1979). Ototoxicity, In V Goodhill (ed), *Ear Diseases, Deafness, and Dizziness* (New York: Harper and Row).

Sicklick, MJ and Rubinstein, A (1992). Types of HIV infection and the course of the disease. In AC Crocker, HJ Cohen, and TA Kastner (eds), (1992), *HIV Infection and Developmental Disabilities: A Resource for Service Providers* (Baltimore: PH Brookes Publishing).

Siegel-Sadewitz, V and Shprintzen, R (1982). The relationship of communication disorders to syndrome identification. *J Speech Hear Dis* 47:338–354.

Silman, S and Silverman, CA (1991). *Auditory Diagnosis: Principles and Applications* (New York: Academic Press).

Simmons, FB and Russ, FN (1974). Automated newborn hearing screening: The crib-o-gram. *Arch Otolaryn* 100:1–7.

Simonds, RJ and Rogers, MF (1992). Epidemiology of HIV in children and other populations, In AC Crocker, HJ Cohen, and TA Kastner (eds), (1992). *HIV Infection and Development Disabilities: A Resource for Service Providers* (Baltimore: Paul H. Brookes Publishing).

Simons, MR (1979). Acoustic impedance tests, In V Goodhill (ed), *Ear Diseases, Deafness, and Dizziness.* (New York: Harper and Row).

Smith, ME and Canalis, RF (1989). Otologic manifestations of AIDS: The otosyphilis connection. *Laryng* 99:365–372.

Sooy, CD, Oleske, J, and Williams, MA (1987). The impact of AIDS on Otolaryngology, In EN Myers (ed), *Advances in Otolaryngology* (Chicago: Yearbook Medical Publisher).

Spear, JH (1984). On the road again: A mental health map to the mainstreamed hearing impaired. In RG Stoker and JH Spear, (eds), *Hearing-Impaired Perspectives on Living in the Mainstream* (Washington, DC: AG Bell Association).

Stein, LK and Boyer, KM (1994). Progress in the prevention of hearing loss in infants. *Ear and Hearing* 15:116–125.

Stephens, SDG (1980). Evaluating the problems of the hearing impaired. *Audiology* 19:205–220.

Stern, JC, Lin, P-T, and Lucente, FE (1990). Benign nasopharyngeal masses and human immunodeficiency virus infection. *Arch Otolaryn* 116:206–208.

Stevens, SS and Davis H (1938). *Hearing: Its Psychology and Physiology* (New York: John Wiley and Sons).

Stevens, SS and Volkmann, J (1940). The relation of pitch to frequency: A revised scale. *Am J Psych* 53:329–353.

Stool, SE and Houlihan, R (1977). Otolaryngologic management of craniofacial anomalies. *Otolaryn Clin N Am* 10:41–44.

Stout, G and Windle, J (1986). *Developmental Approach to Successful Listening II (DASL II).* (Englewood, Colo: Resource Point).

Strauss, M and Fine, E (1991). Aspergillus otomastoiditis in acquired immunodeficiency syndrome. *Am J Otol* 12:49–53.

Strome, M (1977). Sudden fluctuating hearing losses. In BF Jaffe (ed), *Hearing Loss in Children* (Baltimore: University Park Press).

Strutz, J (1991). Non-neoplastic central hearing loss: A review. *HNO* 39:332–338.

Suter, A (1985). The development of federal standards and damage risk criteria, In D Lipscomb (ed), *Hearing Conservation in Industry, Schools, and the Military* (Austin, Texas: Pro-Ed).

Sweetow, RW and Barrager, D (1980). Quality of comprehensive audiological care: A survey of parents of hearing-impaired children. *Asha* 22:841–847.

Talmi, YP, Finkelstein, Y, and Zohar, Y. (1989). Postirradiation hearing loss. *Audiology* 28:121–126.

Taylor, L (1969). A language analysis of the writing of deaf children. Unpublished doctoral dissertation, Florida State University, Tallahassee.

Tell, L (1976). Personal communication.

Theissing, G and Kittel, G (1962). Die Bedeutung der Toxoplasmose in der Atiologie der connatalen und früh erworbenen Hörstorungen. *Arch Ohr-Nas und Keh*, Heilk. 180:219.

Thomsen, J, Terkildsen, K and Osterhammel, P, (1978). Auditory brainstem responses in patients with acoustic neuromas. *Scan Aud* 7:179–183.

Tietz, W (1963). A syndrome of deaf-mutism associated with albinism showing dominant autosomal inheritance. *Am J Hum Gen* 15:259–264.

Tillman, T and Carhart, R (1966). An expanded test for speech discrimination utilizing CNC monosyllabic words. Northwestern University Auditory Test No. 6 (Technical Report No. SAM-TR-66– 55).

Timon, CI and Walsh, MA (1989). Sudden sensorineural hearing loss as a presentation of HIV Infection. *J Laryng Otol* 103:1071–1072.

Tooley, W (1973). Hyperbilirubinemia and respiratory distress syndrome. In 65th Ross Conference (Columbus: Ross Laboratories).

Top, FH and Wehrle, PE (1976). *Communicable and Infectious Diseases*, 8th ed. (St. Louis: The C.V. Mosby Co.).

Tullio, P (1929). *Das Ohr* (Berlin: Urban & Schwarzenberg).

Tye-Murray, N (1991). Repair strategy usage by hearing-impaired adults and changes following communication therapy. *J Speech Hear Res* 34:921–928.

Tye-Murray, N and Kelsay, DMR (1993). A communication training program for parents of cochlear implant users. *Volta Rev* 95:21–31.

Tye-Murray, N, Tyler, RS, Bong, B, and Nares, T (1988). Computerized laser videodisc programs for training speechreading and assertive communication behaviors. *J Acad Rehab Aud* 221:143–152.

United States Air Force (1966). *Risk Test to Evaluate Equilibrium in Broadband Noise* (Dayton, Ohio: Wright-Patterson Air Force Base).

United States Navy (1957). *Nystagmus Elicited by High Intensity Sound* (Pensacola, Fla.: Navy Research Lab.).

Utley, J (1946). A test of lipreading ability. *J Speech Hear Dis* 11:109–116.

Uziel, A, Romand, R, and Marot, M (1979). Electro-physiological study of ototoxicity of kanamycin during development in Guinea pigs. *Hear Res* 1:203–212.

Van der Hulst, RJAM, Dreschler, WA, and Urbanus, NAM (1988). High frequency audiometry in prospective clinical research of ototoxicity due to platinum derivatives. *Ann Otol Rhino Laryng* 97: 133–137.

Vartianinen, E, Karjalainen, S, and Karji, J (1985). Vestibular disorders following head injury in children. *Intl J Ped Otorhinol* 9:135–141.

Ventry, I and Schiavetti, N (1980). *Evaluating Research in Speech Pathology and Audiology: A Guide for Clinicians and Students* (Menlo Park, Calif.: Addison-Wesley).

Ventry, I and Weinstein, BE (1982). The hearing handicap inventory for the elderly: A new tool. *Ear and Hearing* 3:128–134.

Visencio, LH and Gerber, SE (1979). Effects of hemodialysis on pure-tone thresholds and blood chemistry measures. *J Speech Hear Res* 22: 756–764.

von Békésy, G (1956). Current status of theories of hearing. *Science* 123:779–783.

von Békésy, G (1960). *Experiments in Hearing* (New York: McGraw-Hill).

Waardenburg, PJ (1951). A new syndrome combining developmental anomalies of the eyelids, eyebrows, and nose root with pigmentary defects of the iris and head hair and with congenital deafness. *Am J Hum Gen* 3:195–253.

Wada, J and Rasmussen, T (1960). Intracarotid injection of sodium amytal for the lateralization of cerebral speech dominance: Experimental and clinical observations. *J Neurosur* 17:266–282.

Walden BE, Demorest ME, and Hepler, EL (1984). Self-report approach to assessing benefit derived from amplification. *J Speech Hear Res* 27:49–56.

Walden, BE and Grant, KW (1993). Research needs in rehabilitative audiology. In JG Alpiner and PA McCarthy (eds.), *Rehabilitative Audiology: Children and Adults*, 2nd ed. (Baltimore: Williams & Wilkins).

Wallace, SP, Prutting, CA, and Gerber, SE (1990). Degeneration of speech, language, and hearing in a patient with mucopolysaccharidosis VII. *Intl J Ped Otorhinol* 19:97–107.

Ward, WD (1973). Adaptation and fatigue, In J Jerger (ed), *Modern Developments in Audiology*, 2nd ed. (New York: Academic Press).

Weaver, CB and Bradley-Johnson, S (1993). A national survey of school psychological services for deaf and hard of hearing students. *Amer Ann Deaf* 138: 267–274.

Weaver, M and Northern JL (1976). The acoustic tumor. In JL Northern (ed), *Hearing Disorders* (Boston: Little, Brown).

Weaver, M and Staller, SJ (1984). The acoustic nerve tumor, In JL Northern (ed), *Hearing Disorders*, 2nd ed. (Boston: Little, Brown).

Wechsler, D (1974). *Manual for Wechsler Intelligence Scale for Children-Revised* (New York: The Psychological Corporation).

Wechsler, D (1981). *Manual for the Wechsler Adult Intelligence Scale-Revised* (New York: The Psychological Corporation).

Welch, BL and Welch, AS (eds), (1970). *Physiological Effects of Noise* (New York: Plenum Press).

Welkoborsky, HJ and Lowitzsch, K (1992). ABR in patients with human immunotropic virus infections of different stages. *Ear and Hearing* 13:55–57.

Weller, TH and Hanshaw, JB (1962). Virologic and clinical observations of cytomegalic inclusion disease. *N Eng J Med* 266:1233–1244.

West, JJ and Weber, JL (1974). A phonological analysis of the spontaneous language of a four-year-old hard-of-hearing child. *J Speech Hear Dis* 38:25–35.

Wilbur, RB (1987). *American Sign Language: Linguistic and Applied Dimensions* (San Diego: College-Hill Press).

Willeford, J (1977). Assessing central auditory behavior in children: A test battery approach. In RW Keith (ed), *Central Auditory Dysfunction* (New York: Grune & Stratton).

Williams, MA (1987). Head and neck findings in pediatric Acquired Immune Deficiency Syndrome. *Laryng* 97:713–716.

Williams, WT, Ghorayeb, BY, and Yeakly, JW (1992). Pediatric temporal bone fractures. *Laryng* 102: 600–603.

Wilson, J (1984). The global challenge of avoidable disablement. Paper presented to the XVII International Congress of Audiology, Santa Barbara, California.

Wilson, J (1985). Deafness in developing countries. *Arch Otol* 111:2–9.

World Health Organization (1967). *The Early Detection and Treatment of Handicapping Defects in Young Children*. Report of a working group convened by the Regional Office for Europe of the World Health Organization.

Wylde, M (1987). Psychological and counseling aspects of the adult remediation process. In JG Alpiner and PA McCarthy (eds), *Rehabilitative Audiology: Children and Adults* (Baltimore: Williams & Wilkins).

Yacobacci-Tam, P (1987). Interacting with the culturally different family. *Volta Rev* 89:46–59.

Ying, E (1990). Speech and language assessment: Communication evaluation. In M. Ross (ed), *Hearing-Impaired Children in the Mainstream*. (Parkton, Md.: York Press).

Zenner, H-P (1993). Possible roles of outer hair cell d.c. movements in the cochlea. *Brit J Aud* 27:73–77.

Zondek, B and Tamari, I (1960). Effects of audiogenic stimulation on genital function and reproduction. *Am J Ob Gyn* 80:1041–1048.

# Index